Springer Japan KK

S. Sasayama (Ed.)

New Horizons for Failing Heart Syndrome

With 97 Figures, Including 3 in Color

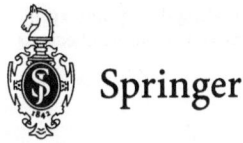 Springer

SHIGETAKE SASAYAMA, M.D.
Department of Cardiovascular Medicine
Kyoto University Graduate School of Medicine
54 Shogoin Kawahara-cho,
Sakyo-ku, Kyoto, 606 Japan

ISBN 978-4-431-66947-0   ISBN 978-4-431-66945-6 (eBook)
DOI 10.1007/978-4-431-66945-6

Library of Congress Cataloging-in-Publication Data
New horizons for failing heart syndrome / S. Sasayama (ed.).
      p.   cm.
    Includes bibliographical references and index.

    1. Heart failure.   I. Sasayama, Shigetake, 1937–
    [DNLM: 1. Heart Failure, Congestive.   2. Heart—physiopathology.
    3. Myocardial Contraction—physiology.   WG 370 N533 1996]
    RC685.C53N485   1996
    616.1′29—dc20

                                                            95-44936

Printed on acid-free paper

© Springer Japan 1996
Originally published by Springer-Verlag Tokyo in 1996.

Typesetting: Best-set Typesetter Ltd., Hong Kong

Preface

Left ventricular dysfunction is caused by all forms of heart disease and leads to the syndrome of heart failure. However, "heart failure" is not the disease name but stands for the pathophysiologic state of the disease; therefore, even its definition has been disputed. A 3-year project for research on heart failure was first organized by the Japanese Circulation Society in 1988. The compilation of the achievements of this project was issued in the monograph entitled *Recent Progress in Failing Heart Syndrome* in 1991.

The second series in heart failure research was started in 1992 and completed in March 1995. During this period, there was further evolution in our understanding of heart failure, and new therapeutic modalities were introduced.

It has become increasingly apparent that heart failure relates not only to cardiac dysfunction but also to the resulting peripheral and neurohormonal responses. Cardiac hypertrophy is the natural response of the heart to an increased mechanical load, but attention has been focused on the mechanisms of transition from compensated hypertrophy to failure. Evidence has accumulated on the structural, biochemical, and functional changes within myocytes of the failing heart and genes that regulate the process of cellular growth, differentiation, and death. The role of the autocrine/ paracrine system in the initiation and the maintenance of a pathologic phenotype has been intensively investigated. More recently, nonlethal alterations of myocytes induced by immune cells and their cytokines have been suggested as a possible cause of heart failure. The failing heart is assumed to be in an energy crisis, and analysis of the energetic state prompted renewed interest in the physiological and biochemical consequences of a decreased energy reserve. Substantial numbers of new drugs have been developed for the management of heart failure. However, the eventual status of cardiotonic agents remains controversial.

The second series of research project was organized in an attempt to elucidate all of these aspects of heart failure. The present volume is a state-of-the-art overview of the current research carried out in Japan. It is the editor's wish that this book will provide readers with additional new insights in the syndrome of heart failure.

Shigetake Sasayama

Contents

Part 3 Energetics and Exercise

Part 4 Medical Treatment of Heart Failure

List of Contributors

Araki J. 133
Asanoi H. 209
Endoh M. 187
Fujii W. 133
Goto Y. 165
Hata K. 165
Honda H. 117
Hori M. 45
Inoko M. 105
Inoue M. 45
Ishizaka S. 209
Ito H. 133
Jones C.J.H. 69
Kameyama T. 209
Kawaguchi H. 27
Kihara Y. 105

Koiwa Y. 117
Komuro I. 3
Kondoh Y. 69
Matsubara H. 133
Matsui S. 219
Matsumori A. 219
Nagai R. 3
Naya T. 117
Ohzono K. 79
Sasayama S. 105, 209, 219
Sato H. 45
Shin W.S. 27
Shioi T. 219
Shiojima I. 3
Shirato K. 117
Suga H. 133

Sugawara M. 69
Sugimachi M. 175
Sunagawa K. 175
Takaki H. 175
Takaki M. 133
Tomoike H. 79
Toyo-oka T. 27
Uchida K. 69
Urabe Y. 79
Yamada T. 219
Yamaguchi S. 79
Yamazaki T. 3
Yasuhara S. 133
Yazaki Y. 3
Zhao L.Y. 133

Part 1
Molecular Mechanism of Heart Failure

Molecular Aspects of Mechanical Stress-Induced Cardiac Hypertrophy and Failure

ICHIRO SHIOJIMA, TSUTOMU YAMAZAKI, ISSEI KOMURO, RYOZO NAGAI, and YOSHIO YAZAKI

Abstract. Studies have demonstrated that hypertensive left ventricular hypertrophy (LVH) simultaneously exhibits physiological and pathological aspects, suggesting that LVH is not a simple adaptation to an increased external load. Many investigators have extensively studied the activation of a novel program of gene expression in the heart induced by pressure overload (i.e., the transient induction of immediate early genes and the reexpression of fetal-type genes of both contractile and noncontractile proteins), which has been shown to be important as an adaptation to maintain cardiac function. Using an in vitro model system of mechanical stress-induced cardiac hypertrophy, we have demonstrated that the external stimuli imposed on cardiomyocytes are transduced into the nucleus through activation of the protein kinase cascade of phosphorylation: passive stretch of cultured cardiomyocytes stimulates the activation of protein kinase C, which leads to the successive phosphorylation of the mitogen-activated protein (MAP) kinase cascade including MAP kinase kinase kinase, MAP kinase, kinase, MAP kinase, and S6 kinase. Furthermore, we have demonstrated that the endogenous angiotensin II (Ang II) partially mediates mechanical stretch-induced cardiomyocyte hypertrophy, indicating that the cardiac tissue renin–angiotensin system plays an important role in the formation of hypertensive LVH. The precise mechanisms by which the sustained increase in external load leads to the impairment of cardiac function remain unclear, although impairment of diastolic function has been detected during the early stage of load-induced hypertrophy when there is no sign of reduced contractility. Using an in vivo model of hypertensive LVH, we noted previously that the depressed function of sarcoplasmic reticulum and the accumulation of interstitial collagen fibers may be responsible for the impaired diastolic function in stressed hearts. Here we review recent work on mechanical stress-induced cardiac hypertrophy and failure, especially bringing into focus the molecular mechanisms by which external load induces cellular hypertrophy of cardiac myocytes and impairment of the diastolic properties of the myocardium.

Key words. Left ventricular hypertrophy—Pressure overload—Immediate early gene—Mitogen-activated protein kinase—Renin-angiotensin system

Department of Medicine III, University of Tokyo School of Medicine, 7-3-1 Hongo, Bunkyo-ku, Tokyo 113, Japan

Introduction

Left ventricular hypertrophy (LVH) has been regarded as a secondary adaptation to a sustained increase in hemodynamic workload [1]. Studies, however, have now demonstrated that LVH has simultaneous physiological and pathological aspects. That is, hypertrophied heart has impaired contractile and relaxing functions and reduced coronary reserve following transient ischemia, both of which lead to the high mortality associated with heart failure and ischemic heart disease [2]. Therefore it is imperative in cardiovascular research to understand the mechanisms of the development of LVH and to establish effective measures to prevent it.

The first topic of this review is the molecular aspects of the cardiac cellular hypertrophy induced by external load. It has been controversial as to whether an initiator for cardiac hypertrophy is mechanical stress itself or concurrent activation of neural or humoral factors. Previous studies have shown that the activation of adrenoreceptors accompanies cardiac hypertrophy induced by hemodynamic overload [3]. However, evidence presented below suggests that the mechanical stress itself is an initiating factor for cardiac hypertrophy in response to hemodynamic overload. First, hemodynamic overload induces cardiac hypertrophy even after blocking of adrenoreceptors or sympathectomy [4]. Second, the mechanical overload increases protein synthesis in isolated hearts [5]. Furthermore, stretch of cultured cardiomyocytes stimulates protein synthesis and specific gene expression without participation of systemic neural or humoral factors [6–8]. Accordingly, to investigate the mechanisms by which LVH develops we must clarify how mechanical stimuli mediate cardiomyocyte hypertrophy.

From such a biochemical point of view, there are many examples that external physical (mechanical) stimuli have important effects on the cell interior (e.g., sound: hair cells of the ear; shear stress: endothelial cells of the vasculature). Cardiac hypertrophy is one of the most important prototypes, and the myocardium is in particular an excellent model system with which to address the broad biological questions as to how extracellular mechanical stimuli are converted to intracellular signals that provoke various cellular responses. There should be some "receptors," "transducers," and "effectors" for mechanical stimuli in the signaling pathways, and an understanding of these molecules will likely elucidate the mechanisms of cardiac hypertrophy and failure.

The second topic of this review is the molecular aspects of the control of myocardial relaxation in the presence of LVH. Impairment of diastolic function can be detected during the early stage of load-induced hypertrophy when there is no sign of reduced contractility [9]. Diastolic dysfunction has two characteristics: slowing of relaxation and an increase in chamber stiffness. Relaxation of myocardium has been shown to be associated with intracellular calcium handling regulated by cardiac sarcoplasmic reticulum (SR) [10], and chamber stiffness has been demonstrated to be determined by collagen fiber accumulation in the extracellular matrix [11]. Therefore to reveal the mechanisms by which the diastolic properties are impaired in pressure-overloaded hearts, it is important to know how SR function is altered and how abnormal accumulation of fibrillar collagen in the extracellular space is induced by mechanical stress. In the present review, we discuss mechanical stress-induced cardiac hypertrophy and failure, especially bringing into focus the molecular mechanisms by which external load induces the hypertrophy of cardiac myocytes and impairment of the diastolic properties of the myocardium.

Hypertrophy of Cardiac Myocytes

Regulation of Cardiac Gene Expression by Mechanical Stress

Genes Responsive to Mechanical Stress

The heart responds to increased work load by an increase in muscle mass and by changes in gene expression. Activation of a new program of gene expression in the overloaded heart has been shown to be important as an adaptation to maintain cardiac function. Many lines of evidence have accumulated over the last several years for identifying the genes responsive to mechanical stress in the heart [12]. These genes can be divided into two classes. One is called immediate early genes (IEGs), whose transcription is activated rapidly and transiently within minutes after extracellular stimulation [13, 14]. This transcription induction is independent of new protein synthesis, but subsequent shutoff of transcription requires new protein synthesis [15, 16]. The tightly controlled expression of IEGs suggests a regulatory role for their protein products during the cellular response to external stimuli. The other group is the late response genes, whose expression is induced more slowly, over hours, and requires new protein synthesis. In pressure-overloaded hearts, induction of the latter type of gene is observed, for the most part, as reexpression of fetal-type genes.

Induction of IEGs by Mechanical Stress

As a model for the induction of IEGs by mechanical stress, an increase in the mRNA level of the proto-oncogenes such as c-*fos* and c-*myc* by aortic constriction was first reported in rat hearts [17–19]. Their mRNA levels peaked at 3–8h and returned to the baseline within 24h to 10 days. These delayed, persistent expression kinetics are different from those of other cell systems stimulated by growth factors and suggest the involvement of multiple factors, such as mechanical, humoral (e.g., renin–angiotensin system), or neural factors (e.g., catecholamines). Bauters et al. [20] demonstrated the expression of proto-oncogenes c-*fos* and c-*myc* in an isolated, coronary perfused heart of adult rats. When coronary flow was augmented, the expression of c-*fos* and c-*myc* was both sequentially and transiently increased in a beating heart but not in an arrested heart, and the expression levels paralleled the coronary flow. In another experiment, the induction of c-*fos* expression was observed in an isolated beating heart, and its level was proportional to the magnitude of the peak LV systolic wall stress [21]. Thus although the factors that induce expression of proto-oncogenes in the heart are still controversial, these results suggest that mechanical stress can directly induce the expression of IEGs.

Reexpression of Fetal-Type Genes of Contractile Proteins by Mechanical Stress

The contraction unit of the myocardium is the sarcomere. The sarcomere is constituted by seven major proteins: myosin heavy chain (MHC), myosin light chain (MLC), tropomyosin (TM), troponin (Tn) complex (TnT, TnI, and TnC), and actin, as well as several minor ones. All of these major proteins have multiple isoforms generated by alternative pre-mRNA splicing [22] (α- and β-TM, TnT, and MLC) and by a multigene family [23] (MHC, MLC, actin, TM, TnT, TnI, and TnC). The expression of each member of this multigene family is regulated at the transcriptional level in a tissue-specific and developmentally regulated manner. With cardiac hypertrophy, some of these contractile protein genes, which are ordinarily expressed in the embryonic heart but not in the adult heart, are selectively activated at the alternative pre-mRNA splicing level (β-TM) [17] and the transcriptional level (β-MHC, smooth and akeletal α-actin) [24–26]. Hypertrophy provoked by loading in adult myocardium recapitulates at least in part the embryonic program of gene expression observed during cardiac development.

The reexpression of fetal isoforms in cardiac hypertrophy mimics the mitogenic response of many differentiated cell types, such as hepatocytes. During liver regeneration the fetal proteins (e.g., α-fetoprotein) are up-regulated, whereas the proteins of adult phenotype (e.g., albumin) are down-regulated. As a later event caused by hemodynamic overload, isoform transition of MHC has been best studied at the physiological and molecular levels [27, 28]. In a variety of models of cardiac hypertrophy, the Ca^{2+}-activated myosin ATPase activity is reduced, which has been demonstrated to be due to the shift from the V1 isoform (homodimer of α-MHC) to the V3 isoform (homodimer of β-MHC) [28]. The transition from V1 to V3 decreases the initial speed of shortening but improves the efficiency of contraction for an equivalent amount of work [27], suggesting that it might be the "adaptation" of the cardiac muscle. This change occurs at least in part at the pretranslational level. In other contractile proteins, α-actin is next well characterized. Smooth and skeletal α-actin mRNA is induced in the heart by hemodynamic overload [26]. Because generation of the force results from the interaction of myosin and actin, and one amino acid replacement of actin significantly affects the kinetics of force generation, these changes in actin during hypertrophy may have some effect on cardiac contraction or relaxation. A precise, systematic comparison of these α-actins by reconstruction studies or in vitro motility assays may clarify this question.

Reexpression of Fetal-Type Genes of Noncontractile Proteins by Mechanical Stress

The reprogramming of gene expression in the heart by hemodynamic overload is not limited to the contractile proteins. Atrial natriuretic peptide (ANP) is expressed in the ventricle as well as in the atrium during the embryonic stage, but after birth the expression of ANP is restricted to the atrium, being hardly detectable in the normal adult ventricle. In the overloaded ventricle, however, ANP is abundantly expressed [29, 30]. Taking into account the relative muscle volume, the total amount of ANP in hypertrophic ventricle can thus be more than that in the atrium. Because ANP has potent natriuretic, diuretic, and vasodilatory effects, the induction of ANP in the ventricle in response to hemodynamic overload might be interpreted as an adaptational response to reduce the increased wall stress.

Induction of ANP gene expression during hypertrophy may be regulated by protooncogenes c-fos and c-jun. ANP gene expression has been known to be regulated by a variety of stimuli, such as hormones and physical stretch of myocardial tissue [29, 31]. As an intracellular second messenger, activation of protein kinase C (PKC) has been demonstrated to induce secretion of ANP as well as expression of the ANP gene [32]. PKC has been shown to activate target gene expression through a number of mechanisms. One of the best studied involves the transcription complex AP-1: PKC stimulates the expression of both c-fos and c-jun genes transcriptionally and activates target gene expression via the AP-1 complex, the Fos/Jun heterodimer. In the 5' flanking region of ANP gene, there are three potential AP-1 binding sites. The Fos/Jun complex has been shown to interact with this region, and selective mutation of this site has been demonstrated to suppress the basal activity of the ANP promoter [33]. These results indicate that two proto-oncogenes, c-*fos* and c-*jun*, may be the potential "second messengers" that link the environmental stimuli with reprogramming of the gene expression in cardiac hypertrophy.

In contrast to those up-regulated genes, some genes are down-regulated by hemodynamic overload. One of these genes is for SR Ca^{2+}-ATPase. The mRNA level of Ca^{2+}-ATPase is gradually decreased by pressure overload in the animal model [34, 35], and reduced expression of Ca^{2+}-ATPase was observed in the failing human heart [36]. The down-regulation of Ca^{2+}-ATPase is induced not only by mechanical stress but also by some growth factors [37], and it is also observed during the fetal stage [34]. The down-regulation of specific genes such as those that encode albumin, cytochrome P450 R-17, apoA-1, and apoE are also observed during liver regeneration. These results indicate that the changes in pretranslational regulation of specific genes during cardiac hypertrophy reflect an alteration of the phenotype to an earlier state of cardiocyte differentiation. In addition, these phenomena suggest the existence of common signal transduction pathways in the fetal heart and the hypertrophied heart.

Development of an In Vitro Model System for Cardiac Hypertrophy

Because the heart consists of a variety of cells, such as neural, vascular, endothelial, interstitial, and muscle cells [38], it is impossible to evaluate the exact role of mechanical stress in cardiac hypertrophy even in the isolated perfused heart. Moreover, because it has been demonstrated that not only mechanical stress but also neural or humoral factors can induce hypertrophy of cardiac myocytes and the expression of IEGs [1, 39, 40], it remains unknown if mechanical stress directly regulates gene expression and protein synthesis without the participation of neural or humoral factors. To overcome these problems, an in vitro model of mechanical stress-induced cardiac hypertrophy has been established [6–8]. It has been shown using a Langendorf preparation that stretching the ventricular wall accompanied by increased aortic pressure is the mechanical stimulus most closely related to an increase in protein synthesis in the heart [5]. Therefore we cultured neonatal rat cardiocytes in deformable silicone dishes and imposed a mechanical load on the adherent cells by stretching the culture dishes.

Liquid silicone rubber was purchased from Shin Etsu Chemical Co. (Tokyo, Japan), and elastic culture dishes ($2 \times 4 \times 1$ cm) were prepared by vulcanizing liquid silicone rubber consisting of methylvinyl polysiloxane and dimethyl hydrogen silicone resin using platinum as a catalyst. The bottom of the dish is 1 mm thick and is highly transparent because of no inorganic filler in either component. Primary cultures of cardiac myocytes were prepared from the ventricles of 1-day-old Wistar rats essentially according to the method of Simpson and Savion [41]. Trypsinization was performed with 0.05% trypsin-EDTA at 37°C for 10 min. Cells from the first treatment were discarded, and the procedure was repeated until all tissues were dissociated (about five times). To reduce the number of contaminating nonmuscle cells, dissociated cells were preplated on 100-mm culture dishes in Dulbecco's modified Eagle's medium (DMEM) with 10% fetal calf serum for 1 h. Cells not attached to the preplated dishes were plated on laminin-coated (20 mg/ml) silicone dishes at a field density of 1×10^5 cells/cm² (cardiac myocyte-rich fraction). A nonmuscle cell-rich fraction was obtained from cells attached to the preplated

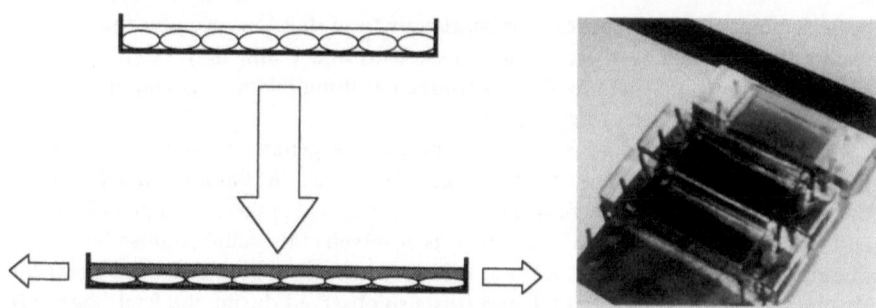

FIG. 1. Deformable silicone culture dishes. Mechanical stress on cardiac cells is applied by gently pulling the dish 10%–20% in the longitudinal axis and hanging it on pegs

dishes. Cardiac myocytes were maintained at 37°C in humidified air with 5% CO_2 in order to achieve a final pH of 7.35–7.40 in the medium. At 24 h after seeding, the culture medium was changed to a serum-free chemically defined solution consisting of DMEM. At this point, more than 90% and fewer than 10% of the cells were beating in the cardiac myocyte-rich and the nonmuscle cell-rich fractions, respectively. It has been confirmed that a 10% change in the length of the dish results in a $9.3 \pm 0.9\%$ ($n = 100$) change in the length of the cell along a single axis (Fig. 1) [6].

Stretch of myocytes stimulated the expression of IEGs (e.g., c-fos, c-myc, c-jun, Egr-1) in a stretch length-dependent manner, followed by an increase in amino acid incorporation into proteins (Fig. 2) [6, 7]. The induction of c-fos was most prominent (more than 20-fold increase in mRNA levels after stretch) among these IEGs, and the expression kinetics of c-fos were similar to those of other cells stimulated by growth factors: The c-fos mRNA was enhanced within 15 min by stretch, peaked at 30 min, and declined to undetectable levels by 240 min. The c-fos induction was observed more abundantly in the myocyte-rich fraction than in the nonmyocyte-rich fraction, suggesting that there is heterogeneity in the response to mechanical stress among cell types. The induction of IEGs and increased protein synthesis indicates that this in vitro model well mimics the in vivo model of stress-induced cardiac hypertrophy and

A Phenylalanine Incorporation

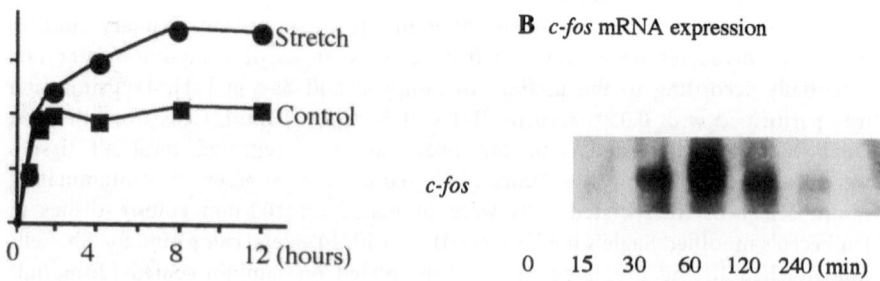

B c-fos mRNA expression

FIG. 2. Mechanical stretch induces an increase in protein synthesis (**A**) and transient c-fos mRNA expression (**B**) in cultured cardiomyocytes

is a useful experimental system for investigating load-induced cardiac cellular hypertrophy without the effects of systemic humoral or neural factors.

To determine whether the increase in c-*fos* mRNA levels by mechanical stress is due to the transcriptional activation or the increase in mRNA stability, nuclear runoff transcription experiments were performed. New RNA transcripts are not initiated in this assay, but transcripts that are already initiated are faithfully elongated, giving a reasonably accurate measure of the level of transcription at the time of cell lysis. The nuclear runoff assay showed that c-*fos* expression was regulated at least in part at the transcriptional levels [7]. These results indicate that mechanical stress directly regulates the gene expression in cardiomyocytes. In other words, the primary response to the mechanical stimuli in the terminal differentiated cardiomyocytes mimics early events of cell division induced by growth factors in a variety of cell types.

Intracellular Signaling Pathway Mediating Stretch-Induced Cardiomyocyte Hypertrophy

Acceleration of protein synthesis in the heart by mechanical stimuli was reportedly first done by stretching quiescent papillary muscle in vitro [42]. Elevation of aortic pressure in perfused hearts also caused an increase in protein synthesis [43], and the papillary muscle whose tendon was cut to be released from the tension did not exhibit hypertrophy even during aortic constriction, whereas the neighboring intact papillary muscle showed marked hypertrophy [4]. In addition, specific gene expression was induced by mechanical stress during cardiac hypertrophy. To elucidate the molecular mechanisms of load-induced cardiac hypertrophy, we must clarify how the mechanical stress in converted to biochemical signals that result in the induction of specific load-responsive genes and the increase in protein synthesis. Because the c-*fos* expression by stretch was significant and rapid, we used the c-*fos* expression as a molecular marker to examine the signal transduction pathways from mechanical stress to specific gene expression.

Phospholipase C-PKC

To elucidate the mechanisms of c-*fos* induction by stretch, the promoter activity of the c-*fos* gene was examined. The transfected chloramphenicol acetyltransferase (CAT) gene linked to upstream sequences of the c-*fos* gene indicated that the sequences containing a serum response element (SRE) were required for efficient transcription by stretch, and that sequences containing a cAMP/calcium response element was not sufficient for the c-*fos* response to stretch [7]. It was shown also that the stretch response element maps to SRE using a c-*fos*-CAT construct that has point mutations in the SRE [44]. These results suggest the involvement of PKC in the c-*fos* expression by mechanical stress, a notion supported by pharmacological studies. The c-*fos* induction was suppressed by the inhibitors for PKC and by the down-regulation of PKC, but it was not inhibited by high concentrations of streptomysin and gadolinium (blocker of the stretch-activated ion channels [45, 46]), amilorides (blocker of the Na^+/H^+ pump), terazosin and yohimbine (α_1- and α_2-adrenergic antagonists, respectively), propranolol (β-adrenergic antagonist), tetrodotoxin (Na^+ channel blocker), nifedipine, diltiazem, and nicardipine (Ca^{2+} channel blockers), pertussis toxin (Gi protein inhibitor), and short exposure to EDTA. The c-*fos* expression was observed even in Na^+-free medium (replaced by Li^+) or Ca^{2+}-free medium [6, 7]. These pharmacological data suggest that c-*fos* induction by stretch in the cardiomyocytes depends on PKC activation but not on Ca^{2+} or Na^+ ions, and that adrenergic receptors or Gi protein may not be involved in this signal transduction pathway. To examine whether mechanical stress can activate PKC activity, inositol phosphate levels were measured in the cardiocytes in the presence or absence of mechanical stress. Myocyte stretching slightly but significantly increased inositol phosphate levels, suggesting the production of 1,2-diacylglycerol (DG) and inositol-1,4,5-triphosphate (IP3) by virtue of phospholipase C activation [7, 44]. Activation of PKC by phorbol esters or DG stimulated the expression of proto-oncogenes (e.g., c-*fos* and c-*jun*) and fetal genes such as skeletal α-actin and ANP. Moreover, PKC was shown to activate β-MHC, MLC-2, and ANP transcription by co-transfection of constitutively activated PKC and reporter genes [47]. Taken together, these results strongly suggest that PKC might be the second messenger in the signaling pathway between external mechanical stress and intracellular gene regulation. Because PKC is a serine/threonine kinase, it may regulate gene expression through phosphorylation of transcription factors or other regulators.

Mitogen-Activated Protein Kinase Cascade

A large number of intracellular signals are transduced into a nucleus through protein kinase cascades of phosphorylation [48]. Among them, the mitogen-activated protein kinase (MAPK) cascade has been most extensively investigated because it was demonstrated to be involved in the cellular responses to various external stimuli such as those provoked by growth factors [49–51]. Therefore we examined MAPK activity in total cell lysates of cardiac myocytes before and after stretching using myelin basic protein (MBP) as an exogenous substrate [52]. The MBP kinase activity of cardiomyocyte lysates was induced maximally 10 min after stretch by approximately 1.8-fold. The MAPK activity was partially suppressed by the inhibitors for PKC or by the down-regulation of PKC, suggesting that MAPK activation is partially dependent on PKC, and that PKC may be situated upstream of MAPK.

The upstream activator of MAPKs is reported to be MAPK kinase (MAPKK) [53–55], which is a dual-specificity protein kinase that phosphorylates MAPKs on both threonine and tyrosine residues within a conserved TEY motif [56]. In addition, MAPKK is also activated by phosphorylation of two serine residues [57]. Current candidates for the MAPKK kinase (MAPKKK) in mammalian cells are the proto-oncogene product Raf-1 [58] and MAPK/ERK (extracellular signal-regulated kinase) kinase kinase (MEKK) [59]. Raf-1 has been reported in many cell types to be activated through PKC-dependent and PKC-independent pathways [60]; and MEKK has been suggested to mediate primary signals originating from receptors via G proteins or PKC [59]. Activated MAPKs translocate into the nucleus and activate nuclear transcription factors such as c-*jun*, NF-IL6, and Elk-1 [61]. Moreover, 90-kDa ribosomal S6 kinase (p90^{rsk}) is reported to be a downstream enzyme of MAPKs [49] and to phosphorylate nuclear lamins [62]. These observations suggest that MAPKs and p90^{rsk} play vital roles in transducing signals into the nucleus. By in-gel assays using specific antibodies and substrates, we have demonstrated that stretching of myocytes sequentially activated MAPKKKs, MAPKK, MAPKs, and p90^{rsk} [T. Yamazaki et al., unpublished observation], suggesting that this sequential signaling pathway induced by mechanical stretch may play an important role in transducing an extracellular signal to the nuclear events (Fig. 3).

In various cell types the MAPK cascade has been demonstrated to play critical roles in cell growth and differentiation. Thiophosphorylated MAPK has been shown to

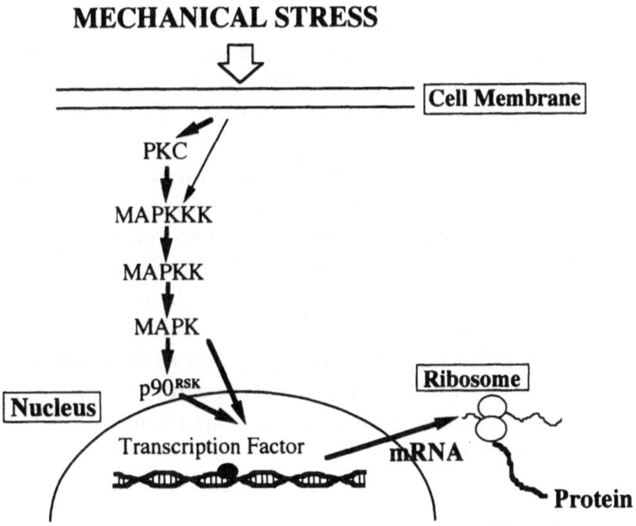

MECHANICAL STRESS

FIG. 3. Molecular mechanisms of cardiac hypertrophy. Sequential activation of protein kinases, including the MAPK cascade, is involved in the development of cardiomyocyte hypertrophy provoked by mechanical stretch

arrest *Xenopus* oocyte maturation [63], and interfering mutants of MAPK inhibited fibroblast proliferation [64]. Furthermore, Cowley et al. [65] have shown that the activated mutants of MAPKK stimulated PC12 cell neuronal differentiation and transformed NIH 3T3 cells, and that the interfering mutants inhibited growth factor-induced PC12 differentiation and reversed v-*src*- and *ras*-transformed cells. However, it is still controversial as to whether the MAPK cascade is involved in the stretch-induced hypertrophic responses. Thorburn et al. [66] showed that phenylephrine treatment results in activation of MAPKs, but that inhibition of MAPKs does not prevent phenylephrine-induced organization of actin filaments. Additional studies are needed to clarify the precise roles of the MAPK cascade in cardiac hypertrophy, although we hypothesize that the MAPK cascade may, at least in part, participate in the development of cardiomyocyte hypertrophy induced by mechanical stress.

Mechanisms That Convert Mechanical Stimuli to Intracellular Signals

Because cardiomyocytes respond to external mechanical stress, there should be some "mechanosensors" or "mechanoreceptors." Although some candidates may sense and transduce the extracellular stimuli into intracellular signaling molecules as discussed below, the precise mechanism of mechanoreception by cardiomyocytes remains uncertain.

Stretch-Sensitive Ion Channels

Many cells respond to a variety of environmental stimuli by ion channels in the plasma membrane. Mechanosensitive ion channels have been observed with single-channel recordings in more than 30 cell types of prokaryotes, plants, fungi, and all animals so far examined [67]. The activation of stretch-sensitive channels has been proposed as the transduction mechanism between load and protein synthesis with cardiac hypertrophy [68]. The stretch-sensitive channels allow passage of the major monovalent physiological cations Na^+ and K^+ and the divalent cation Ca^{2+}. With the use of Ca^{2+}-binding fluorescent dye, fluo3, and the patch-clamp technique, Ca^{2+} influx through stretch channels was shown to lead to waves of calcium-induced calcium release [69].

When an Na^+ ionophore (monensin or veratridine) was added to cultured cardiomyocytes, c-*fos* expression was observed, possibly because of increased Ca^{2+} uptake by the Na^+/Ca^{2+} exchange mechanism [70]. However, the expression of fetal-type genes was not induced by an Na^+ increase. Moreover, the blockers of stretch-activated channels, Na^+ channels, and Na^+/Ca^{2+} exchanger did not affect c-*fos* expression [7, 70, 71]. Although ion influx through stretch-sensitive channels may play some role, such as inducing arrhythmias [72], and we cannot rule out the existence of the inhibitor-insensitive stretch channels in cardiomyocytes, an opening of the stretch-sensitive ion channels alone cannot explain the many biochemical events evoked by stretch of cardiomyocytes.

Extracellular Matrix and Cytoskeleton

External stimuli are usually transduced into the cell interior through plasma membranes where a number of functionally important organs such as ion channels, transporters, receptors, and a variety of enzymes are embedded in lipid bilayers. Because these membrane organs are associated with the cytoskeleton by which the cell shape is maintained, it is reasonable to speculate that mechanical stress may alter the characteristics of these membrane organs by reorganizing the cytoskeleton.

There are many data indicating that external mechanical stress is transduced into the cell interior from the sites at which cells attach to extracellular matrix (ECM) [73]. Therefore transmembrane ECM receptors, such as the integrin family, are good candidates for mechnoreceptors. A large extracellular domain of the integrin–receptor complex binds to various ECM proteins, and a short cytoplasmic domain has been shown to interact with the cytoskeleton in the cell [74]. Integrins are known to transmit the extracellular signals not only by organizing the cytoskeleton but also by altering biochemical properties of cytoplasmic proteins [73]. Furthermore, because cytoskeleton proteins can potentially regulated plasma membrane proteins such as enzymes, ion channels, and ion exchangers, mechanical stress may modulate these membrane-associated proteins and stimulate second messenger systems through the cytoskeleton. The importance of the interaction of ECM–integrin–cytoskeleton on mechanotransduction was demonstrated by Wang et al. [75]. To directly apply mechanical load to specific cell surface molecules without producing large-scale changes in cell shapes, these authors bound spherical ferromagnetic microbeads coated with specific receptor ligands and then magnetized these surface-bound beads in one direction; they then applied a second weaker magnetic field oriented at 90 degrees, by which they were able to twist the beads in place and exert a controlled shear stress on bound cell surface receptors. Using this system they showed that integrin β1 not only induced focal adhesion formation but also supported a force-dependent stiffening response, and that an increase in cytoskeletal stiffness in response to the applied stress required an intact cytoskeleton. These results suggest that mechanical stress may be first received by integrin, and integrin-linked actin microfilaments transduce mechanical stress in concert with microtubules and intermediated filaments, or that the change in the cytoskeleton may alter the sorting and secreting of growth factors or cytokines. These experiments were performed using endothelial cells, and it remains unknown whether these mechanisms are applicable to other cell types including cardiomyocytes.

Autocrine and Paracrine Mechanisms

Many cells produce a variety of growth factors and cytokines through autocrine or paracrine mechanisms (or both), and second messenger cascades activated by mechanical stress in cardiomyocytes are similar to those evoked by growth factors or cytokines. Therefore it is possible that cardiomyocytes and nonmyocytes, such as fibroblasts, endothelial cells, and smooth muscle cells, secrete some hypertrophy-promoting factors following mechanical stretch. Mechanical stress on cardiomyocytes has been reported to increase the synthesis of some growth-promoting factors [76]. So far, many growth factors, including acidic and basic fibroblast growth factor (FGF), transforming growth factor (TGF) β1, and insulin-like growth factors (IGFs) I and II, have been reported to exist in the heart, and some can induce cardiac hypertrophy and specific gene expression in cultured cardiomyocytes: When cardiocytes were stimulated with basic FGF or TGF-β1, the reexpression of fetal genes was observed [37]. However, it remains uncertain whether these growth factors are involved in the development of mechanical stress-induced cardiac hypertrophy. On the other hand, as discussed in detail in the next section, angiotensin II (Ang II) has been demonstrated to be a candidate that mediates stretch-induced cardiomyocyte hypertrophy as an autocrine/paracrine-released cardiac growth factor. Endothelin-1 (ET-1) is another candidate hypertrophy-promoting factor released by an autocrine/paracrine mechanism. ET-1 has been shown to stimulate hypertrophy of cultured cardiomyocytes [77, 78] and ETA receptor antagonist has been demonstrated to block the load-induced cardiac hypertrophy during the early phase [79], although it remains uncertain whether ET-1 is produced or secreted in cardiomyocytes by mechanical stress. These results suggest that a variety of growth factors released by autocrine/paracrine mechanisms might participate in the development of cardiac hypertrophy induced by mechanical stress.

Involvement of the Cardiac Renin–Angiotensin System in Stretch-Induced Cardiomyocyte Hypertrophy

Renin–Angiotensin System and Cardiac Hypertrophy

Clinical studies indicate that the degree of LVH is not necessarily related quantitatively to the level of hypertension. This finding suggests that factors other than blood pressure modify the development of LVH in response to hypertension. Studies have demonstrated that angiotensin II acts as a growth factor on cardiac myocytes and that there is a strong similarity between the signaling pathway induced by mechanical load and that induced by Ang II: Both accelerate phosphatidyl inositol turnover and activate PKC, which increases the activity of MAPK; and these signals finally lead to enhanced protein synthesis and specific gene expression in cardiomyocytes [80–82]. Furthermore, angiotensin-converting enzyme (ACE) inhibitors have been shown to induce regression of LVH in experimental animal models [83–85] and hypertensive patients [86–88]. These results suggest the putative role of the renin–angiotensin system (RAS) in the formation of LVH. Of course, both mechanical and humoral factors have been implicated in the development of LVH, and the effects of ACE inhibitors antagonizing the growth-promoting influence of Ang II can never be disso-ciated from the concomitant systemic hemodynamic effects of these agents. However, a previous study indicating that even nonantihypertensive doses of an ACE inhibitor reversed LVH in thoracic aorta-constricted rats [89] strongly suggests the involve-ment of the RAS in the pathogenesis of LVH. Furthermore, a growing body of evi-dence supports the existence of a tissue RAS in individual organs and suggests the potential relevance of a cardiac RAS to cardiovascular homeostasis [90, 91]. One study showed that Ang II content in the hypertrophied left ventricle (LV) of spontaneously hypertensive rats (SHR) correlated with LV weight [92]. Furthermore, it has been shown that mRNA levels of angiotensinogen and ACE are increased in cardiac tissue subjected to pressure overload [93, 94]. These results suggest that the cardiac tissue RAS is activated by increased external load and that the endogenous Ang II, rather than the circulating one, plays a more important role than previously believed in the development of LVH.

Regression of LVH by Type1 Ang II Receptor Antagonist

Because we cannot exclude the possibility that the antihypertrophic effect of ACE inhibitors is due to the increase in the amount of bradykinins, the effect of type 1 Ang II (AT1) receptor antagonist TCV-116 [95] on LVH was investigated to confirm the contribution of the RAS in the development of pressure-overload LVH [96]. Treat-ment of SHR with TCV-116 induced regression of LVH in a dose-dependent manner, indicating involvement of the RAS in the development of hypertensive LVH in vivo. Moreover, TCV-116 treatment reduced the isozymic transition of MHC from V1 to V3 and inhibited the accumulation of collagen fibers in the extracellular space of the myocardium [96], which is comparable to the effect of ACE inhibitors on hypertro-phy-associated ventricular remodeling [97, 98]. These results suggest that the RAS may contribute to the hypertrophy of cardiomyocytes and to remodeling of the myocardium associated with pressure-overload LVH.

Inhibition of Intracellular Signaling Pathway of Stretch-Mediated Cardiomyocyte Hypertrophy by AT1 Receptor Antagonist

Although antagonizing AT1 receptors induced the regression of stress-induced cardiac hypertrophy in vivo, we cannot dissociate the antihypertrophic effect of this agent from its concomitant antihypertensive effect. Thus to elucidate the relation between mechanical load and endogenous Ang II in the development of cardiac hypertrophy, we cultured cardiac myocytes and imposed a mechanical load on them after treatment with AT1 receptor antagonist CV-11974, an active metabolite of TCV-116 [96]. This in vitro study revealed that antagonizing the AT1 receptors partially inhibited the intracellular signaling induced by stretching cardiomyocytes: pretreat-ment with CV-11974 partially inhibited the activation of MAPK, the induction of c-fos gene expression, and an increase in protein synthesis (Fig. 4). These results suggest that the autocrine/paracrine Ang II secretion partially mediates the stretch-induced cardiomyocyte hypertrophy via AT1 receptor subtype. On the other hand, Sadoshima et al. indicated that induction of the stretch-induced c-fos gene is completely inhibited by the AT1 receptor antagonist [99]. To elucidate this dis-crepancy, we extensively examined the relation between mechanical stress and Ang II using three Ang II receptor antagonists: saralasin (antagonist of type 1 and type 2 Ang II receptors), CV-11974 (type 1 receptor-specific antagonist), and PD123319 (type 2 receptor-specific antagonist) [T. Yamazaki et al., unpublished observation]. The mechanical stretch-induced activation of MAPK was significantly but only partially inhibited by pretreatment with saralasin and CV-11974 but not with PD123319. Furthermore, activation of MAPK induced by the conditioned medium of stretched silicone dishes was completely suppressed by saralasin or CV-11974 but not by PD123319. These results indicate that Ang II plays an important role in inducing the hypertrophic response to mechanical stress as an autocrine/paracrine-released cardiac growth factor via AT1 receptor subtype, although there also exist Ang II-independent pathways that mediate the stretch-induced cardiomyocyte hypertrophy (Fig. 5).

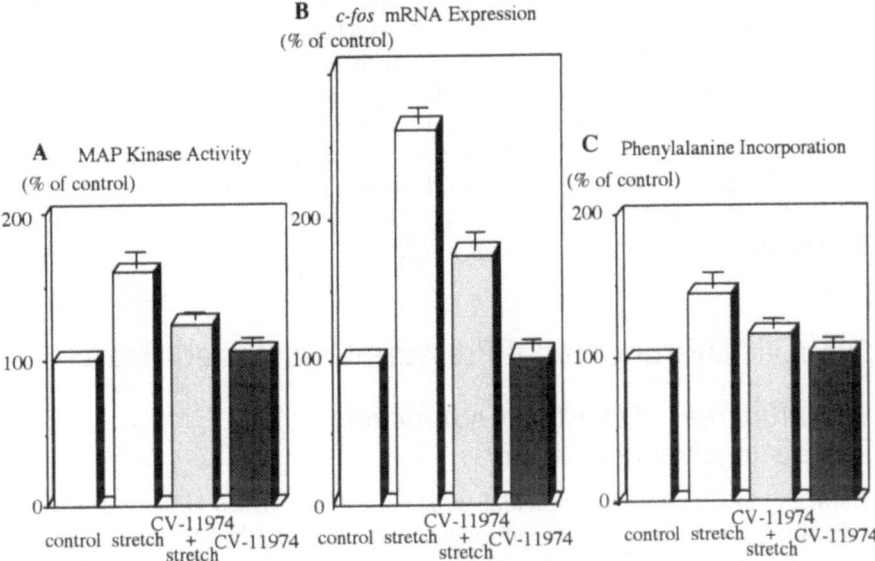

FIG. 4. AT1 receptor antagonist CV-111974 partially inhibits the activation of MAPK (A), c-fos mRNA expression (B), and an increase in protein synthesis (C) provoked by mechanical stretch

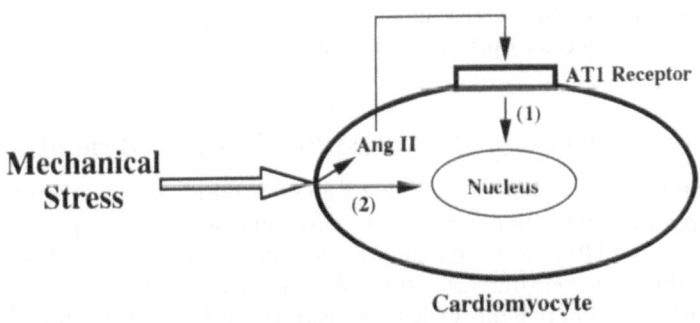

FIG. 5. Hypothetical role of AII in stretch-induced cardiac cellular hypertrophy. There are at least two pathways, that mediate stretch-induced cardiomyocyte hypertrophy: (1) a secreted Ang II-dependent one via the AT1 receptor; and (2) an Ang II-independent one. Ang II, angiotensin II; AT1, type 1 Ang II

The secretion of Ang II from cardiac myocytes by stretch has been reported by Sadoshima et al. [99]. The mechanism by which Ang II is released into the culture medium is then open to question. Because Ang II was reported to exist in a small granular compartment [99], Ang II should be secreted from cardiac myocytes by regulated mechanisms. Accumulated evidence suggests that an increase in intracellular calcium and PKC activity plays an important role in regulated secretion. It is known that the stretch of cardiomyocytes induces the entrance of extracellular Ca^{2+} into cells, which then induces Ca^{2+} release from Ca^{2+} stores in the myocytes [69]. Although stretch-induced activation of MAPKs is partially dependent on trans-sarcolemmal influx of Ca^{2+} [52], the chelation of extracellular Ca^{2+} with EDTA basically had no effect on stretch-induced c-*fos* gene expression [70, 100]. In contrast, c-*fos* gene expression induced by mechanical stress was completely blocked by PKC inhibitors and by the down-regulation of PKC [7]. These results suggest that PKC may be directly activated by mechanical stress, which may subsequently induce Ang II secretion. Hence mechanical stress may directly activate the protein kinase cascade of phosphorylation, including PKC and MAPK; and the activated PKC may induce secretion of Ang II, which in turn may amplify the signals evoked by mechanical stress. Further investigation, however, is necessary to understand the mechanisms by which mechanical stress stimulates Ang II secretion and to prove this hypothesis.

Diastolic Dysfunction of Pressure-Overloaded Hearts

Two Properties of Diastolic Dysfunction in Pressure-Overloaded Hearts

Slowing of myocardial relaxation and an increase in ventricular stiffness are detectable during the early stage of load-induced hypertrophy when there is no sign of reduced contractility [9]. The impaired relaxation is thought to be due mainly to the depressed function of the SR, and increased chamber stiffness is believed to be a result of collagen accumulation in the extracellular matrix. These two properties might account for the diastolic dysfunction in hypertrophied left ventricle [10, 11]. To ascertain the molecular mechanism of impaired diastolic properties in cardiac hypertrophy, we examined the altered function of the SR and the interstitial myocardial fibrosis in LVH induced by pressure overload.

Depressed Function of SR in Pressure-Overloaded Hearts

Cardiac SR is the major determinant that sequesters intracellular calcium and influences myocardial relaxation and tension development. Calcium uptake by SR is driven by Ca^{2+}-ATPase, a membrane protein with a molecular weight of approximately 100 kDa that constitutes 35–40% of the protein in SR [101, 102]. Many studies have reported the abnormalities of diastolic relaxation to be consistent with depressed Ca^{2+}-ATPase content and calcium uptake by SR in hypertrophied hearts [103, 104]. To investigate the mechanism of altered SR function in stressed hearts, we examined the regulation of Ca^{2+}-ATPase in an experimental model of cardiac hypertrophy induced by pressure overload [34].

Gene Expression of SR Ca[21]-ATPase in Pressure-Overloaded Hearts

As already discussed, expression of the Ca^{2+}-ATPase gene was markedly decreased by pressure overload in abdominal aorta-constricted rat hearts [34, 35]: The decrease was first detectable at 4h after the operation and gradually progressed. Densitometer scanning revealed that the mRNA level at 1 month after the operation was $32 \pm 7\%$ compared with that of the control group. The developmental change of Ca^{2+}-ATPase was also examined [34]. The expression of Ca^{2+}-ATPase was significantly low during the early embryonic period and steeply increased beginning at 2 days before birth. These results indicate that mechanical stimuli reduce the expression of the SR Ca^{2+}-ATPase gene, which reflects the fetal-type expression of this gene.

Ca[21]-ATPase Content and Calcium Uptake by SR in Pressure-Overloaded Hearts

To clarify whether reduced mRNA expression of the SR Ca^{2+}-ATPase gene affects SR Ca^{2+}-ATPase protein content or SR function, SR was isolated from hearts of control, sham-operated, and abdominal aorta-constricted rats; the yield of the SR fraction, the protein content of SR Ca^{2+}-ATPase, and the calcium uptake by SR were then measured. There was no significant change in the yield of SR protein in aorta-constricted rats compared to that in the sham-operated group. However, the Ca^{2+}-ATPase content and calcium uptake by SR were significantly decreased in rats that underwent pressure overload for 1 month compared to sham-operated rats [34].

Altered Function of SR and Impaired Diastolic Function in Stressed Hearts

The process of myocardial relaxation is regulated by cellular mechanisms that restore cytosolic calcium to a low concentration during diastole. Calcium uptake by SR Ca^{2+}-ATPase is thought to be foremost among these mechanisms. The results mentioned above demonstrate that (1) the expression of Ca^{2+}-ATPase is regulated by hemodynamic load and developmental stage at the mRNA level, and (2) the function of SR is reduced in pressure-overload hypertrophy. Such altered function of SR in the presence of cardiac hypertrophy may be regarded as a compensatory mechanism because depressed calcium sequestration by SR may reduce calcium release during systole and thus suppress oxygen consumption by hypertrophied myofibrils. At the same time, reduced SR function may cause an insufficient decrease of intracellular calcium during diastole and induce slowing of ventricular relaxation.

Cardiac SR also contains a unique low-molecular-weight integral protein, phospholamban. The phosphorylation of phospholamban by cyclic AMP-dependent protein kinase increases calcium uptake by accelerating the turnover rate of SR Ca^{2+}-ATPase [105]. Studies have indicated that the mRNA level of phospholamban is decreased in load-induced hypertrophy [35]. Taken together, these data suggest that the depressed function of SR regulated at the mRNA level of SR Ca^{2+}-ATPase may be responsible for the impaired diastolic function in pressure-overloaded hearts.

Interstitial Fibrosis of Myocardium in Pressure-Overloaded Hearts

The existence of an extracellular collagen matrix in the mammalian heart has been delineated [106], and the major part of the collagenous network is proposed to be produced by cardiac fibroblasts possibly in concert with myocytes. Previous studies have reported that hypertrophied postmortem left ventricles obtained from patients with systemic hypertension are associated with significant accumulation of fibrillar collagen within the extracellular space [107–109], and that this reactive fibrosis might be responsible for the increased ventricular stiffness [11]. We examined the formation of myocardial fibrosis in pressure-overloaded rat hearts in vivo and collagen synthesis of cardiac fibroblasts in vitro.

Abnormal Accumulation of Fibrillar Collagen in Cardiac Interstitium

Hearts from abdominal aorta-constricted and sham-operated rats were examined histologically 4 weeks after operation. Interstitial collagen fibers were studied by means of Azan staining. In sham-operated rats hearts, a slight amount of collagen was detected just around the vessel walls. With pressure-overload hypertrophy, on the other hand, significant collagen accumulation was observed within the interstitium as well as in the perivascular area. The amount of collagen in pressure-overloaded hearts examined by measuring the content of hydroxyproline was about twofold greater than that of sham-operated controls [110], demonstrating that the degree of interstitial fibrosis is greater than that of cardiomyocyte hypertrophy in this experimental animal model.

Expression of Collagen Genes in Pressure-Overloaded Hearts

Cardiac collagen fibers are composed predominantly of type I and type III collagen: about 80% and 15%, respectively [111]. The mRNA levels of both types of collagen gene have been demonstrated to increase progressively after abdominal aorta constriction [110, 112]. Other investigators previously reported that the relative amount of type III collagen to type I collagen is increased in pressure-overload hypertrophy [113]. These results suggest that both qualitative and quantitative changes in the extracellular matrix of hypertrophied heart are induced by hemodynamic overload and contribute to the increased chamber stiffness in pressure-overloaded hearts.

Effects of TGF-,1 and Ang II on Collagen Synthesis

Studies have demonstrated that collagen synthesis is regulated by many growth factors, cytokines, and other humoral factors such as TGF-β1 and Ang II. TGF-β1 is a 25-kDa homodimeric peptide that controls cell growth and differentiation in various kinds of cell types; it has also been known to regulate the abundance and composition of extracellular matrix [114, 115]. Ang II has been shown to have stimulative effects on connective tissue formation in vascular smooth muscle cells [116]. Because cardiac fibroblasts, rather than myocytes, are thought to be primarily responsible for collagen production in cardiac tissue [117], the effects of TGF-β1 and Ang II on collagen synthesis of cultured cardiac fibroblasts were examined.

An in vitro analysis using cultured cardiac fibroblasts and radiolabeled proline demonstrated that TGF-β1 stimulates collagen synthesis of cardiac fibroblasts in a dose-dependent manner [110], and an increase in TGF-β1 mRNA levels has been reported in rat hearts overloaded by aortic banding [70, 112]. Although it is unlikely that TGF-β1 is an initial mediator for cardiac hypertrophy because the increase in TGF-β1 mRNA is recognized 12h after banding, it is possible that TGF-β1 induces interstitial fibrosis in pressure-overloaded hearts. Furthermore, Ang II was demonstrated to stimulate collagen synthesis of cardiac fibroblasts in vitro [110]. These results, together with the fact that the cardiac tissue RAS is activated by hemodynamic overload, suggest that both TGF-β1 and endogenously produced Ang II contribute to the accumulation of extracellular collagen matrix and to the increase in ventricular chamber stiffness of pressure-overloaded myocardium.

Remodeling of Cardiac Interstitium and Ventricular Stiffness in Pressure-Overloaded Hearts

The collagenous matrix of cardiac interstitium provides a framework for myocytes. The remodeling of extracellular matrix by pressure overload can be an adaptational phenomenon because accumulation of collagen fibers might be necessary to support the hypertrophied myofibrils so they have effective force generation. Such abnormal interstitial fibrosis, however, increases chamber stiffness and may be an important cause of impaired diastolic function in stressed hearts. Our results suggest that the augmented production of TGF-β1 and Ang II may contribute to the formation of interstitial fibrosis in pressure-overloaded hearts. Increased plasma aldosterone has been shown to potentiate myocardial fibrosis [118]; thyroid hormone, on the other hand, was reported to suppress collagen matrix formation [119], suggesting that various kinds of humoral factors may be involved in the fibrotic response of the myocardium to hemodynamic overload. Furthermore, passive mechanical stretch has been demonstrated to stimulate collagen synthesis in cultured cardiac fibroblasts in vitro [120]. Although the precise mechanism of stretch-induced collagen synthesis is unknown at present, this finding suggests that mechanical stimuli may directly regulate collagen gene expression in cardiac fibroblasts.

Mechanism of Impaired Diastolic Function in Pressure-Overloaded Hearts

Various qualitative and quantitative changes in myocytes and extracellular components occur during the development of pressure-overloaded cardiac hypertrophy. Many of these changes serve as compensatory mechanisms at least during the early stage of ventricular hypertrophy, but under the condition of sustained hemodynamic overload they may be pathological and lead to diastolic dysfunction.

As already discussed, diastolic dysfunction has two aspects: slowing of relaxation and increased chamber stiffness. Depressed SR function might be responsible for delayed relaxation, whereas the accumulation of interstitial collagen is thought to contribute to the increase in ventricular stiffness. These two properties may play important roles in the mechanism of impaired diastolic function in stressed hearts.

Conclusions and Future Directions

Studies including ours have demonstrated that mechanical stress directly induces specific gene expression as well as protein synthesis in cardiac myocytes. IEGs are first induced, and then fetal-type genes are reinduced. Mechanical stress can also evoke a variety of biochemical signals in cardiomyocytes, and the molecules involved in the signal transduction pathway of mechanical stress are similar to those that play important roles in many other cells stimulated by growth factors, suggesting that the signal transduction pathways might be common among many cell types once extracellular stimuli are received and converted to intracellular signals.

It has also been demonstrated that the autocrine/paracrine effects of endogenous growth factors, such as Ang II and TGF-β1, may play critical roles in the pathogenesis of load-induced cardiac hypertrophy. Hence the interaction between cardiac myocytes and nonmyocytes or between cardiac cells and extracellular matrix is essential to the development of pressure-overloaded cardiac hypertrophy.

Although many of the biochemical events that occur in cardiomyocytes subsequent to mechanical stretch have been clarified, an intriguing question concerns how external mechanical stress is converted to intracellular biochemical signals. This question remains unanswered. In addition, the precise mechanisms by which external load induces release of endogenous growth factors and the sites at which these growth factors are produced are also still unknown. Furthermore, in pheochromocytoma-derived PC12 cells, both nerve growth factor (which acts as a neuronal differentiation factor) and epidermal growth factor (which acts as a growth-promoting factor) activate the MAPK cascade, although these two growth factors induce completely different phenotypes [121–123]. This finding suggests that a signaling pathway other than the MAPK cascade specifies the cellular response induced by different stimuli including mechanical stress. Additional studies are required to identify specific signaling molecules, including mechanoreceptors, mechanotransducers, and intracellular signaling molecules that are specific for stress-induced cardiomyocyte hypertrophy. The characterization of these signaling components will promote our understanding of the mechanisms by which adaptive cardiac hypertrophy deteriorates into congestive heart failure.

References

1. Morgan H, Gordon E, Kita Y, Chua B, Russo L, Peterson C, McDermott P, Watson P (1987) Biochemical mechanisms of cardiac hypertrophy. Annu Rev Physiol 49:533–543
2. Levy D, Garrison RJ, Savage DD, Kannel WB, Castelli WP (1990) Prognostic implications of echocardiographically determined left ventricular mass in the Framingham heart study. N Engl J Med 322:1561–1566
3. Zark R (ed.) (1984) Factors controlling cardiac growth: growth of the heart in health and disease. Raven, New York, 165–185
4. Cooper G, Kent R, Uboh C, Thompson E, Marino T (1985) Hemodynamic versus adrenergic control of cat right ventricular hypertrophy. J Clin Invest 75:1403–1414
5. Kira Y, Kochel P, Gordon E, Morgan H (1984) Aortic perfusion pressure as a determinant of cardiac protein synthesis. J Physiol (Lond) 246:C247–C258
6. Komuro I, Kaida T, Shibazaki Y, Kurabayashi F, Takaku F, Yazaki Y (1990) Stretching cardiac myocytes stimulates proto-oncogene expression. J Biol Chem 265:3595–3598
7. Komuro I, Katoh Y, Kaida T, Shibasaki Y, Kurabayashi M, Takaku F, Yazaki Y (1991) Mechanical loading stimulates cell hypertrophy and specific gene expression in cultured rat cardiac myocytes. J Biol Chem 266:1265–1268
8. Mann DL, Kent RL, Cooper G (1989) Load regulation of the properties of adult feline cardiocytes: growth induction by cellular deformation. Circ Res 64:1079–1090
9. Grossman W, Mclaurin LP (1976) Diastolic proterties of the left ventricle. Ann Intern Med 84:316–326
10. Gwathmey JK, Morgan JP (1985) Altered calcium handling in experimental pressure-overload hypertrophy in the ferret. Circ Res 57:836–847
11. Jalil JE, Doering CW, Janicki JS, Shroff SG, Weber KT (1989) Fibrillar collagen and myocardial stiffness in the intact hypertrophied rat left ventricle. Circ Res 64:1041–1050

12. Komuro I, Yazaki Y (1993) Control of cardiac gene expression by mechanical stress. Annu Rev Physiol 55:55–75
13. Greenberg ME, Greene LA, Ziff EB (1985) Nerve growth factor and epidermal growth factor induce rapid transient changes in protooncogene transcription in PC12 cells. J Biol Chem 260:14101–14110
14. Komuro I, Shibazaki Y, Kurabayashi M, Takaku F, Yazaki Y (1990) Molecular cloning of gene sequences from rat heart rapidly responsive to pressure overload. Circ Res 66:979–985
15. Boheler KR, Dillman WH (1988) Cardiac response to pressure overload in the rat: the selective alteration of in vitro directed RNA translation products. Circ Res 63:448–456
16. Castellucci VF, Kennedy TE, Kandel ER, Goelet P (1988) A quantitative analysis of 2-D gels identifies proteins in which labeling is increased following long-term sensitization in Aplysia. Neuron 1:321–328
17. Izumo S, Nadal-Ginard B, Mahdavi V (1988) Proto-oncogene induction and reprogramming of cardiac gene expression produced by pressure overload. Proc Natl Acad Sci USA 85:339–343
18. Komuro I, Kurabayashi M, Takaku F, Yazaki Y (1988) Expression of cellular oncogenes in the myocardium during the developmental stage and pressure overload hypertrophy of the rat heart. Circ Res 62:1075–1079
19. Mulvagh SL, Michael LH, Perryman MB, Roberts R, Schneider MD (1987) A hemodynamic load in vivo induces cardiac expression of the cellular oncogene, c-myc. Biochem Biophys Res Commun 147:627–636
20. Bauters C, Moalic JM, Bercovici J, Mouas C, Emanoil Ravier R, Schaffino S, Swynghedauw B (1988) Coronary flow as a determinant of c-myc and c-fos proto-oncogene expression in an isolated adult rat heart. J Mol Cell Cardiol 20:97–101
21. Schunkert H, Jahn L, Izumo S, Apstein CS, Lorell BH (1992) Localization and regulation of c-fos and c-jun protooncogene induction by systolic wall stress in normal and hypertrophied rat hearts. Proc Natl Acad Sci USA 88:11480–11484
22. Breitbert RE, Andreadis A, Nadal-Ginard B (1987) Alternative splicing: a ubiquitous mechanism for the generation of multiple protein isoforms from single genes. Annu Rev Biochem 56:467–495
23. Swynghedauw B (1986) Developmental and functional adaptation of contractile proteins in cardiac and skeletal muscles. Physiol Rev 66:710–771
24. Izumo S, Lompre A-M, Matuoka R, Koren G, Schwartx K, Nadal-Ginard B, Mahdavi V (1987) Myosin heavy chain messenger RNA and protein isoform transitions during cardiac hypertrophy. J Clin Invest 79:970–977
25. Black FM, Parker TG, Michael LH, Roberts R, Schwartz RJ, Schneider MD (1991) The vascular smooth muscle α-actin gene is reactivated during cardiac hypertrophy provoked by load. J Clin Invest 88:1581–1588
26. Schwartz K, de la Bastie D, Bouveret P, Oliviero P, Alonso S, Buckingham M (1986) α-Skeletal muscle actin mRNAs accumulate in hypertrophied adult rat hearts. Circ Res 59:551–555
27. Alpert NR, Mulieri LA (1982) Increased myothermal economy of isometric force generation in compensated cardiac hypertrophy induced by pulmonary artery constriction in the rabbit: a characterization of heat liberation in normal and hypertrophied right ventricular papillary muscles. Circ Res 50:491–500
28. Lompre A-M, Schwartz K, D'Albis A, Lacombe G, Thiem NV (1979) Myosin isoenzyme distribution in chronic heart overload. Nature 282:105–107
29. Day ML, Schwartz D, Wiegand RC, Stockman PT, Brunnert SR, Tolunay HE, Currie MG, Standaert DG, Needleman P (1987) Ventricular atriopeptin: unmasking of messenger RNA and peptide synthesis by hypertrophy or dexamethasone. Hypertension 9:485–491
30. Lattion AL, Michel JB, Arnauld E, Corvol P, Soubrier F (1986) Myocardial recruitment during ANF mRNA, increase with volume overload in the rat. Am J Physiol 251:H890–H896

31. Gardner DG, Gertz BJ, Hane S (1987) Thyroid hormone increases rat atrial natriuretic peptide messenger ribonucleic acid accumulation in vivo and in vitro. Mol Endocrinol 1:260–265
32. La Pointe MC, Deschepper CF, Wu J, Gardner DG (1990) Extracellular calcium regulates expression of the gene for atrial natriuretic factor. Hypertension 15:20–28
33. Kovacic-Milivojevic B, Gardner DG (1992) Divergent regulation of the human atrial natriuretic peptide gene by c-fos and c-jun. Mol Cell Biol 12:292–301
34. Komuro I, Kurabayashi M, Shibazaki Y, Takaku F, Yazaki Y (1989) Molecular cloning and characterization of a $Ca^{2+} + Mg^{2+}$-dependent adenosine triphosphatase from rat cardiac sarcoplasmic reticulum. J Clin Invest 83:1102–1108
35. Nagai R, Zarain-Herzberg A, Brandl CJ, Fujii J, Tada M (1989) Regulation of myocardial Ca^{2+}-ATPase and phospholamban mRNA expression in response to pressure overload and thyroid hormone. Proc Natl Acad Sci USA 86:2966–2970
36. Mercadier JJ, Lompre AM, Cuc P, Boheler KR, Fraysse JB (1990) Altered sarcoplasmic reticulum Ca^{2+}-ATPase gene expression in the human ventricle during end-stage heart failure. J Clin Invest 85:305–309
37. Parker T, Schneider M (1991) Growth factors, protooncogenes, and plasticity of the cardiac phenotype. Annu Rev Physiol 53:179–200
38. Zak R (1973) Cell proliferation during cardiac growth. Am J Cardiol 31:211–219
39. Chien KR, Knowlton KU, Zhu H, Chien S (1991) Regulation of cardiac gene expression during myocardial growth and hypertrophy: molecular studies of an adaptive physiologic response. FASEB J 5:3037–3046
40. Margan HE, Baker KM (1991) Cardiac hypertrophy; mechanical, neural, and endocrine dependence. Circulation 83:13–25
41. Simpson P, Savion, S (1982) Differentiation of rat myocytes in single cell cultures with and without proliferating non-myocardial cells. Circ Res 50:101–116
42. Peterson MB, Lesch M (1972) Protein synthesis and amino acid transport in isolated rabbit right ventricular muscle. Circ Res 31:317–327
43. Takala T (1981) Protein synthesis in the isolated perfused rat heart: effects of mechanical workload, diastolic ventricular pressure, and coronary flow on amino acid incorporation and its transmural distribution into left ventricular protein. Basic Res Cardiol 76:44–61
44. Sadoshima J, Izumo S (1993) Mechanical stretch rapidly activates multiple signal transduction pathways in cardiac myocytes: potential involvement of an autocrine/paracrine mechanism. EMBO J 12:1681–1692
45. Ohmori H (1985) Mechano-electrical transduction currents in isolated vestibular hair cells of the chick. J Physiol (Lond) 359:189–217
46. Yang XC, Sachs F (1989) Block of stretch-activated ion channels in Xenopus oocytes by gadolinium and calcium ions. Science 243:1068–1071
47. Kariya K, Karns LR, Simpson PC (1991) Expression of a constitutively activated mutant of the β-isozyme of protein kinase C in cardiac myocytes stimulates the promoter of the β-myosin heavy chain isogene. J Biol Chem 266:10023–10026
48. Cantley L, Auger K, Carpenter C, Duckworth B, Graziani A, Kapeller R, Soltoff S (1991) Oncogenes and signal transduction. Cell 64:281–302
49. Sturgill TW, Ray LB, Erickson E, Maller JL (1988) Insulin-stimulated MAP-2 kinase phosphorylates and activates ribosomal protein S6 kinase II. Nature 334:715–718
50. Tobe K, Kadowaki T, Tamemoto H, Ueki K, Hara K, Koshio O, Momomura K, Gotoh Y, Nishida E, Akanuma Y, Yazaki Y, Kasuga M (1991) Insulin and 12-O-tetradeca-noylphorbol-13-acetate activation of two immunologically distinct myelin basic protein/microtubule-associated protein 2 (MBP/MAP2) kinases via de novo phosphorylation of threonine and tyrosine residues. J Biol Chem 266:24793–24803
51. Boulton TG, Nye SH, Robbins DJ, Nancy YI, Radziejewska E, Morgenbesser SD, DePinho RA, Panayotatos N, Cobb MII, Yancopoulos GD (1991) ERKs: a family of protein-serine/threonine kinases that are activated and tyrosine phosphorylated in response to insulin and NGF. Cell 65:663–675

52. Yamazaki T, Tobe K, Hoh E, Maemura K, Kaida T, Komuro I, Tamemoto H, Kadowaki T, Nagai R, Yazaki Y (1993) Mechanical loading activates mitogen-activated protein kinase and S6 peptide kinase in cultured rat cardiac myocytes. J Biol Chem 268:12069–12076

53. Gomez N, Cohen P (1991) Dissection of the protein kinase cascade by which nerve growth factor activates MAP kinases. Nature 353:170–173

54. Ahn NG, Seger R, Bratlien RL, Diltz CD, Tonks NK, Krebs EG (1991) Multiple components in an EGF-stimulated protein kinase cascade: in vitro activation of a MBP/MAP2 kinase. J Biol Chem 266:4220–4227

55. Matsuda S, Kosako H, Takenaka K, Moriyama K, Sakai H, Akiyama T, Gotoh Y, Nishida E (1992) Xenopus MAP kinase activator: identification and function as a key intermediate in the phosphorylation cascade. EMBO J 11:973–982

56. Nishida E, Gotoh Y (1993) The MAP kinase cascade is essential for diverse signal transduction pathways. Trends Biochem Sci 18:128–131

57. Zheng CF, Guan KL (1994) Activation of MEK family kinase requires phosphorylation of two conserved Ser/Thr residues. EMBO J 13:1123–1131

58. Kyriakis JM, App H, Zhang X, Banerjee P, BrautiganDL, Rapp UR, Avruch J (1992) Raf-1 activates MAP kinase-kinase. Nature 358:417–421

59. Lange-Carter CA, Pleiman AM, Blumer KJ, Johnson GL (1993) A divergence in the MAP kinase regulatory network defined by MEK kinase and Raf. Science 260:315–319

60. Wood KW, Sarnecki C, Roberts TM, Blenis J (1992) Ras mediates nerve growth factor receptor modulation of three signal-transducing protein kinases: MAP kinase, Raf-1 and RSK. Cell 68:1041–1050

61. Davis DJ (1993) The mitogen-activated protein kinase signal transduction pathway. J Biol Chem 268:14553–14556

62. Ward GE, Kirschner MW (1990) Identification of cell cycle-regulated phosphorylation sites on nuclear lamin C. Cell 61:561–577

63. Haccard O, Sarcevic B, Lewellin A, Hartley R, Roy L, Izumi T, Erikson E, Maller JL (1993) Induction of metaphase arrest in cleaving Xenopus embryos by MAP kinase Science 262:1262–1265

64. Pages G, Lenormand P, L'allemain G, Chambard JC, Meloche S, Pouyssegur J (1993) Mitogen-activated protein kinases p42^{mapk} and p44^{mapk} are required for fibroblast proliferation. Proc Natl Acad Sci USA 90:8319–8323

65. Cowley S, Paterson H, Kemp, Marshall PCJ (1994) Activation of MAP kinase kinase is necessary and sufficient for PC12 differentiation and for transformation of NIH 3T3 cells. Cell 77:841–852

66. Thorburn J, Frost JA, Thorburn A (1994) Mitogen-activated protein kinases mediate changes in gene expression, but not cytoskeletal organization associated with cardiac muscle cell hypertrophy. J Cell Biol 126:1565–1572

67. Morris C (1990) Mechanosensitive ion channels. J Membr Biol 113:93–107

68. Kent R, Hoober K, Cooper G (1989) Load responsiveness of protein synthesis in adult mammalian myocardium: role of cardiac deformation linked to sodium influx. Circ Res 64:74–85

69. Sigurdson W, Ruknudin A, Sachs F (1992) Calcium imaging of mechanically induced fluxes in tissue-cultured chick heart: role of stretch-activated ion channels. Am J Physiol 262:H1110–H1115

70. Komuro I, Katoh Y, Hoh E, Takaku F, Yazaki Y (1991) Mechanisms of cardiac hypertrophy and injury: possible role of protein kinase C activation. Jpn Circ J 55:1149–1157

71. Sadoshima J, Takahashi T, Jahn L, Izumo S (1992) Role of mechano-sensitive ion channels, cytoskeleton, and contractile activity in stretch-induced immediate-early gene expression and hypertrophy of cardiac myocytes. Proc Natl Acad Sci USA 89:9905–9909

72. Hansen D, Borganelli M, Stacy G, Taylor L (1991) Dose-dependent inhibition of stretch-induced arrhythmias by gadolinium in isolated canine ventricles: evidence for a unique mode of antiarrhythmic action. Circ Res 69:820–831

73. Juliano R, Haskill S (1993) Signal transduction from the extracellular matrix. J Cell Biol 120:577–585

74. Hynes R (1992) Integrins: versatility, modulation and signaling in cell adhesion. Cell 69:11–25
75. Wang N, Butler JP, Ingber DE (1993) Mechanotransduction across the cell surface and through the cytoskeleton. Science 260:1124–1127
76. Hammond GL, Wieben E, Market CL (1979) Molecular signals for initiating protein synthesis in organ hypertrophy. Proc Natl Acad Sci USA 76:2455–2459
77. Ito H, Hirata Y, Hiroe M, Tsujino M, Adachi S, Takamoto T, Nitta M, Taniguchi K, Marumo F (1991) Endothelin-1 induces hypertrophy with enhanced expression of muscle-specific genes in cultured neonatal rat cardiac myocytes. Circ Res 69:209–215
78. Ito H, Hirata Y, Adachi S, Tanaka M, Tsujino M, Koike A, Nogami A, Marumo F, Hiroe M (1993) Endothelin-1 is an autocrine/paracrine factor in the mechanism of angiotensin II-induced hypertrophy in cultured rat cardiac myocytes. J Clin Invest 92:398–403
79. Ito H, Hiroe M, Hirata Y, Fujisaki H, Adachi S, Akimoto H, Ohta Y, Marumo F (1994) Endothelin ETA receptor antagonist blocks cardiac hypertrophy provoked by hemodynamic overload. Circulation 89:2198–2203
80. Baker KM, Aceto JF (1990) Angiotensin II stimulation of protein synthesis and cell growth in chick heart cells. Am J Physiol 259:H610–H618
81. Katoh Y, Komuro I, Shibasaki Y, Yamaguchi H, Yazaki Y (1989) Angiotensin II induces hypertrophy and oncogene expression in cultured cardiac myocytes. Circulation 80(suppl II):450
82. Sadoshima J, Izumo S (1993) Molecular characterization of angiotensin II-induced hypertrophy of cardiac myocytes and hyperplasia of cardiac fibroblasts: critical role of the AT1 receptor subtype. Circ Res 73:424–438
83. Sen S (1983) Regression of cardiac hypertrophy: experimental animal model. Am J Med 75(suppl 6A):87–93
84. Sen S, Tarazi RC, Bupus FM (1983) Effect of converting enzyme inhibitor (SQ 14225) on myocardial hypertrophy in spontaneously hypertensive rats. Hypertension 2:169–176
85. Pfeffer JM, Pfeffer MA, Mirsky I, Braunwald E (1983) Prevention of the development of heart failure and the regression of cardiac hypertrophy by captopril in the spontaneously hypertensive rats. Eur Heart J 4:143–148
86. Dunn FG, Oigman W, Ventura HO, Messeri FH, Kobrin I, Frohlich ED (1984) Enalapril improves systemic and renal hemodynamics and allows regression of left ventricular mass in essential hypertension. Am J Cardiol 53:105–108
87. Nakashima Y, Fouad FM, Tarazi RC (1984) Regression of left ventricular hypertrophy from systemic hypertension by enalapril. Am J Cardiol 53:1044–1049
88. Garavaglia GE, Messeri FH, Nunez BD, Schmieder RE, Frohlich ED (1988) Immediate and short-term cardiovascular effects of a new converting enzyme inhibitor (lisinopril) in essential hypertension. Am J Cardiol 62:912–916
89. Scholkens BA, Linz W, Martorana PA (1991) Experimental cardiovascular benefits of angiotensin-converting enzyme inhibitors: beyond the blood pressure. J Cardiovasc Pharmacol 18(suppl II):26–30
90. Dzau VJ (1988) Cardiac renin-angiotensin system: molecular and functional aspects. Am J Med 84(suppl 3A):22–27
91. Lindpaintner K, Ganten D (1991) The cardiac renin-angiotensin system: an appraisal of present experimental and clinical evidence. Circ Res 68:905–921
92. Mizuno K, Tani M, Hashimoto S, Niimura S, Sanada H, Watanabe H, Ohtsuki M, Fukuchi S (1992) Effects of losartan, a nonpeptide angiotensin II receptor antagonist, on cardiac hypertrophy and tissure angiotensin II content in spontaneously hypertensive rats. Life Sci 51:367–374
93. Baker KM, Chernin MI, Wixson SK, Aceto JF (1990) Renin-angiotensin system involvement in pressure-overload cardiac hypertrophy in rats. Am J Physiol 259:H324–H332
94. Schunkert H, Dzau VJ, Tang SS, Hirsch AT, Apstein CS, Lorell BH (1990) Increased rat cardiac angiotensin converting enzyme activity and mRNA expression in pressure overload left ventricular hypertrophy: effect on coronary resistance, contractility, and relaxation. J Clin Invest 86:1913–1920

95. Noda M, Shibouta Y, Inada Y, Ojima M, Wada T, Sanada T, Kubo K, Kohara Y, Naka T, Nishimawa K (1993) Inhibition of rabbit aortic angiotensin II (AII) receptor by CV-11974, a new nonpeptide AII antagonist. Biochem Pharmacol 46:311–318

96. Kojima M, Shiojima I, Yamazaki T, Komuro I, Zou Y, Wang Y, Mizuno T, Ueki K, Tobe K, Kadowaki T, Nagai R, Yazaki Y (1994) Angiotensin II receptor antagonist TCV-116 induces regression of hypertensive left ventricular hypertrophy in vivo and inhibits the intracellular signaling pathway of stretch-mediated cardiomyocyte hypertrophy in vitro. Circulation 89:2204–2211

97. Childs TJ, Adams MA, Mak AS (1990) Regression of cardiac hypertrophy in spontaneously hypertensive rats by enalapril and the expression of contractile proteins. Hypertension 16:662–668

98. Brilla CG, Janicki JS, Weber KT (1991) Cardioprotective effects of lisinopril in rats with genetic hypertension and left ventricular hypertrophy. Circulation 83:1771–1779

99. Sadoshima J, Xu Y, Slayter HS, Izumo S (1993) Autocrine release of angiotensin II mediates stretch-induced hypertrophy of cardiac myocytes in vitro. Cell 75:977–984

100. Komuro I, Yazaki Y (1994) Intracellular signaling pathways in cardiac myocytes induced by mechanical stress. Trends Cardiovasc Med 4:117–121

101. Tada M, Yamamoto T, Tonomura Y (1978) Molecular mechanism of active transport by sarcoplasmic reticulum. Physiol Rev 58:1–79

102. MacLennan DH, Holland PC (1975) Calcium transport in sarcoplasmic reticulum. Annu Rev Biophys Bioeng 4:377–404

103. Suko J, Vogel JHK, Chidsey CA (1970) Intracellular calcium and myocardial contractility. III. Reduced calcium uptake and ATPase of sarcoplasmin reticulum fraction prepared from chronically failing calf hearts. Circ Res 27:235

104. Sordahl LA, McCollum WB, Wood WG, Schwartz A (1973) Mitochondria and sarcoplasmic reticulum function in cardiac hypertrophy and failure. Am J Physiol 224:497–502

105. Tada M, Katz AM (1982) Phosphorylation of the sarcoplasmic reticulum and sarcolemma. Annu Rev Physiol 44:401–423

106. Caulfield JB, Borg TK (1979) The collagen network of the heart. Lab Invest 40:364–372

107. Caspari PG, Newcomb M, Gibson K, Harris P (1977) Collagen in the normal and hypertrophied human ventricle. Cardiovas Res 11:554–558

108. Anderson KR, St John Sutton MG, Lie JT (1979) Histopathological types of cardiac fibrosis in myocardial disease. J Pathol 128:79–85

109. Pearlman ES, Weber KT, Janicki JS, Pietra G, Fishman AP (1982) Muscle fiber orientation and connective tissue content in the hypertrophied human heart. Lab Invest 46:158–164

110. Shiojima I, Komuro I, Yamazaki T, Nagai R, Yazaki Y (1994) Molecular aspects of the control of myocardial relaxation: diastolic relaxation of the heart. In: Lorell BH, Grossman W (eds) Diastolic relaxation of the heart. Kluwer, Boston, pp. 25–32

111. Medugorac I, Jacob R (1983) Characterization of left ventricular collagen in the rat. Cardiovasc Res 17:15–21

112. Villarreal FJ, Dillmann WH (1992) Cardiac hypertrophy-induced changes in mRNA levels for TGF-β1, fibronectin and collagen. Am J Physiol 262:H1861–H1866

113. Weber KT, Janicki JS, Shroff SG, Pick R, Chen RM, Bashey RI (1988) Collagen remodeling of the pressure-overloaded hypertrophied nonhuman primate myocardium. Circ Res 62:757–765

114. Ignotz RA, Massageu J (1986) Transforming growth factor-β stimulates the expression of fibronectin and collagen and their incorporation into the extracellular matrix. J Biol Chem 261:4337–4345

115. Sporn MB, Roberts AB, Wakefield LM, de-Crombrugghe B (1987) Some recent advances in the chemistry and biology of transforming growth factor-beta. J Cell Biol 105:1039–1045

116. Kato H, Suzuki H, Tajima S, Ogata Y, Tominaga T, Sato A, Saruta T. Angiotensin II stimulates collagen synthesis in cultured vascular smooth muscle cells. J Hyperten 9:17–22

117. Eghbali M, Czaja MJ, Zeyclel M, Weiner FR, Zern MA, Seifter S, Blumenfeld OO (1988) Collagen chain mRNAs in isolated heart cells from young and adult rats. J Moll Cell Cardiol 20:267–276

118. Brilla CG, Pick R, Tan LB, Janicki JS, Weber KT (1990) Remodeling of the rat right and left ventricles in experimental hypertension. Circ Res 67:1355–1364
119. Yao J, Eghbali M (1992) Decreased collagen gene expression and absence of fibrosis in thyroid hormone-induced myocardial hypertrophy: response of cardiac fibroblasts to thyroid hormone in vitro. Circ Res 71:831–839
120. Carver W, Nagpal ML, Nachtigal M, Borg KT, Terracio L (1991) Collagen expression in mechanically stimulated cardiac fibroblasts. Circ Res 69:116–122
121. Traverse S, Gomez N, Paterson H, Marshall C, Cohen P (1992) Sustained activation of the mitogen-activated protein (MAP) kinase cascade may be required for differentiation of PC12 cells: comparison of the effects of nerve growth factor and epidermal growth factor. Biochem J 288(Pt 2):351–355
122. Nguyen TT, Scimeca JC, Filloux C, Peraldi P, Carpentier JL, Van Obberghen E (1993) Co-regulation of the mitogen-activated protein kinase, extracellular signal-regulated kinase 1, and the 90-kDa ribosomal S6 kinase in PC12 cells: distinct effects of the neurotrophic factor, nerve growth factor, and the mitogenic factor, epidermal growth factor. J Biol Chem 268:9803–9810
123. Peraldi P, Scimera JC, Filloux C, Van Obberghen E (1993) Regulation of extracellular signal-regulated protein kinase 1 (ERK-1 or p44/mitogen-activated protein kinase) by epidermal growth factor and nerve growth factor in PC12 cells: implication of ERK1 inhibitory activities. Endocrinology 132:2578–2585

Calcium-Activated Neutral Proteases and Myocardial Protein Catabolism

Teruhiko Toyo-oka, Hiroyuki Kawaguchi, and Wee Soo Shin

Abstract. Calcium-activated neutral protease (CANP, calpain) has many unique characteristics different from the lysosomal proteases (cathepsins) in myocardial cells. Its basic aspects have been clarified regarding biochemical profile, autoactivation, isoforms, subunit structure, functional domain, gene structure, and amino acid sequence deduced from cDNA. Its in vitro characteristics and interaction with endogenous inhibitor (calpastatin) specific to CANP was also studied in detail. However, its physiological and pathological aspects in vivo are still obscure. Several findings reported earlier suggest a grave and significant role in protein turnover in myocardial hypertrophy and its regression or irreversible protein degradation during the process of myocardial cell breakdown. We present an overview of the function of CANP and indicate a promising direction for research, restricting the scope of our investigation to the cardiovascular system.

Key words. Calpain—Calcium-activated neutral protease—Calpastatin—Myocardial degradation—Essential hypertension

Introduction

The net protein content in a cell depends on the balance of protein synthesis (anabolism) and degradation (catabolism). Protein metabolism in heart is directly related to many physiological aspects including cardiac hypertrophy, remodeling, apoptosis, and regression. Advances in molecular biology have made it possible to establish the mechanism of protein biosynthesis, whereas other aspects of protein catabolism are still unresolved, mainly because of the difficulty of analysis.

Most proteolytic enzymes are included in lysosomes and digest cytosolic proteins after incorporation into lysosomes [1]. Calcium-activated neutral protease (CANP; EC 3.4.22.17), also termed calpain, has four unique characteristics; (1) It is contained in the cytosolic fraction and may be the protease that initially degrades the highly organized architecture of the myocardial sarcomere or membrane proteins. (2) It requires Ca^{2+} for activation at micromolar or millimolar levels. (3) It is active at neutral pH, different from most cathepsins. (4) It is categorized as a cysteine (or thiol) protease, the active site of which contains cysteine; and it requires dithiothreitol

The Second Department of Internal Medicine, Health Service Center, Tokyo University Hospital, University of Tokyo, Hongo 7-3-1, Bunkyo-ku, Tokyo, 113 Japan

TABLE 1. Features of CANP in myocardial cells

1. Classified as thiol protease, which demands cysteine in the active site.
2. Requires millimolar or micromolar concentrations of Ca^{2+} for activation. High concentration of Ba^{2+} or Sr^{2+}, but not Mg^{2+}, replaces the role of Ca^{2+}.
3. Included in the cytoplasm of myocardial cells but not in lysosomes, such as cathepsins.
4. Degrades Z disks in the sarcomere. Accordingly, it makes it possible to morphologically identify the proteolytic action.
5. Inactivated by antibiotics (leupeptin, antipain), synthetic exoxysuccinate (e.g., NCO-700), and endogenous protein inhibitors (calpastatin I, calpastatin II).

CANP, calcium-activated neural proteases.

(DTT) or β-mercaptoethanol for full activation. CANP was first discovered in 1966 by Drummond and Duncan as a factor that activates phosphorylase b kinase during glycogen metabolism [2] and was accordingly designated the kinase-activating factor (KAF). It was later identified as a protease by Huster and Krebs [3] and finally purified from porcine skeletal muscle [4, 5] and then several tissues including heart muscle [6, 7]. As with other proteinases, CANP must be under continuous spatial and temporal control, and the structural and functional properties of the natural CANP inhibitor, calpastatin, must be considered (Table 1).

The CANP–calpastatin (an endogenous inhibitor of CANP) system is the functional proteolytic unit that may control the activity of the intracellular proteolytic system, which is related to the control of calcium homeostasis and to transmembrane signaling. There have been several excellent reviews on CANP [8–11]. Focusing mainly on the contribution of CANP to the cardiovascular system, we discuss here concepts concerning both the basic and clinical significance of this protease, which requires more convincing data obtained from sophisticated experiments for verification. We also address a promising methodology that may precisely elucidate the physiological significance of this unique enzyme.

Basic Enzymology

The CANPs and calpastatins are ubiquitously present in mammalian cells. There is emerging evidence of their importance in the turnover of myofibrillar proteins [4–6, 12, 13] and membrane-associated proteins [14]. CANP that is activated at millimolar concentrations of Ca^{2+} (mCANP) was first isolated using column chromatography. Purified enzyme revealed an 80-kDa protein band with [4] or without an extra 26-kDa subunit, according to sodium dodecyl sulfate polyacrylamide gel electrophoresis (SDS-PAGE) [6, 7]. The 80-kDa subunit was found to be stoichiometrically bound to the 26-kDa subunit but is not essential for the proteolytic action of CANP [6, 15]. The 26-kDa subunit may serve to translocate with the 80-kDa subunit on membrane systems in cells (e.g., sarcolemma and sarcoplasmic reticulum). The complex formation between the 80- and 26-kDa subunits is not tight and has been easily dissociated in high concentrations of urea, suggesting a hydrophobic bond between the two subunits [6] (Table 2).

When a portion of mCANP was autodigested, it became active in a micromolar concentration of Ca^{2+} [9]. It is activated by phospholipid and is associated with membrane systems [16]. Calpastatin not only inhibits CANP activity but also makes CANP attach to membranes. The translocation characteristics of CANP are similar to those of protein kinase C. Interestingly, protein kinase C is hydrolyzed by CANP and loses its ability to be regulated by Ca^{2+} and diacylglycerol. Protein kinase C is then permanently activated. It is uncertain if this uncontrolled activation occurs in vivo. With respect to their structure–function relation and enzyme activity regulation, CANPs are regarded as proenzymes that can be activated at the cell membrane in the presence of Ca^{2+} and phospholipid; they presumably regulate the functions of membrane-associated proteins after limited proteoysis [16]. The regulatory mechanism of CANP activity is shown in Fig. 1.

Thereafter μCANP, which is active at $10\,\mu M$ Ca^{2+}, was isolated from cardiac muscle by Mellgren [17]. The Ca^{2+} concentration required for μCANP activation was much lower than that for mCANP and might be much closer to physiological $[Ca^{2+}]_i$ $(0.1–1.0\,\mu M)$ [18]. Though μCANP was more relevant to $[Ca^{2+}]_i$ for proteolysis than mCANP, the Ca^{2+} concentration needed for full activation was still high $(1–10\,\mu M)$ in cardiac muscle [19]. Accordingly, some potentiating mechanism must exist to fill the gap between optimal Ca^{2+} concentration for enzyme activation and $[Ca^{2+}]_i$, as described below.

A full-length cDNA clone for the large subunit of mCANP from human tissues has been isolated [20, 21]. The primary structure of mCANP [relative molecular mass (Mr) 80 kDa; 705 amino acids] contains four distinct domains (Fig. 2), with a marked similarity between the second and papain-like thiol proteases and marked similarity between the fourth domain and calmodulin-like calcium-binding proteins. This

TABLE 2. CANP family identified by protein chemistry or molecular biology

Isoform	Structure
mCANP	80 kDa (+ 26 kDa)
Autolyzed mCANP	Partially hydrolyzed 80 kDa
μCANP	80 kDa (+ 26 kDa)
New CANP	90 kDa, in rabbit skeletal muscle (not in cardiac musle?)

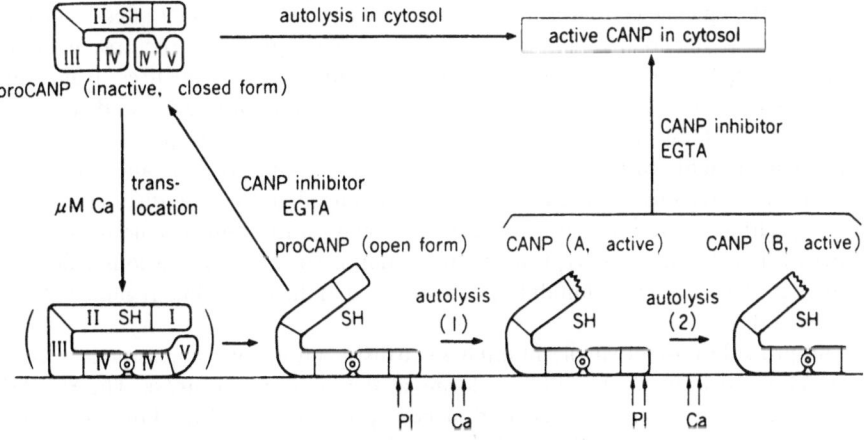

FIG. 1. Regulation of calcium-activated neural protease (*CANP*) activity. Several pathways to control mCANP are presented, including autodigestion and translocation between cytosol and the inner side of the sarcolemma. *PL*, phospholipid; *roman numerals*, domain; *SH*, cysteine residue at active site

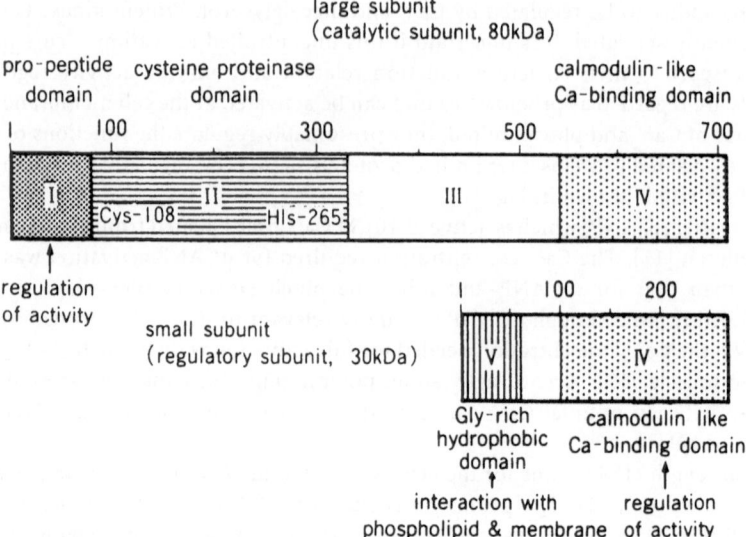

FIG. 2. Domain structure of CANP

finding suggests that calcium protease arose from the fusion of genes for proteins of completely different function and evolutionary origin. The deduced protein has essentially the same structural features as those revealed previously for the large subunits of μCANP [22].

The complete amino acid sequence of the large (catalytic) subunit of human μCANP was also deduced from its cDNA base sequence [20]. It is composed of 714 amino acid residues. Human μCANP has a clear four-domain structure. The role of each domain in Ca^{2+} sensitivity and protease activity of CANP was similar on the basis of sequence comparison [22]. Two sets of clones were identified as cDNA clones for μCANP and mCANP from a comparison of the primary structures deduced from the nucleotide sequences with partial amino acid sequences from the two isozymes. The cDNA clones for the 80-kDa subunits of μCANP and mCANP contained, in total, about 1.5- and 2.2-kb cDNA inserts, respectively, which correspond roughly to the C-terminal halves of the coding regions and the entire 3'-noncoding regions. The two isozymes are encoded by two distinct mRNA species, although the amount of mRNA significantly differs among tissues. Four E-F hand structures, typical calcium-binding structures in various calcium-binding proteins such as calmodulin, were detected in the C-terminal regions of both CANPs [23].

Autoproteolysis of the small subunit has two distinct functional consequences, each of which is associated with different forms of the autolyzed protease. The 80 kDa/ 26 kDa form of mCANP represents an inactive proenzyme, and the initial Ca^{2+}-dependent cleavage of the 26-kDa subunit results in activation of the protease. The activated enzyme hydrolyzes protein substrates with a Ca^{2+} concentration requirement of 350 μM for half-maximal rates. Further autoproteolysis, which results in formation of the 80 kDa/17 kDa heterodimer, serves to reduce the Ca^{2+} concentration requirement for protease activity 25-fold. Thus specific roles of the small subunit were identified during the regulation of mCANP activity [24].

Furthermore, a novel member of the CANP large subunit family was isolated from human and rat muscle cDNA libraries. The encoded protein (designated p94) consists of 821 amino acid residues (Mr 94 084 daltons) and shows significant sequence homology with both human μCANP and mCANP large subunits. p94 was divided into four domains (I–IV). Domains II and IV are potential cysteine protease and calcium-binding domains, respectively, and have sequences homologous to the corresponding domains of other CANP large subunits. However, domain I of p94 is significantly different from the others. In contrast to the ubiquitous expression of μCANP and mCANP, Northern blot analysis revealed that the mRNA for p94 exists in skeletal muscle, but none was detected in other tissues including heart muscle and smooth muscle [25].

Activation Mechanisms

Autoproteolysis

The proenzyme form of the Ca^{2+}-requiring neutral proteinase of human erythrocytes (proCANP) is converted to the active CANP by low concentrations of Ca^{2+} in the presence of appropriate substrates such as β-hemoglobin or heme-free β-globin chains. The conversion of proCANP to CANP is accompanied by a small decrease in the molecular mass of the catalytic subunit, from 80 kDa to 75 kDa; however, activation is not accelerated by addition of a small quantity of CANP. The autocatalytic inactivation of active CANP is related to disappearance of the 75-kDa subunit and the formation of smaller peptide fragments [26].

Activation of the Ca^{2+}-dependent neutral proteinase of human erythrocytes in the presence of Ca^{2+} and a digestible substrate is promoted by phospholipids (phosphatidylcholine, phosphatidylinositol, and phosphatidylserine). The presence of unsaturated fatty acid chains is essential, and metabolic derivatives are ineffective [15].

Phospholipids

The most effective promoter was a freshly prepared mixture of phospholipids from human erythrocyte membranes. Activation, which involves conversion of the 80-kDa proenzyme (proCANP) subunit to the 75-kDa active proteinase, is irreversible. Phospholipids act by producing a large decrease in the concentration of Ca^{2+} required for conversion of proCANP to active CANP [16]. Pontremoli's group has presented evidence that the exocytosis response is mediated by membrane-bound protein kinase C: (1) it is blocked by inhibitors of protein kinase C; and (2) it is enhanced in cells preloaded with leupeptin, which prevents proteolysis of protein kinase C and its subsequent dissociation from the cell membrane. Exocytosis promoted by either a high concentration of phorbol myristate acetate (PMA) or N-formyl-methionyl-leucyl-phenylalanine (fMLP) is inhibited by leupeptin, indicating that it is due to the action of an intracellular CANP, either directly or by conversion by CANP of membrane-bound protein kinase C to the soluble Ca^{2+}/diacylglycerol (DAG)-independent form. Intracellular mobilization of Ca^{2+} is also observed after stimulation with either PMA or fMLP, but only the latter results in a net increase in the intracellular concentration of free Ca^{2+}; under these conditions maximum exocytosis of granule contents is observed [27]. Stimulation of human neutrophils with PMA or fMLP results in translocation to the plasma membrane of 25–40% of the cellular CANP activity. In the membrane-bound form the Ca^{2+} requirement for proteolytic activity is substantially reduced. An anti-CANP antibody internalized by stimulated neutrophils is recovered in the same subcellular fraction that contains the membrane-bound CANP, apparently in the form of pinocytotic vesicles. When both antibody and CANP were present in these vesicles, membrane-bound proteinase activity was markedly inhibited, providing an explanation for the inhibitory effect of the antibody on intracellular CANP activity and the concomitant inhibition of granule exocytosis. The activated CANP associated with the plasma membrane compartment is therefore identified as the form specifically involved in mediating the physiological responses [28]. When this mechanism is working in the release of atrial natriuretic peptide (ANP) in normal atrial cells and in ventricular cells under overload, CANP would be regarded as a "converting enzyme" from proANP to active ANP.

Other Potentiators

An endogenous activator of the CANP has been identified in human neutrophils. In the presence of the activator, the affinity of CANP for Ca^{2+} is increased by more than 100-fold, and maximum catalytic activity is observed with a Ca^{2+} concentration below 1 µM (i.e., physiological range). The activator is a heat-stable protein with an apparent molecular mass of approximately 40 kDa. It appears to be associated with the cytoskeletal fraction of human neutrophils. Neutrophils also contain calpastatin. The effects of the activator and inhibitor appear to be antagonistic and may constitute a physiological mechanism for modulating intracellular CANP activity [29].

Isovalerylcarnitine (IVC), a product of the catabolism of L-leucine, is a potent activator of CANP in human neutrophils, rat skeletal muscle, and cardiac muscle [30–32]. At Ca^{2+} concentrations in the low micromolar range, activation was 12- to 15-fold, and the activity exceeded that observed with millimolar Ca^{2+} concentrations in the absence of the activator (an increase in V_{max} 1.3- to 1.6-fold above the values observed with the native enzymes at saturating Ca^{2+}). Of the acylcarnitine derivatives tested, IVC was most active. IVC did not increase the activity of CANP, which was fully activated by an endogenous cytoskeleton-associated activator protein; but at low concentrations of the latter, synergistic effects of the two activators were observed. IVC is also a potent activator of rat mCANP from heart muscle, with increasing affinity of CANP for Ca^{2+}. The increased affinity for Ca^{2+} results in an increased rate of autoproteolysis of mCANP. Activation by IVC is additive to that promoted by association to phospholipid vesicles [16] and may operate as a selective activator of CANP in the cytosol and the membrane fraction [31]. Of the two CANP isozymes present in muscle, the activator was identified and discovered to be specific for mCANP. It promotes activation of the proteinase by reducing the Ca^{2+} requirement for maximum catalytic activity of the proteinase from the millimolar to the micromolar level. Competition experiments revealed that the proteinase contains distinct sites for the activator [32].

Human erythrocytes contain a CANP activator protein with a molecular mass of approximately 40 kDa. The activator is present in association with the plasma membrane and promotes expression of CANP activity at a Ca^{2+} concentration close to physiological values. The initial step of the activating mechanism involves association of the activator with CANP, followed by autoproteolytic activation of the proteinase in the presence of 1 µM Ca^{2+}, at a rate identical to that induced by 1 mM Ca^{2+}. In a reconstituted system, the activator binds to erythrocyte membranes. In its membrane-associated form, the activator was selectively associated with CANP, thus favoring interaction of the proteinase with the inner surface of plasma membranes [33].

Rat skeletal muscle contains similar CANP activator protein characterized by a high specificity for mCANP. The activator protein increases the rate of intramolecular conversion of the native 80-kDa catalytic subunit of CANP to the autolyzed 75-kDa form, with the maximal rate at a Ca^{2+} concentration approximately 25-times lower than that required by the native mCANP. The activator protein interacts with native mCANP, forming a stoichiometric complex; interaction does not occur with the fully activated form, produced by autoproteolysis. Even after immobilization to membranes, the activator binds to CANP, which then undergoes sequential activation and release from its bound form. The activator is itself resistant to digestion by mCANP, whereas it increases the rate at which homologous calpastatin is degraded by the proteinase [34].

Calpastatin Isoform

Drummond and Duncan have identified an endogenous inhibitor (calpastain) for CANP in cardiomyocytes [2]. Calpastatin was purified, and the cDNA was cloned with a synthetic oligodeoxynucleotide probe based on the partial amino acid sequence of the purified protein. The deduced amino acid sequence contains 718 amino acid residues (Mr 76964), and the mature protein corresponds to the deduced sequence from the 80th residue of the primary translation product (resultant Mr 68 113). This deduced molecular weight is significantly lower than that determined by SDS-PAGE, suggesting that the inhibitor is posttranslationally modified. The sequence of the mature inhibitor contains four consecutive internal repeats, approximately 140 amino acid residues long, each of which might be responsible for the inhibitory activity [35].

From subcloning of restriction fragments of the cDNA corresponding to each of the four domains (encoding 104–156 amino acid residuces of the total 718 residues), the following two conclusions were drawn: (1) each of the four repeating units of the CANP inhibitor (about 140 amino acid residues) is a functional unit and can inhibit CANP activity independently; and (2) domains corresponding to well conserved sequences of about 30 amino acid residues containing a consensus Thr-Ile-Pro-Pro-X-Tyr-Arg sequence that is essential for the inhibitory activity [36].

Myocardial calpastatin appears to be associated in part with intracellular membranes, where it may effectively block the activity of mCANP on membrane-associated proteins [37]. Immunoelectron microscopic studies suggest that myocardial CANP and calpastatin are associated with a number of membranous organelles [38]. After increasing the $[Ca^{2+}]_i$ by Ca ionophore, calpastatin II is converted to calpastatin I in rat heart, whereas the reverse reaction is induced by the addition of cyclic AMP. Both interconversions preserved μCANP in a permanently inactive state. In contrast, expression of mCANP activity is significantly repressed as a result of a profound increase or decrease in the mCANP level [39].

Two calpastatins, calpastatin I and II, have been isolated from rat heart and displayed distinct inhibitory efficiency with μCANP and mCANP, respectively. Though the level of calpastatin I always exceeds that of μCANP, the level of calpastatin

II appears to be more closely correlated to the level of mCANP. As previously shown for skeletal muscle, the two inhibitor proteins can be interconverted by a phosphorylation-dephosphorylation reaction; the enzyme responsible for phosphate incorporation in calpastatin I is identified in cAMP-dependent protein kinase (A kinase). The presence of two interconvertible calpastatin forms provides the cells with a highly sensitive mechanism of regulation of the Ca^{2+}-dependent proteolytic system [40].

Bovine myocardial calpastatin could bind to SR preparations at neutral pH and low ionic strength. Even in the presence of 100–200 mM KCl, 4–5 µg of calpastatin was bound per milligram of membrane. Although calpastatin is found associated with bovine myocardial sarcolemma, neither canine nor human erythrocyte calpastatins were present in isolated erythrocyte membrane preparations. The bovine myocardial calpastatin, but not human erythrocyte calpastatin, could associated with purfied phospholipid vesicles at low ionic strength. Thus phospholipids appear to be involved in the binding of calpastatin to membranes [41].

Localization of mCANP Activity

More than 60% of brain mCANP activity was present in the particulate fraction, with only 30% in cytosol. In contrast, particulate fractions of liver, kidney, muscle, and heart contained about 8–12% of tissue mCANP activity in the particulate fraction, with 88% present in cytosol [37]. Adhesion plaques—specialized regions of the plasma membrane where a cell contacts its substratum—are dynamic structures. Little is known, however, about how protein–protein interactions are controlled at adhesion plaques. One mechanism by which a cell might modulate its associations with the substratum is by selective, regulated proteolysis of an adhesion plaque component. The catalytic subunit of mCANP is localized in adhesion plaques of several cell types (BS-C-1, EBTr, MDBK). Beckerle et al. have compared the susceptibility of the adhesion plaque constituents vinculin, talin, and α-actinin to calcium-dependent proteolysis in vitro and have found talin to be the preferred substrate for mCANP. The co-localization of a calcium-requiring proteolytic enzyme and talin in adhesion plaques raises the possibility that calcium-dependent proteolytic activity provides a mechanism for regulating some aspect of adhesion plaque physiology and function via cleavage of talin [42].

Degradation of Myocardial Proteins In Vivo

Concerning the physiological and pathological processes of myocardial protein catabolism, we have presented evidence that CANP is involved especially in irreversible breakdown of myocardial proteins (Table 3). During myocardial autolysis the amount of CANP at various organelles decreases, but the amount of calpastatin decreases to an even greater extent. Thus there may be a high CANP–calpastatin balance during heart ischemia at these sites. mCANP aggregation may contribute to localization of the proteinase at sites of high Ca^{2+} concentration within cells [43].

The Ca^{2+} sensitivity of natural actomyosin (NAM) isolated from both the intact left ventricle and an area of acute myocardial infarction (AMI) was analyzed by a superprecipitation response 2 to 48 h after left anterior descending coronary artery

TABLE 3. Pathophysiological actions of CANPs

Catabolism of protein
Irreversible breakdown of myocardial proteins during myocardial infarction
Platelet aggregation
Run-down of Ca^{2+} channels in sarcolemma
Impairment of Ca^{2+} release channel in sarcoplasmic reticulum
Irreversible activation of protein C kinase

ligation in the dog. NAM from the intact tissue showed normal superprecipitation and normal Ca^{2+} sensitivity. At 4 h after coronary ligation, Ca^{2+} sensitivity was lowered only in the endocardial half of the AMI region; it was markedly decreased in both the epicardial and endocardial halves at 6 h and was completely lost at 24 and 48 h. A superprecipitation response was demonstrated in all samples, however, indicating that both myosin and action preserved their functions during the course of the AMI. With SDS-PAGE, NAM from the AMI region revealed a moderate decrease in the tropomyosin-binding subunit of troponin (TN-T) and the Ca^{2+}-binding subunit of troponin (TN-C) as well as a drastic decrease in the inhibitory subunit of troponin (TN-I). This reaction resulted in the formation of extra bands of low molecular weight. These results suggest that degradation of troponin subunits occurs at 4 h after coronary artery occlusion and from the endocardial half of the AMI region. This degradation may be caused by one or several proteases that preferentially degrade the regulatory proteins among myofibrillar proteins [6, 19]. Furthermore, we have shown that CANP isolated from bovine heart selectively degrades both TN-T and TN-I in vitro [6, 13].

The structures of CANP and calpastatin have novel features with respect to their structure–function relation and enzyme activity regulation. The protease is regarded as a proenzyme that can be activated at the cell membrane in the presence of Ca^{2+} and phospholipid; it presumably regulates the functions of proteins, especially membrane-associated proteins, by limited proteolysis. Protein kinase C is hydrolyzed and activated by CANP at the cell membrane to a cofactor-independent form. These results suggested the possible involvement of CANP in signal transduction [44].

Calpastatin from skeletal and cardiac muscles of muscular dystrophic hamsters (UMX 7.1) was compared with that from normal control animals at 4 and 10 weeks of age by Western blotting using antibody raised against calpastatin. Fragmented calpastatin was found in dystrophic skeletal muscles in all cases at both ages, whereas intact inhibitor was detected only in the skeletal muscle of the normal hamsters. In contrast, there was little difference in CANP inhibitor from heart between dystrophic and control hamsters at 4 weeks. However, fragmentation similar to that in skeletal muscle was seen in the heart inhibitor in a few of the 10-week-old dystrophic hamsters [45].

Suppression of Myocardial Protein Degradation by a Synthetic Inhibitor

The CANP activity is inhibited by antibiotics including leupeptin and antipain [46] and the synthetic reagent NCO-700 with the chemical formula bis[ethyl(2R,3R)-3-[(S)-methyl-1-[4-(2,3,4-trimethoxyphenyl-methyl)piperazine-1-ylcarbonyl]-

butylcarbonyl]oxiran-2-carboxylate] sulfate [47, 48], whose analogues were synthe-sized against CANP. Among these compounds, NCO-700 most potently reduced the size of the AMI, which had been produced by coronary artery ligation in rabbits in vivo, although it showed less powerful action for inhibiting CANP activity in vitro. Thus NCO-700 might be a promising agent for reducing the size of AMIs and may be beneficial in clinical studies because it does not reduce cardiac muscle contractility, compared with β-antagonists or Ca^{2+} entry blockers. NOC-700 suppressed the activi-ties of both CANP and cathepsin B isolated from cardiac muscle. A kinetics study using ^{14}C-labeled NCO-700 suggested its incorporation into cultured myocardial cells. Under both aerobic and hypoxic conditions, the reagent dose-dependently inhibited peptide release from cultured myocardial cells. The amino acid release from heart slices of the adult rabbit was also blocked by the drug under hypoxic and glucose-depleted conditions. These data and the AMI size-reducing action of NCO-700 support the view that NCO-700-sensitive protease(s), CANP, and cathepsin B are working to induce an irreversible proteolysis during the process of myocardial cell degradation.

Intravenous administration of NCO-700 before or after coronary ligation (or both) significantly and dose-dependently reduced the necrotic mass in the rabbit left ventri-cle and prevented creatine phosphokinase loss in the ischemic myocardium up to 3 h but not at 6 h after the ligation. The activities of both CANP and cathepsin B in the subendocardial and subepicardial layers of the ischemic, marginal, or control myocardium of the dog were inhibited by NCO-700 administration after coronary ligation. A hemodynamic study using a heart-lung preparation of the dog dem-onstrated dose-dependent coronary dilatation with weak and transient negative inotropic and chronotropic effects. These data suggested that NCO-700-sensitive proteases are included in the process of myocardial cell degradation, and that NCO-700 temporarily salvages the myocardium, which is important for percutaneous transluminal coronary recanalization [49].

Ischemic heart (stunned myocardium) was reperfused after global ischemia for 15 min at 37°C. Recovery of developed pressure during reperfusion in hearts treated with 50 μM leupeptin was significantly greater than that in untreated hearts. Activa-tion of proteases by Ca^{2+} overload is suggested to play a significant role in myocardial stunning [50].

Human Platelet Aggregation and NCO-700 Effect

Platelet aggregation is related to blood clotting, coronary circulation, and coronary spasm after release of potent vasoconstrictors (e.g., thromboxane A_2, serotonin, adenosine diphosphate). Platelets secrete platelet-derived growth factor (PDGF), which promotes cell proliferation and migration of smooth muscle cells or fibroblasts, resulting in the initial event of arteriosclerosis or atherosclerosis. To clarify the physiological role of CANP in human platelets, we loaded platelets with a Ca^{2+}-sensitive fluorescent dye, fura-2, and measured the degree of aggregation, cytosolic $[Ca^{2+}]_i$, and proteolysis by SDS-PAGE. At physiological concentrations of Ca^{2+} (1 mM) in the incubation medium, $[Ca^{2+}]_i$ was less than 0.5 μM and there was no platelet aggregation. Ionomycin (0.15 μM) or collagen (50 μg/ml), but not ADP (10 μM), sharply enhanced the $[Ca^{2+}]_i$ to near 1 μM and caused aggregation. A calcium entry blocker, verapamil, completely abolished both the $[Ca^{2+}]_i$ rise and the aggregation.

NCO-700, a membrane-permeable inhibitor against cysteine proteases (including CANP), dose-dependently blocked the aggregation but did not change the $[Ca^{2+}]_i$ transient.

With SDS-PAGE, filamin, talin, and 70-kDa protein were seen to be degraded when platelets were aggregated by ionomycin or collagen; proteolysis was not observed when the aggregation was blocked by verapamil or NCO-700. These data provided evidence that Ca^{2+} entry exceeding $0.5\,\mu M$ is essential but not sufficient for platelet aggregation per se; and that activation of cysteine protease, most likely CANP, is involved in platelet aggregation by collagen or calcium ionophore [51]. Accordingly, the beneficial effect of NCO-700 on AMI during myocardial ischemia [47, 48] might be explained by the antiplatelet action. Fox has presented evidence that the shedding of microvesicles from the surface of platelets mixed with physiological agonists also involves activation of CANP, which cleaves components of the membrane skeleton and dissociates it from the plasma membrane GPIb–IX complex [52].

Essential Hypertension and Calpastatin

With regard to CANP in red blood cells or renal cells of hypertensive rat strains and humans, Pontremoli's group has presented an attractive ideal [53–63]. The presence of low levels of calpastatin activity in erythrocytes of hypertensive rats affects the regulation of CANP activity so it is highly susceptible to activation within physiological fluctuations of Ca^{2+}. When exposed to progressive and limited increases in $[Ca^{2+}]_i$, erythrocytes from hypertensive rats, but not those from normotensive rats, show a high degree of fragility that can be restored to normal values by inhibition of CANP. Within fluctuations in $[Ca^{2+}]_i$ close to physiological values, regulation of CANP activity is efficiently accomplished in normal erythrocytes but is completely lost in cells from hypertensive animals. Regulation is of critical importance for maintaining normal structural and functional properties of selective red blood cell (RBC) membrane and cytoskeletal proteins, among which band 3 and Ca^{2+}-ATPase appear to be the substrates with the highest susceptibility to digestion by CANP [53].

Human RBCs also include large amounts of mCANP and calpastatin. There is no difference of CANP activity in the RBCs of patients with essential hypertension regarding the boundary type and the distinct type. The amount of calpastatin measured by immunoactivity, however, was obviously diminished in the hypertensive group, and CANP activity predominated. In addition, the $[Ca^{2+}]_i$ concentration in platelets from patients with essential hypertension was reported to be high compared to that of normal subjects. Although it is not clear whether this phenomenon directly causes hypertension, more information is needed, as an elevated $[Ca^{2+}]_i$ was identified in platelets of hypertensive subjects [54].

During isolation of CANP from the human heart, we identified two new calcium-activated neutral hydrolases. One is an esterase of molecular weight 300 kDa that required millimolar concentrations of Ca^{2+} and hydrolyzed Ac-Tyr-OEt H_2O (optimal pH 7.0). The other is an amidase with a molecular weight of 70 kDa; it also required millimolar concentrations of Ca^{2+} and hydrolyzed a synthetic substrate for chymotrypsin, suc-Leu-Leu-Val-Tyr-MCA (optimal pH 7.2). Neither enzyme degraded casein or myofibrillar proteins (myosin, actin, troponin, tropomyosin). Their activities were not inhibited by exogenous protease inhibitors, leupeptin, antipain, monoiodoacetic acid, or chymostatin, whereas amidase activity was selectively blocked by the endogenous inhibitor against CANP. Thus their characteristics are different from those of chymotrypsin or CANP, and they seem to be new hydrolases in the human heart [55]. At present, the physiological and pathological significance of these hydrolases is not clear. It would be reasonable to assume that they contribute to the progression of myocardial cell breakdown during ischemia, when $[Ca^{2+}]_i$ increases concomitantly with CANP or Ca^{2+}-sensitive phospholipases [56].

Calpastatin activity, significantly reduced in erythrocytes of patients with essential hypertension, was restored to normal by appropriate treatment in parallel with a decline in blood pressure; it was degraded in human and rat RBCs by homologous CANP. Thus increased proteolytic degradation catalyzed by CANP could explain both the decrease in the amount of calpastatin activity and the profound difference between the intracellular level of the calpastatin observed in erythrocytes from patients with essential hypertension [57]. The presence in erythrocytes from hypertensive patients of an uncontrolled intracellular CANP-mediated proteolytic system accompanied by increased phosphorylation of band 3 protein(s) suggested molecular alteration, which is associated with the hypertensive state [58] and an unbalanced proteolytic system [59].

Digestion of Membrane-Associated Proteins in Myocytes by CANP and Modulation of Ionic Flow

Multicatalytic proteinase, which is known to degrade a large number of oxidized proteins, did not affect the native or oxidized forms of Na^+/K^+-ATPase. During oxidative stress there may be accelerated degradation of the oxidatively damaged Na^+/K^+-ATPase, either through internalization and transport to lysosomes or by the action of CANPs at the membrane; those isoforms of the enzyme that are more sensitive to oxidants are more susceptible to degradation by the above processes [64]. The covalent modification at the specific sulfhydryl residues in sarcoplasmic reticulum (SR) ATPase may mark the enzyme for degradation by intracellular proteinases, such as CANP [65]. Yoshida et al. have shown that a destructive process leading to the degradation of Ca^{2+}-ATPase in SR is activated by reperfusion but not by ischemia per se, and that CANP is not implicated in the degradation of Ca^{2+}-ATPase in SR [66].

The triad junction is important for efficient coupling between membrane excitation and muscle contraction. The triads are a composite mixture of breakage-susceptible (weak) and breakage-resistant (strong) triads to CANP digestion. The transverse tubules of strong triads contain a relatively high number of dihydropyridine receptors compared to those of weak triads [67].

Run-Down Phenomenon of Ca^{2+} Channels

The ATP-sensitive K^+ channels may contribute to increased cellular K^+ efflux and shortening of the action potential duration (APD) during metabolic inhibition, hypoxia, and ischemia in the heart. Inside-out membrane patches excised from control nonmetabolically inhibited myocytes were also exposed to various proteases, phospholipases, and other reagents that may be activated during metabolic inhibition. μCANP had no apparent effect on dissociation [68].

The Ca^{2+} channels and ryanodine receptor are co-purified with the 400- to 450 kDa high-molecular-weight protein of cardiac and skeletal junctional SR. mCANP selectively degrades the high-molecular-weight protein in cardiac and skeletal muscle SR vesicles. Degradation of this protein was associated with the appearance of 315-kDa and 150-kDa proteolytic fragments and with a change in the ultrastructure of the "feet" (extravesicular projections that protrude from the junctional SR membrane).

Proteolysis did not alter the unitary channel conductances but did increase the percentage of channel open times. After proteolysis, channel opening remained dependent on micromolar concentrations of cis-Ca^{2+}. Proteolysis of the Ca^{2+} release channels in SR with mCANP selectively impairs their inactivation, leaving their unitary conductance and the requirement for micromolar concentrations of Ca^{2+} intact [69].

The Ca^{2+} channels comprise the main influx pathway, which relates directly to the excitation-contraction coupling of myocytes. Because these channels are easily inactivated during patch-clamp experiments, it is usually difficult to perform the experiment over an extended time. This phenomenon was designated the run-down phenomenon. The inactivation rate is dependent on the Ca^{2+} concentration, relatively slow in the presence of the Ca^{2+} chelator EGTA, and accelerated when CANP is added in the presence of Ca^{2+}. The run-down phenomenon was inhibited when calpastatin was added to the incubation mixture. Accordingly, CANP was suspected to be a responsible factor for inactivating Ca^{2+} channels.

Conclusion

The structures of CANP and calpastatin have novel features with respect to their structure–function relation and enzyme activity regulation. The protease is regarded as a proenzyme that can be activated at the cell membrane in the presence of Ca^{2+} and phospholipid; it presumably regulates the functions of proteins, especially membrane-associated proteins, by limited proteolysis. Protein kinase C is hydrolyzed and activated by CANP at the cell membrane to become a cofactor-independent form. These results suggest the possible involvement of CANP in signal transduction [44].

Some CANP studies are still under way. Many factors, including adjustment of $[Ca^{2+}]_i$, the existence of two or three isoforms of CANP, an activation mechanism that includes autodigestion for each CANP, the potentiating action of phospholipids, translocation of each CANP, and endogenous and exogenous inhibitors add to the complexity of the enzyme. CANP is likely involved in transmembrane signal transduction and intracellular processing of biologically inert prosubstances to active substances. It is essential to develop a completely new strategy in order to gain insight into the physiological and pathophysiogical significance of CANP.

Acknowledgments. This study was financially supported in part by: the Ministries of Education, Science, and Culture, and of Health and Welfare, Japan; Ca Signal Workshop in Cardiovascular Systems funded by the Research Foundation of Sankyo Life Science for Clinical Pharmacology and for Basic Study on Cardiac Hypertrophy;

Uehara Memorial Foundation; and Fukuda Memorial Foundation. The authors thank Ms. M. Kataoka for her secretarial assistance.

References

1. De Duve C, Wattiau R (1966) Function of lysosomes. Annu Rev Physiol 28:435–492
2. Drummond GI, Duncan L (1966) The action of calcium ion on cardiac phosphorylase b kinase. J Biol Chem 241:3097–3103
3. Huston RB, Krebs EG (1968) Activation of skeletal muscle phosphorylase kinase by Ca^{2+}: identification of the kinase activating factor as a proteolytic enzyme. Biochemistry 7:2116–2122
4. Dayton WR, Goll DE, Zeece MG, Robson RM, Reville WJ (1976) A Ca^{2+}-activated protease possibly involved in myofibrillar protein turnover: purification from porcine muscle. Biochemistry 15:2150–2158
5. Dayton WR, Reville WJ, Goll DE, Stromer MH (1976) A Ca^{2+}-activated protease possibly involved in myofibrillar protein turnover: partial characterization of the purified enzyme. Biochemistry 15:2159–2167
6. Toyo-oka T, Masaki T (1979) Calcium-activated neutral protease from bovine ventricular muscle: isolation and some of its properties. J Mol Cell Cardiol 11:769–786
7. Croall DE, DeMartino GN (1983) Purification and characterization of calcium-dependent proteases from rat heart. J Biol Chem 258:5660–5665
8. Pontremoli S, Melloni E (1986) Extralysosomal protein degradation. Annu Rev Biochem 55:455–481
9. Suzuki K, Imajoh S, Emori Y, Kawasaki H, Minami Y, Ohno S (1988) Regulation of activity of calcium activated neutral protease. Adv Enzyme Regul 27:153–169
10. Mellgren RL, Renno WM, Lane RD (1989) The non-lysosomal, calcium-dependent proteolytic system of mammalian cells. Rev Biol Celular 20:139–159
11. Mellgren RL, Renno WM, Lane RD (1989) The non-lysosomal, calcium-dependent proteolytic system of mammalian cells. Rev Biol Celular 20:139–159
12. Toyo-oka T (1980) Increased activity of intramuscular proteases in hyperthyroid state. FEBS Lett 117:1224
13. Toyo-oka T (1982) Phosphorylation with cyclic adenosine 3'5' monophosphate-dependent protein kinase renders bovine cardiac troponin sensitive to the degradation by calcium-activated neutral protease. Biochem Biophys Res Commun 107:44–50
14. Melloni E, Pontremoli S (1989) The calpains. Trends Neurosci 12:438–444
15. Suzuki K, Emori Y, Ohno S, Imahori S, Kawasaki H, Miyake S (1986) Structure and function of the small (30K) subunit of calcium-activated neutral protease (CANP). Biomed Biochim Acta 45:1487–1491
16. Pontremoli S, Melloni E, Sparatore B, Salamino F, Michetti M, Sacco O, Horecker BL (1985) Role of phospholipids in the activation of the Ca^{2+}-dependent neutral proteinase of human erythrocytes. Biochem Biophys Res Commun. 129:389–395
17. Mellgren RL (1980) Canine cardiac calcium-dependent proteases: resolution of two forms with different requirements for calcium. FEBS Lett 109:129–133
18. Ebashi S (1980) Regulation of muscle contraction: a Croonian lecture. Proc R Soc Lond [Biol] 201:258–286
19. Toyo-oka T, Ross J Jr (1981) Ca^{2+} sensitivity change and troponin loss in cardiac natural actomyosin after coronary occlusion. Am J Physiol 240:H704–708
20. Ohno S, Emori Y, Imajoh S, Kawasaki H, Kisaragi M, Suzuki K (1984) Evolutionary origin of a calcium-dependent protease by fusion of genes for a thiol protease and a calcium-binding protein? Nature 312:566–570
21. Imajoh S, Aoki K, Ohno S, Emori Y, Kawasaki H, Sugihara H, Suzuki K (1988) Molecular cloning of the cDNA for the large subunit of the high-Ca^{2+}-requiring form of human Ca^{2+}-activated neutral protease. Biochemistry 27:8122–8128
22. Aoki K, Imajoh S, Ohno S, Emori Y, Koike M, Kosaki G, Suzuki K. (1986) Complete

amino acid sequence of the large subunit of the low-Ca^{2+}-requiring form of human Ca^{2+}-activated neutral protease (μCANP) deduced from its cDNA sequence. FEBS Lett 205:313–317

23. Emori Y, Kawasaki H, Sugihara H, Imajoh S, Kawashima S, Suzuki K (1986) Isolation and sequence analyses of cDNA clones for the large subunits of two isozymes of rabbit calcium-dependent protease. J Biol Chem 261:9465–9471

24. DeMartino GN, Huff CA, Croall DE (1986) Autoproteolysis of the small subunit of calcium-dependent protease II activates and regulates protease activity. J Biol Chem 261:12047–12052

25. Sorimachi H, Imajoh OS, Emori Y, Kawasaki H, Ohno S, Minami Y, Suzuki K (1989) Molecular cloning of a novel mammalian calcium-dependent protease distinct from both m- and μ-types: specific expression of the mRNA in skeletal muscle. J Biol Chem 264:20106–20111

26. Pontremoli S, Sparatore B, Melloni E, Michetti M, Horecker BL (1984) Activation by hemoglobin of the Ca^{2+}-requiring neutral proteinase of human erythrocytes: structural requirements. Biochem Biophys Res Commun 123:331–337

27. Pontremoli S, Melloni E, Michetti M, Sacco O, Salamino F, Sparatore B, Horecker BL (1986) Biochemical responses in activated human neutrophils mediated by protein kinase C and a Ca^{2+}-requiring proteinase. J Biol Chem. 261:8309–8313

28. Pontremoli S, Melloni E, Salamino F, Patrone M, Michetti M, Horecker BL. Activation of neutrophil calpain following its translocation to the plasma membrane induced by phorbol ester or fMet-Leu-Phe. Biochem Biophys Res Commun 160:737–743

29. Pontremoli S, Melloni E, Michetti M, Salamino F, Sparatore B, Horecker BL (1988) An endogenous activator of the Ca^{2+}-dependent proteinase of human neutrophils that increases its affinity for Ca^{2+}. Proc Natl Acad Sci USA 85:1740–1743

30. Pontremoli S, Melloni E, Michetti M, Sparatore B, Salamino F, Siliprandi N, Horecker BL (1987) Isovalerylcarnitine is a specific activator of calpain of human neutrophils. Biochem Biophys Res Commun 148:1189–1195

31. Pontremoli S, Melloni E, Viotti PL, Michetti M, Di LF, Siliprandi N (1990) Isovaleryl-carnitine is a specific activator of the high calcium requiring calpain forms. Biochem Biophys Res Commun 167:373–380

32. Pontremoli S, Viotti PL, Michetti M, Sparatore B, Salamino F, Melloni E (1990) Identification of an endogenous activator of calpain in rat skeletal muscle. Biochem Biophys Res Commun 171:569–574

33. Salamino F, Sparatore B, Melloni E, Michetti M, Viotti PL, Pontremoli S, Carafoli E (1994) The plasma membrane calcium pump is the preferred calpain substrate within the erythro cyte. Cell Calcium 15:28–35

34. Michetti M, Viotti PL, Melloni E, Pontremoli S (1991) Mechanism of action of the calpain activator protein in rat skeletal muscle. Eur J Biochem 202:1177–1180

35. Emori Y, Kawasaki H, Imajoh S, Imahori K, Suzuki K (1987) Endogenous inhibitor for calcium-dependent cysteine protease contains four internal repeats that could be responsible for its multiple reactive sites. Proc Natl Acad Sci USA 84:3590–3594

36. Emori Y, Kawasaki H, Imajoh S, Minami Y, Suzuki K (1988) All four repeating domains of the endogenous inhibitor for calcium-dependent protease independently retain inhibitory activity: expression of the cDNA fragments in Escherichia coli. J Biol Chem 263:2364–2370

37. Banik NL, Chakrabarti AK, Hogan EL (1992) Effects of detergents on Ca^{2+}-activated neural proteinase activity (calpain) in neural and non-neural tissue: a comparative study. 17: 797–802

38. Salamino F, De TR, Mengotti P, Viotti PL, Melloni E, Pontremoli S. Site-directed activation of calpain is promoted by a membrane-associated natural activator protein. Biochem J 290:191–197

39. Pontremoli S, Melloni E, Viotti PL, Michetti M, Salamino F, Horecker BL. Identification of two calpastatin forms in rat skeletal muscle and their susceptibility to digestion by homologous calpains. Arch Biochem Biophys 288:646–652

40. Salamino F, De TR, Michetti M, Mengotti P, Melloni E, Pontremoli S (1994) Modulation of

calpastatin specificity in rat tissues by reversible phosphorylation and dephosphorylation. Biochem Biophys Res Commun 199:1326–1332

41. Mellgren RL (1988) On the mechanism of binding of calpastatin, the protein inhibitor of calpains, to biologic membranes. Biochem Biophys Res Commun 150:170–176

42. Beckerle MC, Burridge K, DeMartino GN, Croall DE (1987) Colocalization of calcium-dependent protease II and one of its substrates at sites of cell adhesion. Cell 51:569–577

43. Toyo-oka T, Morita M, Shin WS, Okaimatsuo Y, Sugimoto T (1991) Contribution of calcium-activated neutral protease to the degradation process of ischemic heart. Jpn Circ J 55:1124–1126

44. Suzuki K, Imajoh S, Emori Y, Kawasaki H, Minami Y, Ohno S (1987) Calcium-activated neutral protease and its endogenous inhibitor: activation at the cell membrane and biological function. FEBS Lett 220:271–277

45. Nakamura M, Imajoh OS, Suzuki K, Kawashima S (1991) An endogenous inhibitor of calcium-activated neutral protease in UMX 7.1 hamster dystrophy. Muscle Nerve 14:701–708

46. Toyo-oka T, Shimizu T, Masaki T (1978) Inhibition of proteolytic activity of calcium activated neutral protease by leupeptin and antipain. Biochem Biophys Res Commun 82:484–491

47. Toyo-oka T, Kamishiro T, Hara K, Nakamura N, Kitahara M, Masaki T (1986) Suppression of myocardial protein degradation by the protease inhibitor bis[ethyl(2R,3R)-3-[(S)-methyl-1-[4-(2,3,4-tri-methoxy-phenyl-methyl) piperazine-1-ylcarbonyl] butyl carbonyl]oxiran-2-carboxylate]sulfate under hypoxia. Arzneimittelforschung 36:190–193

48. Toyo-oka T, Kamishiro T, Gotoh Y, Fumino H, Masaki T, Hosoda S (1986) Temporary (2,3,4-trimethoxyphenyl-methyl) piperazin-1-ylcarbonyl]butyl-carbonyl]oxiran-2-carboxylate]sulfate. Arzneimittelforschung 36:671–675

49. Toyo-oka T, Kamishiro T, Masaki M, Masaki T (1982) Reduction of experimentally produced acute myocardial infarction size by a new synthetic inhibitor, NCO-700, against calcium-activated neutral protease. Jpn Heart J 23:829–834

50. Matsumura Y, Kusuoka H, Inoue M, Hori M, Kamada T (1993) Protective effect of the protease inhibitor leupeptin against myocardial stunning. J Cardiovasc Pharmacol 22:135–142

51. Toyo-oka T, Shin WS, Okai Y, Dan Y, Morita M, Iizuka M, Sugimoto T (1989) Collagen-stimulated human platelet aggregation is mediated by endogenous calcium-activated neutral protease. Circ Res 64:407–410

52. Fox JE (1994) Shedding of adhesion receptors from the surface of activated platelets. Blood Coagul Fibrinolysis 5:291–304

53. Salamino F, De TR, Mengotti P, Viotti PL, Melloni E, Pontremoli S (1992) Different susceptibility of red cell membrane proteins to calpain degradation. Arch Biochem Biophys 298:287–292

54. Erne P, Bolli P, Burgisser E, Buhler FR (1984) Correlation of platelet calcium with blood pressure: effect of antihypertensive therapy. N Engl J Med 310:1084–1088

55. Ikeda U, Toyo-oka T, Hosoda S (1986) Identification of two new calcium dependent hydrolases in the human heart. Biochem Biophys Res Commun 136:773–777

56. Toyo-oka T, Hara K, Nakamura N, Kitahara M, Masaki T (1985) Ca overload and the action of calcium sensitive proteases, phospholipases and prostaglandin E_2 in myocardial cell degradation. Basic Res Cardiol 80:303–315

57. Toyo-oka T, Kamishiro T, Masaki M, Masaki T (1982) Reduction of experimentally produced acute myocardial infarction size by a new synthetic inhibitor, NCO-700, against calcium-activated neutral protease. Jpn Heart J 23:829–834

58. Pontremoli S, Sparatore B, Salamino F, De TR, Pontremoli R, Melloni E (1988) The role of calpain in the selective increased phosphorylation of the anion-transport protein in red cell of hypertensive subjects. Biochem Biophys Res Commun 151:590–597

59. Pontremoli S, Salamino F, Sparatore B, De TR, Pontremoli R Melloni E (1988) Charac-

terization of the calpastatin defect in erythrocytes from patients with essential hypertension. Biochem Biophys Res Commun 157:867–874

60. Pontremoli S, Melloni E, Salamino F, Sparatore B, Michctti M, Sacco O, Bianchi G (1986) Characterization of the defective calpain-endogenous calpain inhibitor system in erythrocytes from Milan hypertensive rats. Biochem Biophys Res Commun 139:341–347

61. Pontremoli S, Melloni E, Salamino F, Sparatore B, Viotti P, Michetti M, Duzzi L, Bianchi G (1987) Decreased level of calpain inhibitor activity in kidney from Milan hypertensive rats. Biochem Biophys Res Commun 145:1287–1294

62. Pontremoli S, Melloni E, Sparatore B, Salamino F, Pontremoli R, Tizianello A (1987) Increased phosphorylation in red cell membranes of subjects affected by essential hypertension. Biochem Biophys Res Commun 145:1329–1334

63. Pontremoli S, Melloni E, Sparatore B, Salamino F, Pontremoli R, Tizianello A, Barlassina C, Cusi D, Colombo R, Bianchi G. Erythrocyte deficiency in calpain inhibitor activity in essential hypertension. Hypertension 12:474–478

64. Zolotarjova N, Ho C, Mellgren RL, Askari A, Huang WH (1994) Different sensitivities of native and oxidized forms of Na$^+$/K$^+$-ATPase to intracellular proteinases. Biochim Biophys Acta 1192:125–131

65. Chung SS, Kwak KB, Lee JS, Ha DB, Chung CH (1990) Preferential degradation of the KMnO$_4$-oxidized or N-ethylmaleimide-modified form of sarcoplasmic reticulum ATPase by calpain from chick skeletal muscle. Biochim Biophys Acta 1041:160-163

66. Yoshida Y, Shiga T, Imai S (1990) Degradation of sarcoplasmic reticulum calcium-pumping ATPase in ischemic-reperfused myocardium: role of calcium-activated neutral protease. Basic Res Cardio. 85:495–507

67. Kim KC, Caswell AH, Brunschwig JP, Brandt NR (1990) Identification of a new subpopulation of triad junctions isolated from skeletal muscle; morphological correlations with intact muscle. J Membr Biol 113:221–235

68. Deutsch N, Weiss JN (1993) ATP-sensitive K$^+$ channel modification by metabolic inhibition in isolated guinea-pig ventricular myocytes. J Physiol (Lond) 465:163–179

69. Rardon DP, Cefali DC, Mitchell RD, Seiler SM, Hathaway DR Jones LR (1990) Digestion of cardiac and skeletal muscle junctional sarcoplasmic reticulum vesicles with calpain II: effects on the Ca^{2+} release channel. Circ Res 67:84–96

Cytoskeletal Changes in the Calcium-Overloaded Heart

Masatsugu Hori, Hiroshi Sato, and Michitoshi Inoue

Abstract. Calcium handling is impaired in the failing heart, causing calcium overload of the heart. Enhanced sympathetic nerve activity during heart failure could accerelate calcium overload by increasing the calcium influx. Calcium overload may also be induced in the ischemic heart, particularly after reperfusion. When intracellular Ca^{2+} cannot be sequestered normally, myofilaments are desensitized to Ca^{2+}, leading to contractile dysfunction. The cytoskeleton is sensitive to intracellular Ca^{2+} concentration. Microtubules, which support the scaffold of cell membranes and intracellular organelles and contribute to the assembly of myofilaments, are disrupted in Ca^{2+}-overloaded hearts and cardiomyocytes. In ischemic-reperfused hearts, several interventions that can attenuate Ca^{2+} influx after reperfusion (e.g., acidotic reperfusion, staged reperfusion, and low Ca^{2+} reperfusion) significantly attenuated microtubule disruption. Potent β-adrenergic stimulation also disrupts microtubules of the myocardium in vitro and in vivo. Although microtubules do not directly contribute to the contractile function of the heart, microtubular disruption may cause cellular dysfunction and could be a precipitating factor for progression of heart failure. Other cytoskeletal abnormalities should be further studied.

Key words. Cytoskeletons—Microtubules—β-adrenergic stimulation—Ca^{2+} overload—failing heart

Introduction

Failing hearts are characterized by impaired contractility of the myocardium, a poor response to sympathetic stimulation, and limited preload reserve. These functional impairments are explained by down-regulation of β-adrenoceptors [1], abnormal intracellular signal transduction [2, 3], and alterations in contractile proteins [4]. In addition to these functional abnormalities, morphological alterations are also observed in the failing heart: hypertrophic changes in cardiomyocytes, dilatation of the heart, and fibrotic changes of the interstitial tissue [5, 6]. These histological changes are called "remodeling" of the heart, and evidence for a detrimental role of remodeling has been accumulating [7, 8]. Although the extracellular collagen matrix

---

First Department of Medicine, Information Science, Osaka University, School of Medicine, 2-2 Yamadaoka, Suita, Osaka 565, Japan

serves an important role in maintaining the dimensions of the heart, accumulation of interstitial collagen matrix may be detrimental for the heart probably through its mechanical impedance and the impaired transport of oxygen and diffusible sub-stances to be supplied from the vessels [9]. Intracellular cytoskeletal abnormalities, however, are given less attention and have not been studied extensively. It is known that the cytoskeleton serves as scaffolding material for the cell structure, maintaining the integrity of the sarcolemma and myofilaments [10, 11]. The connection of myofibrils to Z-bands, maintenance of the organelles in their places, and transport of particles and proteins within the cells are achieved by the cytoskeleton.

Cytoskeletons are classified into three types of filaments: actin filaments, inter-mediate filaments, and microtubules [12]. Actin filaments are mainly involved in contraction of myofilaments as an actin–myosin complex. In the endothelial cell, however, actin filaments are distributed throughout the cytoplasm as a stress fiber, contributing to cell motility and bearing the mechanical stress [13, 14]. Intermediate filaments serve as mechanical integrators of cellular space [15]; desmin filaments connect all Z disks, thereby preventing the sarcomeres from slipping during contrac-tion [16]; and vimentin, mainly observed in mesenchymal tissues, represents a cellu-lar element of the extracellular space [17]. Intermediate filaments also preferentially bind to DNA and histones [18], influencing nuclear morphology and function. Microtubules are involved in maintenance of the cellular structures associated with intermediate filaments, transport of intracellular particles, and cell locomotion [19]. Microtubules are largely located surrounding the nucleus and contribute to protein synthesis and assembly of newly synthesized sarcomeres [20].

These cytoskeletons strongly support the framework of the cells: the scaffolding of the sarcolemmal membranes, holding of the intracellular organelles, assembly of the myofibrils, and connection of the myofilaments to Z-bands. Hence, disruption of the cytoskeletal structure may cause the cell to lose its integrity, rendering it fragile and vulnerable when exposed to a mechanical load. These abnormalities may be induced in the ischemic heart and failing heart, as some components of the cytoskeleton are sensitive to intracellular Ca^{2+} concentrations.

Cytoskeletal Changes in Ischemic Heart

Histological Changes in Ischemic Myocardium

Characteristic structural changes were observed in ischemic myocardium after 30–40 min of coronary occlusion [21]. It is well recognized that 15 min of ischemia does not induce irreversible ischemic injury, and myocardium subjected to 15 min of ischemia shows a histological picture indistinguishable from that of the intact myocardium except for a minimal change in cell volume, relaxed myofibrils, and swollen mitochondria in some cells [22]. At 30–40 min of ischemia, however, myo-cardial cells show marked swelling and amorphous mitochondrial matrix densities, often associated with sarcolemmal bleb formation, which indicates irreversible injury. Electron micrographs of the lethal ischemic myocardium show disruptions of the plasmalemma of the sarcolemma, but the basal lamina usually remains intact [23]. Thus plasma membrane disintegration is a feature of lethal myocardial ischemia. Cell swelling may be a cause of plasma membrane disruption, but preceding oxygen and substrate deprivation is required to increase membrane fragility [24]. Membrane fragility may be caused by the damage to the cytoskeleton due to cytoskeletal Z-line attachment between the plasma membrane and the underlying myofibrils being

FIG. 1. Photomicrograph showing micro-tubular networks of normal canine ventricu-lar myocardium immunohistochemically stained with mouse monoclonal antibodies against β-tubulin. Filamentous fine networks are observed throughout the cytoplasm and around the nucleus. Cytoplasmic micro-tubules are composed of longitudinal and transverse filaments

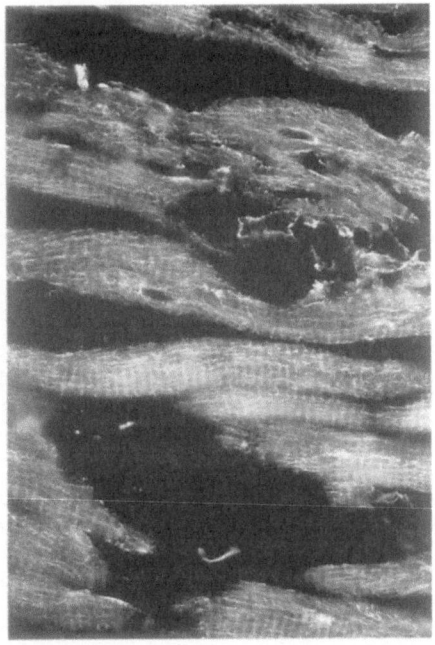

broken at the subsarcolemmal blebs. Steenbergen et al. demonstrated that break-down of the vinculin scaffold underlying the plasma membrane is responsible for weakening and rupture of the sarcolemma as a consequence of cell swelling during ischemia [25].

We also demonstrated that microtubules that support the structural integration of myofibrils and other organelles are disrupted during severe myocardial ischemia prior to the irreversible injury, promoting the irreversible change after reperfusion [26]. In dogs no alterations of immunoreactivities of microtubules were observed with ischemia of less than 20 min. Figure 1 depicts the immunohistochemically stained microtubules of the intact canine heart. A fine filamentous network is observed throughout the cytoplasm; the cytoplasmic microtubules are composed of longitudinal and transverse filaments, and a portion of them forms the circular architecture around the nucleus. Initial detectable changes in microtubules are observed 20 min after coronary occlusion; the immunoreactivities of the transverse filaments are decreased or lost in patchy lesions, and the loss of microtubular struc-tures is progressively increased with the duration of ischemia (Fig. 2). Disruption of microtubules may cause "untethering" of microtubules from sarcolemma-binding sites, leading to irreversible changes because tubulin binds with the anchor proteins (e.g., ankyrin, a 206-kDa plasmalemmal cytoskeletal element [27], and spectrin, located in Z-band-associated striations, binding with microtubules through tau protein [28, 29]); thus disruption of microtubules likely breaks the scaffold of the sarcolemma.

Calcium Overload in Ischemic Reperfused Heart

Postischemic ventricular dysfunction is recognized as "myocardial stunning," which is often observed in the clinical setting after recanalization of an occluded coronary

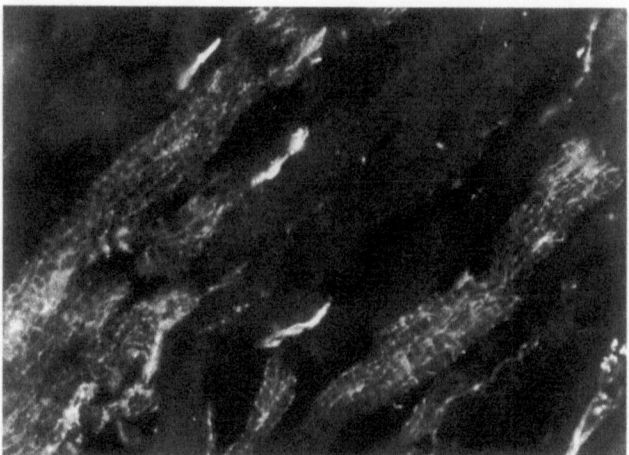

FIG. 2. Photomicrograph showing microtubular filaments at 60 min of ishchemia stained immunohistochemically with mouse monoclonal antibodies against β-tubulin. Patchy loss of microtubular stains is observed, whereas double staining of actin filaments with rhodamine-phalloidin shows intact alignments of actin filaments. (From [26], with permission)

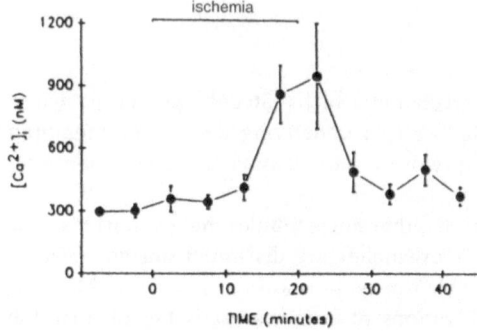

FIG. 3. Serial changes in intracellular Ca^{2+} concentration during 20 min of ischemia and after reperfusion in the Langendorf preparation of the ferret heart. Intracellular Ca^{2+} concentration was measured by ^{19}F nuclear magnetic resonance using ^5F-BAPTA. To exclude the Ca^{2+} buffering effect of ^5F-BAPTA, the extracellular Ca^{2+} concentration was kept at 8 mM. During ischemia $[Ca^{2+}]_i$ was increased after 10 min and further increased immediately after reperfusion. Note that transient but excessive Ca^{2+} loading occurs immediately after reperfusion. (From [33], with permission)

artery [30]. Myocardial stunning is characterized by reversible ischemic injury with minimal histological change. Oxygen free radicals [31], excitation–contraction un-coupling due to abnormal function of sarcoplasmic reticulum [32], Ca^{2+} overload [33, 34], insufficient energy production in mitochondria [35], impaired energy use of myofibrils [36], and blunted sensitivity of myofilaments to calcium [33] have been proposed to explain this reversible functional abnormality. Among these possibilities, Ca^{2+} overload may play a major role in the pathogenesis of contractile dysfunction. Figure 3 displays the average changes in intracellular Ca^{2+} concentration $[Ca^{2+}]_i$ in perfused ferret hearts subjected to 20 min of ischemia followed by reperfusion. During ischemia the time-averaged $[Ca^{2+}]_i$ increased after 10 min of ischemia and reached the threefold level at the end of ischemia. $[Ca^{2+}]_i$ was further increased after reperfusion and thereafter returned to the control level within 10 min. Although the cellular mechanisms of the increase in $[Ca^{2+}]_i$ have not been clarified, several lines of evidence support the hypothesis that Na^+-Ca^{2+} exchange plays an important role in the postischemic increase in Ca^{2+} influx [37]. During ischemia intracellular H^+ accumulates, and subsequently Na^+ influx is increased through Na^+-H^+ exchange. This result is supported by the finding that an early rise in intracellular Na^+ is prevented by the Na^+-H^+ exchange inhibitor EIPA, a derivative of amiloride [38]. Under acidotic conditions, Na^+-Ca^{2+} exchange is relatively inactive, as H^+ inhibits this exchange [39]. Upon reperfusion, however, acidosis is rapidly recovered, and Na^+-Ca^{2+} exchange is activated, leading to an increase in Ca^{2+} influx. Transient Ca^{2+} overload may be induced after reperfusion because calcium pump activity is depressed in the ischemic myocardium.

Calcium overload may induce a number of unfavorable sequelae: The high energy phosphate supply is substantially spent to sequester Ca^{2+} in the sarcoplasmic reticulum during diastole. In the presence of Ca^{2+} overload, mitochondria also

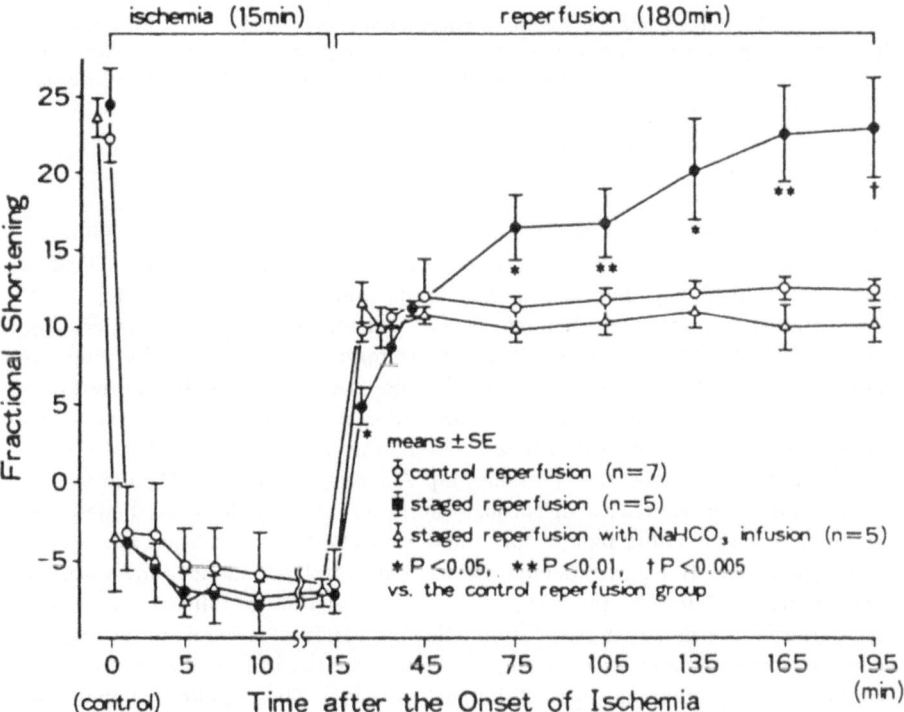

FIG. 4. Serial changes during fractional shortening before, during, and after 15 min of coronary occlusion for control reperfusion (*open circles*), staged reperfusion (*solid squares*), and staged reperfusion with $NaHCO_3$ infusion (*open triangles*). The fractional shortening with staged reperfusion shows the improved contractile function after reperfusion, whereas marked myocardial stunning was observed for the control reperfusion and the staged reperfusion with $NaHCO_3$. These results indicate that gradual recovery of acidosis could prevent myocardial stunning after reperfusion. (From [37], with permission)

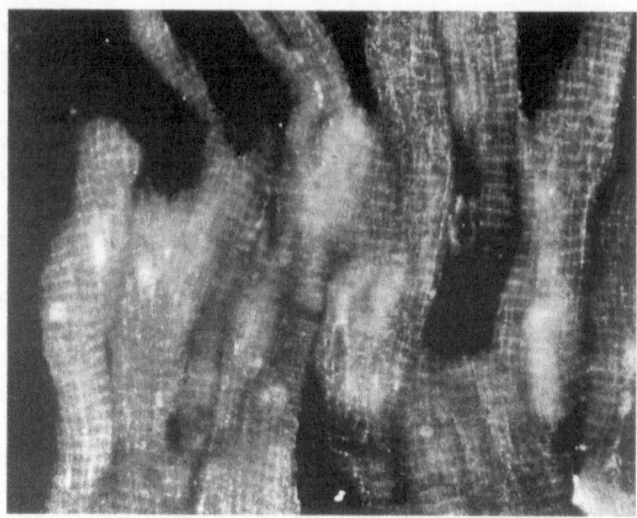

FIG. 5. Photomicrograph showing microtubular staining of canine myocardium reperfused with EDTA after 15 min of ischemia. EDTA dissolved in distilled water (100 mM) and adjusted to pH 7.4 was infused into the coronary artery during the initial 10 min of reperfusion (1.67 μmol/kg body weight per minute) to chelate the calcium in the perfused blood. The microtubular structures are well preserved in both the cytoplasm and around the nucleus. (From [41], with permission)

sequester intracellular Ca^{2+}, thereby decreasing oxidative phosphorylation [40]. An increase in $[Ca^{2+}]_i$ also activates numerous proteolytic enzymes (e.g., Ca^{2+}-activated protease), which may damage the membrane and cytoskeleton [25, 41]. High concentrations of Ca^{2+} may attenuate the Ca^{2+} sensitivity of myofilaments, causing sustained contractile dysfunction [42]. If these mechanisms underlie the stunning after reperfusion, low $[Ca^{2+}]_i$ after reperfusion may attenuate the contractile dysfunction. Indeed, this situation is the case in Langendorf perfused ferret hearts and open-chest dogs [33, 41]. Pretreatment with ryanodine, an inhibitor of cellular Ca^{2+} overload, also attenuates the stunning [43]. Acidotic reperfusion [44] and staged reperfusion (stepwise release of coronary occlusion [37]), both of which slow the recovery of acidosis after reperfusion, could attenuate the postischemic contractile dysfunction (Fig. 4). Figure 5 demonstrates the microtubular stains of myocardium when EDTA (1.67 μmol/kg per minute), a calcium chelator, was infused in the coronary artery for 10 min after reperfusion following 15 min of ischemia in the dog. In contrast, transient perfusion with a high Ca^{2+} solution ($CaCl_2 \cdot 9$ μmol/kg per minute) could mimic the stunning even without ischemia [41]. These findings support the hypothesis that Ca^{2+} overload plays a crucial role in the pathogenesis of sustained contractile dysfunction.

Microtubule Disruption After Reperfusion

Structural changes are minimal in the stunned myocardium; cellular and mitochondrial swelling is observed, but there are no irreversible changes. Therefore histological changes have received less attention than metabolic abnormalities.

However, Zhao et al. reported that damaged extracellular collagen matrix could contribute to mechanical dysfunction in the stunned myocardium [45]. The structural integrity of the microtubules that support the cytoskeletal framework of the cell are also regulated by intracellular $[Ca^{2+}]$ and Ca^{2+}/calmodulin-dependent protein kinase [46, 47]. In our study the anesthetized open-chest dogs were subjected to 15 min of myocardial ischemia by occluding their left anterior descending coronary artery; they were then reperfused for 1 h. The ischemia and reperfused area showed sustained cardiac dysfunction, as evidenced by a marked decrease in regional fractional shortening. In the stunned myocardium, loss of microtubular staining and fragmentation of the microtubules into small sections were observed heterogeneously in the epicardial and endocardial layers (Fig. 6A). The contractile apparatus remained intact; actin filaments labeled with rhodamine phalloidin showed fine cross-striations of the sarcomeres, even in cells with disrupted microtubules (Fig. 6B). In the affected cells, immunoreactive staining of microtubules is not uniform within the cell. In the intact cells perinuclear staining of the microtubules is highly condensed, whereas in the stunned myocardium perinuclear structures are substantially affected, indicating that the microtubules around the nucleus are susceptible to ischemia-reperfusion. It is of interest that the alterations of microtubular staining are distinct from those of ischemic myocardium; in the ischemic myocardium small,

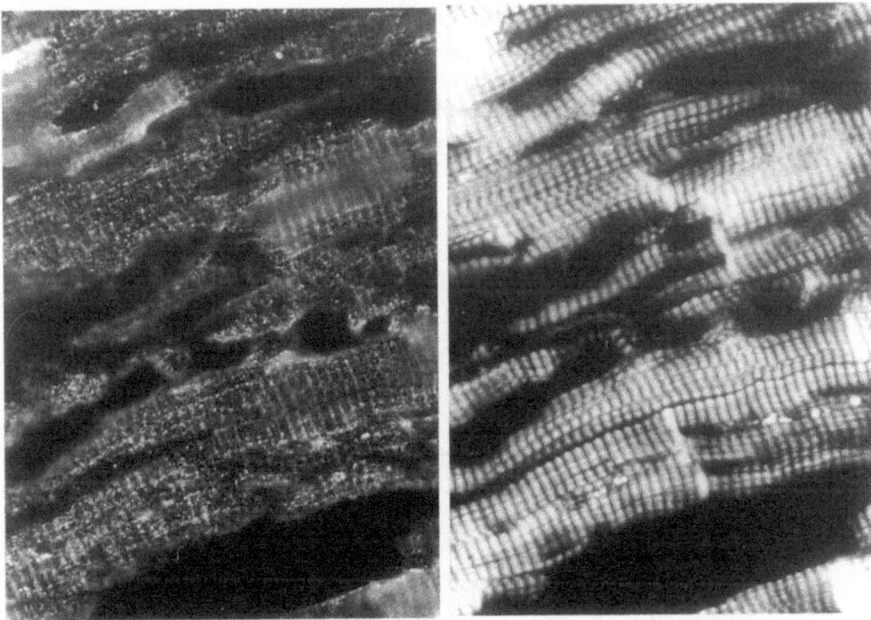

A   B

FIG. 6. Photomicrographs showing double staining of microtubules and actin filaments of the stunned myocardium (1 h after 15 min of ischemia). Microtubules were stained immuno-histochemically with mouse monoclonal antibodies against β-tubulin (A), and actin filaments were stained with rhodamine phalloidin (B). Loss of microtubular staining in the cytoplasm and fragmentation of microtubular filaments are observed in the stunned myocardium, whereas cross-striation of actin filaments is well preserved. (From [41], with permission)

patchy lesions are observed in which the immunoreactivity is decreased, but fragments of immunoreactivity are not observed. This finding is in contrast to reperfusion
injury of microtubules, which often show fragmentation. These differences may
indicate that the underlying mechanisms of microtubular disruption in stunned
myocardium are different from those in ischemic myocardium.

In stunned myocardium, abnormal staining of microtubules is no longer observed
24 hours after reperfusion. The density and intensity of the microtubular staining is
slightly increased over that in the control myocardium. These hyperreactive responses are more prominently observed in longitudinal filaments than in transverse
filaments. Thus the microtubular disruption is restored more or less within 24 h,
preceding the recovery of contractile function. The microtubular structures are even
thicker and more rigid 3 days after reperfusion, and the density of the filaments is
greater than in the control myocardium; but they return to the preischemic state
5 days after reperfusion.

A transient increase in Ca^{2+} influx during ischemia and the postischemic period
may cause the stunning; hence low Ca^{2+} reperfusion could attenuate the systolic
dysfunction. Microtubular immunoreactivity in the EDTA-reperfused myocardium is
well preserved, indicating that microtubular disruption is mediated by Ca^{2+} influx
[41]. In contrast to EDTA reperfusion, intracoronary infusion of a high concentration of Ca^{2+} ($CaCl_2$ 6.7 μmol/kg per minute) for 10 min markedly decreased the
immunoreactivity of microtubules, and the area of microtubular disruption was significantly increased (Fig. 7). This finding supports the hypothesis that Ca^{2+} overload
causes myocardial stunning and microtubular disruption.

Several mechanisms underlying microtubular disruption in ischemia-reperfused
myocardium should be considered. Phosphorylation of tubulin or microtubule-associated proteins by Ca^{2+}/calmodulin-dependent protein kinase may inhibit the polymerization of tubulin [47]. Activation of Ca^{2+}-dependent neural protease may also

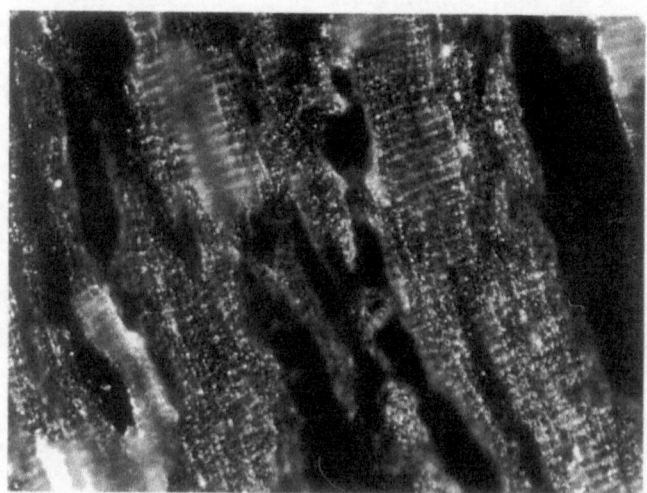

FIG. 7. Photomicrograph showing microtubular structures of canine ventricular myocardium
treated with intracoronary infusion of $CaCl_2$. Microtubules were stained with mouse
monoclonal antibodies against β-tubulin. Microtubular filaments are fragmented, yielding
dotted spots, as observed in the stunned myocardium. (From [41], with permission)

be involved [48–50]. It is possible that Ca^{2+} could accelerate depolymerization of microtubules as observed in an in vitro study [46]. Guanosine triphosphate (GTP) depletion may also affect microtubular assembly, though it is not plausible in stunned myocardium [51]. The precise mechanism of microtubular disruption is not clarified, but there is no question that Ca^{2+} overload immediately after reperfusion may be a primary cause of this cytoskeletal change.

The possibility that microtubular disruption is a cause of stunning may be raised, as there are several lines of evidence to support this hypothesis: (1) Microtubular structures are injured in the stunned myocardium. (2) Reperfusion with blood having a low Ca^{2+} concentration (EDTA reperfusion) attenuates the microtubular disruption as well as the contractile dysfunction. (3) Ca^{2+} overlaod without ischemia ($CaCl_2$ perfusion) induces both microtubular and contractile dysfunction. (4) Restoration of the microtubules after reperfusion precedes recovery of contractile function. However, colchicine, which disassembles the microtubules, does not depress contractile function [52]. Tsutsui et al. claimed that an increase in microtubules in hypertrophied heart deteriorates cardiac function [53]. These findings suggest that it is unlikely that microtubules per se contribute to contractile function, although they do support the cellular architecture, plasma membrane, myofibrils, and other cellular organelles by their filamentous network, and they provide pathways for transporting vesicles (e.g., mitochondria, endoplasmic reticulum, and other membranous organelles) [54, 55]. Hence microtubular disruption may contribute to cellular dysfunction even if not primarily.

Microtubules During β-Adrenergic Stimulation

It is well known that sympathetic nerves are activated during heart failure even in the chronic stable state [56–59]. It manifests as tachycardia, cold skin, and decreased urine volume, which are observed in patients with heart failure. Direct recordings of sympathetic activity by microelectrodes at the peroneal nerves demonstrated marked activation of local sympathetic nerves in patients with heart failure [60]. Activated sympathetic nerves are also reflected by high plasma norepinephrine levels [61]. Augmented sympathetic activity in the resting state has been attributed to decreased inhibitory influences in the vasomotor center from aortic and cardiopulmonary baroreceptors [62, 63]; the baroreceptors are desensitized probably owing to decreased distensibility of the cardiovascular wall of the failing heart. Hence the tonic activities of these afferent nerves mediated by the vagal and glossopharyngeal nerves are decreased in heart failure [64].

Another mechanism that regulates the sympathetic activities during exercise is a somatic reflex originating in the exercising muscles, which serves as a feedback mechanism and regulates the instantaneous sympathetic activity during exercise [65, 66]; receptors with unmyelinated group IV afferent fibers in contracting muscles are involved in the reflex loop that responds to hypoxic and other metabolic stimuli (e.g., bradykinin, prostaglandins, or potassium) [67]. In patients with heart failure perfusion of exercising skeletal muscles is inadequate owing to a decreased cardiac reserve during intense exercise resulting in anaerobic metabolism and a decrease in oxygen content in the local blood. These metabolic stimuli activate chemosensitive muscle afferents, which drive the somatic reflex causing sympathetic activation. Indeed, a clear relation is observed between plasma norepinephrine levels and mixed

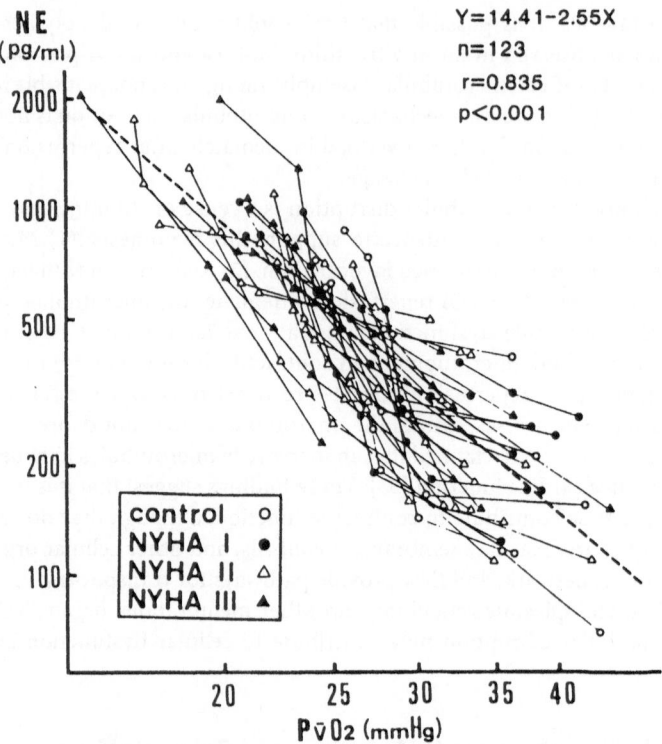

FIG. 8. Relation between venous Po$_2$ (Pvo$_2$) and plasma norepinephrine levels during exercise. With an increase in the intensity of exercise, Pvo$_2$ was decreased and plasma norepinephrine increased. This inverse correlation is not influenced by the severity of the heart failure (NYHA class). (From [68], with permission)

venous oxygen partial pressure (Po$_2$) during exercise (Fig. 8). In patients with heart failure, blood delivery to the exercising skeletal muscles is restricted, and thus anaerobic metabolism is enhanced, causing sympathetic activation through the somatic reflex. The desensitized baroreceptors at rest and the enhanced somatic reflex during exercise are two major mechanisms of sympathetic activation in patients with heart failure.

The increased sympathetic activity serves as a compensatory mechanism during heart failure, increasing the cardiac contractility and heart rate, which maintain blood flow to the essential organs. However, it may also exert harmful influences on the failing heart by increasing myocardial oxygen consumption, precipitating arrhythmia, inducing Ca^{2+} overload, and activating the renin–angiotensin–aldosterone system, which may increase the afterload and preload of the heart. It is also known that β-adrenergic receptor blocker therapy improves cardiac function and prevents functional deterioration during chronic heart failure [69–71]. Several lines of evidence earlier supported the hypothesis that the pathogenesis of catecholamine cardiotoxicity is mainly due to intracellular Ca^{2+} overload through β-adrenoceptor stimulation [72, 73]. The process of cellular damage in the Ca^{2+}-overloaded heart is not fully elucidated.

Microtubular Disruption in Neonatal Cultured Cardiomyocytes

Because the cytoskeletons of the cells support the integrity of the plasma membrane, myofibrils, and intracellular organelles, and some types of cytoskeleton are sensitive to Ca^{2+} [74, 75], it is likely that the Ca^{2+}-sensitive cytoskeletons are injured by intracellular Ca^{2+} overload in failing hearts. We have observed that the microtubular structures of rat cardiomyocytes are disrupted by high Ca^{2+} exposure [76]. Figure 9 shows representative microtubular structures of the cardiomyocytes exposed to 6.0 mM Ca^{2+} for 60 min. In contrast to the normal structures of microtubules in the upper panel, a fine filamentous network of microtubules is fragmented; and in some areas the microtubules are poorly stained, characterized by marked inhomogeneity of the immunoreactive stains.

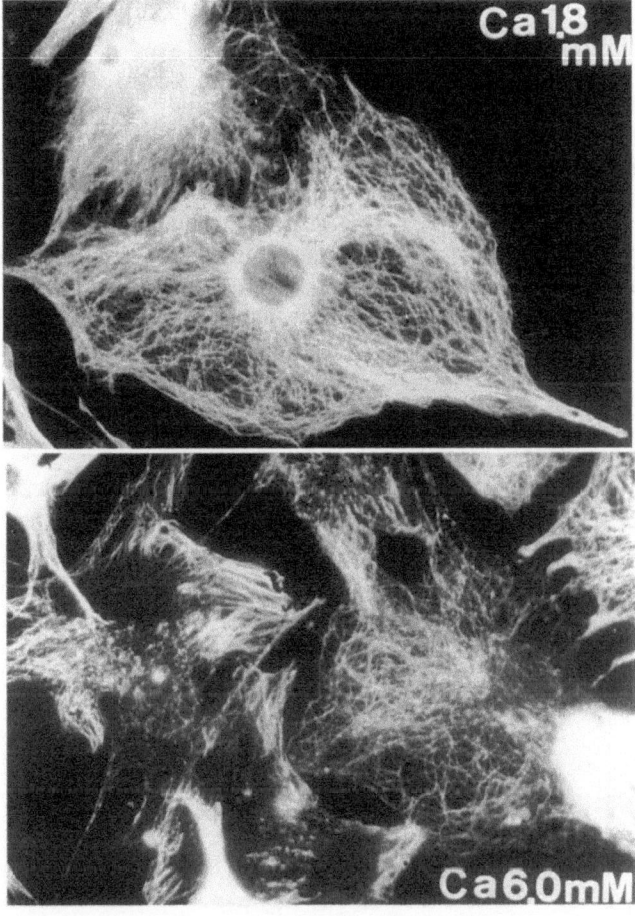

FIG. 9. Photomicrograph (*bottom*) showing microtubular structures of cultured myocytes of rat heart exposed to 6.0 mM Ca^{2+} for 60 min. Fine filamentous structures of the microtubules are partly disrupted and fragmented. Microtubules around the nucleus were susceptible to Ca^{2+} overload. At *top* is the control experiment using 1.8 mM Ca^{2+}

To assess the disruption of microtubular structure, loss of microtubular immunoreactivity was semiquantified according to the grade of microtubular damage: grade 1 (minimal injury), fragmentation of microtubules or loss of staining in fewer than 25% of the total cellular area; grade 2 (moderate injury), microtubular structure not stained in fewer than 50% but more than 25% of the total cellular area; and grade 3 (severe injury), microtubular structure disrupted in more than 50% of the total cellular area. Microscopic views of the cells were photographed, and the extent of microtubular injury was quantified in 100 randomly sampled myocytes. The disruption score in each dish was determined as the sum of $Xn/3$ in 100 cardiomyocytes, where Xn represents the grade in the nth cell studied; thus the disruption score is 100 when the microtubular structure is severely damaged (grade 3) in all 100 cardiomyocytes. Figure 10 depicts the relation between the extracellular Ca^{2+} concentration and the extent of microtubular structures. An increase in extracellular Ca^{2+} concentration augments microtubular disassembly in a dose-dependent manner. The treatment with calcium ionophore A23187 (5 μM) markedly disrupts the microtubules, yielding a high disruption score.

It is of interest that norepinephrine exposure elicits similar changes in microtubular structures in a dose-dependent and time-dependent manner [77]. Treatment with 10 μM norepinephrine partially disrupted microtubular staining as shown in Figure 11. Loss of microtubular staining and fragmentation of microtubular filaments into small dotted spots are heterogeneously observed. These changes were characteristically observed in the perinuclear region and subsequently spread to the surrounding cytoplasm as observed in the stunned myocardium. In contrast to microtubular disruption, actin filaments stained wih rhodamine-phalloidin show the intact cross-striations of sarcomere structures. Thus disruption of microtubules is not associated with damage to the contractile apparatus.

Microtubular disruption increased with the duration of norepinephrine exposure; the microtubular disruption score reaches its maximum after 60 min of exposure. When the cardiomyocytes are exposed to a low dose of norepinephrine (<1 μM), only

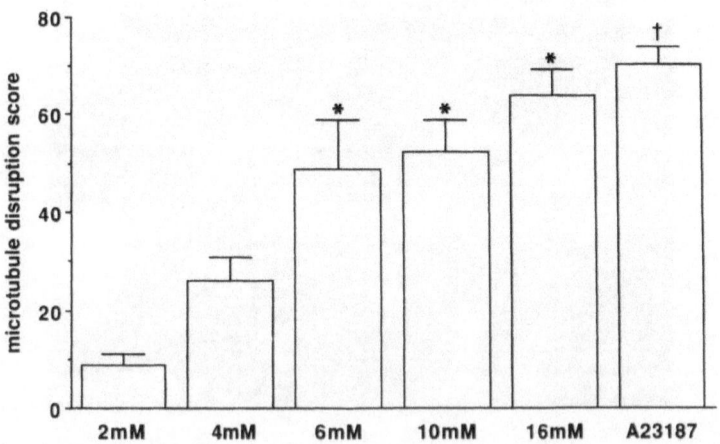

FIG. 10. Microtubular disruptions at various concentrations of extracellular Ca^{2+}. Microtubular disruption scores increased in a dose-dependent manner, and treatment with calcium ionophore A23187 (5 μM/L) markedly disrupted the microtubular structures. (From [37], with permission)

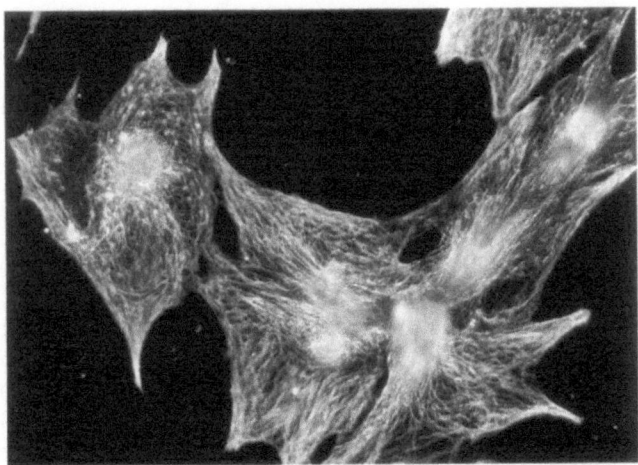

FIG. 11. Micrograph showing microtubular structures of cultured rat cardiomyocytes exposed to norepinephrine (10 μmol/L) for 60 min. Microtubular filaments were immunohistochemically stained with mouse monoclonal antibody against β-tubulin. Partial loss of microtubular staining and fragmentation are observed predominantly around the nucleus. (From [37], with permission)

minimal change was observed in the microtubular structures: Norepinephrine-induced microtubular disruption is mediated by β-adrenoceptors: Propranolol markedly attenuated the microtubular disruption, whereas phentolamine (α-adrenoceptor antagonist) affected it only minimally. This finding is confirmed by the observation that phenylephrine (10–100 μM) minimally disrupted microtubular structures, whereas isoproterenol and denopamine, a β-selective adrenoceptor agonist, disrupted microtubular structures in a dose-dependent manner [77]. As expected, these microtubular insults are cyclic AMP-mediated, as we observed a similar dose-dependent changes of microtubules when the cardiomyocytes were exposed to forskolin and dibutyryl cyclic AMP. It is well known that β-adrenoceptor stimulation increases Ca^{2+} influx through voltage-dependent Ca^{2+} channels. This finding suggests that the β-adrenoceptor-mediated microtubular disruption is intracellular Ca^{2+}-dependent. This hypothesis can be tested if the Ca^{2+} concentration in the medium is lowered when the cardiomyocytes are stimulated by isoproterenol. A decrease in extracellular $CaCl_2$ concentration from 2.0 mM to 0.5 mM during treatment with isoproterenol (10 μM) significantly attenuated the microtubular disruption score. Pretreatment with diltiazem also attenuated the effect of isoproterenol on microtubular disruption. These results support the hypothesis that Ca^{2+} influx during β-adrenergic stimulation is responsible for microtubular disruption.

The cytoskeletal injury can be repaired within 24 h after cessation of β-adrenergic stimulation, suggesting that such injury does not indicate cell death and may be reversible. It is of note, however, that at high concentrations (>10 mM) of $CaCl_2$, the number of contracting cells was decreased, indicating that some of the cells were irreversibly injured by Ca^{2+} overload. Ca^{2+}-induced microtubular disruption was reported in monkey epithelial cells and fibroblasts after microinjection of Ca^{2+} [78, 79]. We have also observed that the microtubules are injured in the stunned myocardium in which Ca^{2+} overload occurs [41]. Previous reports have suggested possible mechanisms of Ca^{2+}-induced microtubular disruption: (1) Ca^{2+}/calmodulin-dependent protein kinase may accelerate the disassembly of microtubules [78]; (2) degradation of microtubular proteins may be induced by a Ca^{2+}-dependent protease [49, 50]; and (3) tubulin polymerization may be inhibited by Ca^{2+}. Schliwa et al. demonstrated that in detergent-extracted monkey kidney cells disassembly induced by micromolar Ca^{2+} is inhibited by calmodulin inhibitors [79]. In our cells, however, calmodulin inhibitors did not attenuate the microtubular injury induced by β-adrenoceptor stimulation. Thus a calmodulin-mediated mechanism is unlikely to be involved in β-adrenergic stimulation in cardiomyocytes. The second possible mechanism is microtubular degradation by Ca^{2+}-dependent protease. Indeed, in nerve tissue culture the neutral protease inhibitor leupeptin inhibits the ischemia-induced microtubular disruption [80]. However, in our cells leupeptin and other several calpain inhibitors did not inhibit microtubular insults. Thus the second mechanism is also unlikely according to our experimental model, which is free of ischemia. The third possible mechanism (i.e., inhibition of tubulin polymerization by Ca^{2+} [47]) may therefore be plausible, although we do not have direct evidence to support this hypothesis.

Microtubular Disruptions in In Vivo Rat Heart

In neonatal cultured cardiomyocytes catecholamine concentrations that induce microtubular disruption are high (1–10 μM of norepinephrine and 1–10 μM of isoproterenol). Although neonatal cardiomyocytes are resistant to catecholamine injury, the findings in neonatal cultured myocytes may not be extended to the in vivo heart.

To determine if administration of norepinephrine to intact animals could injure microtubular structures, we studied the effects of continuous infusion of norepinephrine on the microtubular structures of the rat heart [76]. An osmotic minipump containing norepinephrine and 0.2% ascorbic acid as an antioxidant was implanted in the back of Wistar-Kyoto rats. The osmotic pump allows administration of drug at a constant rate of 1.0 μl/h for more than 3 days, so animals could receive doses of 2, 20, and 200 μg/kg per hour. Continuous infusion of low-dose norepinephrine (2 μg/kg per hour) resulted in increases in plasma norepinephrine from 430 ± 40 pg/ml to 12 600 ± 1700 pg/ml at 24 h. The immunohistochemical studies of microtubules shows small, patchy lesions in which the characteristic filamentous structures were partially lost or fragmented. A large dose of norepinephrine infusion (20 μg/kg per hour) for 6 h demonstrated a similar extent of microtubular changes, at which time the plasma norepinephrine concentration had increased to 14 600 ± 2200 pg/ml. More extensive disruption was observed at 24 h; 40 ± 6% of the area shows microtubular damage, although the cross-striations of actin filaments remained normal. A larger dose of norepinephrine (200 μg/kg per hour) induced more extensive injury of microtubules. Propranolol infusion (500 μg/kg per hour) in the rat markedly attenuated the microtubular disruption, indicating that the effect of norepinephrine is β-adrenoceptor-mediated.

A low dose of norepinephrine (i.e., 2 μg/kg per hour, or 0.067 μg/kg per minute) is used clinically, and the resultant increase in plasma catecholamine level is similar to that observed in patients with pheochromocytoma [81]. This finding suggests that microtubular structures are injured over a long period of uncompensated heart failure in which plasma norepinephrine is markedly increased. It is of interest that the disruption of microtubules during norepinephrine infusion seems morphologically different from that observed during ischemia. In the ischemic heart the immuno-reactivity of microtubules often completely disappears in association with irreversible degeneration of actin filaments. In the catecholamine-loaded heart, micro-tubular disruptions are not associated with irreversible damage of actin filaments, a finding compatible with the same observation in isolated cardiomyocytes exposed to norepinephrine. Thus underlying mechanisms of microtubular disruption in the catecholamine-loaded heart may be different from those seen during ischemia.

Microtubules in Hypertrophied and Failing Hearts

Several lines of evidence have suggested that microtubules contribute to sarco-merogenesis in the developing and the hypertrophied heart [82]. In developing mus-cles, microtubules, intermediate-sized filaments, and striated myofbrils are all oriented to the longitudinal axis of the postmitotic myoblasts or myotubes [83]. Depolymerization of microtubules by colcemid induces cell shape change, and myotubes form multinucleated myosacs [84] where alignment of myofibrils is greatly distorted and the intermediate filaments are aggregated into immense cables [85]. Other investigators have recognized that interaction between myosin and tubulin may be involved in cell motility and cytoplasmic flow, as myosin and tubulin co-precipitate at low ionic strength, and myosin filaments whose cross-bridges are decorated by tubulin aggregate side by side [83, 86]. When the sarcomeres are assembled, the early myofibrils are surrounded by many microtubules, possibly providing a scaffold or a substrate along which myosin monomers polymerize and deliver the nascent thick filaments to either the periphery or the end of a growing myofibril [87]. In the pressure-loaded heart myocardial hypertrophy occurs where microtubules are also involved in sarcomerogenesis. Samuel et al. first reported that microtubules are transiently increased as an early response to pressure overload [88]. According to an earlier hypothesis, the increase in microtubules in the pressure-loaded heart may be an adaptational response to sarcomere synthesis and assembly. More recently re-ported evidence suggests that an increase in microtubules during pressure loading could cause an internal load of myocytes, decreasing the contractile ability (i.e., a decrease in the extent and velocity of shortening) [53]. This point is clearly demon-strated by interventions (e.g., taxol and hypothermia alter the stablilization of the tubulin polymerization). Thus excess microtubules in stress-hypertrophied cells im-pede sarcomere motion. An increase in collage matrix in the hypertrophied heart may increase the stiffness of the myocardium, whereas an increase in intracellular cytoskeletons could increase the impedance of muscle cell shortening rather than alter the stiffness of the sarcomere-sarcolemma connection. What, then, happens in microtubules in the failing heart? This question has not been studied in the animal model. Schaper et al. reported that in biopsied samples of the myocardium from patients with dilated cardiomyopathy the immunoreactivity of microtubules is increased, mostly bound to structural components of the cells, whereas there was a relative paucity of labeling for tubulin (i.e., inhomogeneous immunoreactivity of microtubules) [89]. We also studied morphological changes in microtubules in biopsied myocardium obtained from patients with hypertrophic cardiomyopathy and idiopathic dilated cardiomyopathy [90]. Figure 12 shows representative immunohistochemical staining of microtubules obtained from a patient with dilated

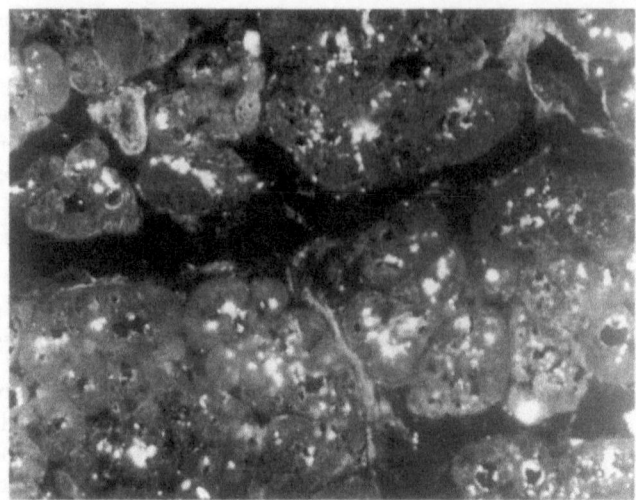

FIG. 12. Micrograph showing microtubular structures of biopsied myocardium from a patient with dilated cardiomyopathy. The immunoreactivity of microtubules is almost completely lost in many cells, whereas condensed microtubular structures are observed sporadically

cardiomyopathy. The aggregation of tubulin is observed, whereas in most cells staining of microtubules was poor or almost nonexistent. Similar observations were obtained in a patient with alcoholic cardiomyopathy. It is of note that microtubules in the hypertrophic cardiomyopathic heart are homogeneously lost, even though this heart is not failing. Abnormal staining of cytoskeletons in the diseased heart should be carefully interpreted because it may be largely influenced by the duration of the disease, the intracellular metabolic state (e.g., Ca^{2+} and other ions and pH), alterations of functionally related proteins (e.g., Ca^{2+}/calmodulin, microtubule-associated proteins, and other enzymes), and morphological changes in the structural proteins that form myofibrils, sarcolemma, and intracellular organelles. However, many cytoskeletal proteins are involved in cellular function. Some are involved in the connections between Z-bands and myofibrils, the scaffolding of the sarcolemma, the support of the intracellular organelles, and the transport of proteins and metabolites; hence their alterations may largely contribute to the functional abnormalities of the diseased heart. Additional studies on cytoskeletal changes in diseased hearts are necessary to elucidate the intracellular remodeling of the heart.

Acknowledgments. This study was supported by a Grant-in-Aid for Scientific Research (06274101) from the Ministry of Education, Science, and Culture, Japan.

References

1. Bristow MR, Ginsburg R, Umans V, Fowler M, Minobe W, Rasmusen R, Zera P, Menlove R, Shah P, Jamieson S, Stinson EB (1986) Beta$_1$- and beta$_2$-adrenergic receptor subpopulations in nonfailing and failing human ventricular myocardium: coupling of both receptor subtypes to muscle contraction and selective beta$_1$-receptor downregulation in heart failure. Circ Res 59:297–309

2. Ishikawa Y, Katsushika S, Kiuchi K, Shannon RP, Komamura K, Sorota S, Vatner DE, Vatner SF, Homcy DJ (1994) Downregulation of adenylylcyclase types V and VI mRNA levels in pacing-induced heart failure in dogs. J Clin Invest 93:2224–2229

3. Feldman AM, Cates AE, Veazey WB, Harshberger RE, Bristow MR, Baughman KL, Baumgartner WA, Van Dop C (1988) Increase of the 40000-mol wt pertussis toxin substrate (G-protein) in the failing human heart. J Clin Invest 82:189–197

4. Mercadier JJ, Lompre AM, Wisnewsky C, Samuel JL, Bercovici J, Swynghedauw B, Schwartz K (1981) Myosin isoenzymic changes in several models of rat cardiac hypertrophy. Circ Res 49:525–532

5. Weber KT, Janicki JS, Shroff SG, Pick R, Chen RM, Bashey RI (1988) Collagen remodeling of the pressure-overloaded, hypertrophied nonhuman primate myocardium. Circ Res 62:757–765

6. Linzbach AJ (1960) Heart failure from the point of view of quantitative anatomy. Am J Cardiol 5:370–382

7. Caulfield JB, Norton P, Weaver RD (1992) Cardiac dilatation associated with collagen alterations. Mol Cell Biochem 118:171–179

8. Janicki JS, Matsubara BB (1993) Myocardial collagen and left ventricular diastolic function. In: Gaasch WH, LeWinter MM (eds) Left ventricular diastolic dysfunction. Lea and Febiger, Philadelphia, pp 125–140

9. Weber KT, Clark WA, Janicki JS, Scroff SG (1987) Physiologic versus pathologic hypertrophy and the pressure-overloaded myocardium. J Cardiovasc Pharmacol 10:S37–S50

10. Pardo JV, Siliciano JD, Craig SW (1983) Vinculin is a component of an extensive network of myofibril-sarcolemma attachment regions in cardiac muscle fibers. J Cell Biol 97:1081–1088

11. Jacobson BS (1983) Interaction of the plasma membrane with the cytoskeleton: an overview. Tissue Cell 15:829–852

12. Bershadsky AD, Vazilliev JM (1988) Cytoskeleton. Plenum, New York

13. Byers HR, White GE, Fujiwara K (1984) Organization and function of stress fibers in cells in vitro and in situ. In: Shay JW (ed) Cell and muscle motility, vol 5. Plenum, New York, pp 83–137

14. Burridge K (1981) Are stress fibers contractile? Nature 294:691–692

15. Lazarides E (1980) Intermediate filaments as mechanical integrators of cellular space. Nature 283:249–256

16. Lazarides E, Granger BL, Gard DL, O'Connor CM, Beekler J, Price M, Danto SI (1982) Desmin- and vimentin-containing filaments and their role in the assembly of the Z disk in muscle cells. Cold Spring Harbour Symp Quant Biol 46:351–378

17. Osborn M, Geisler N, Shaw G, Sharp G, Weber K (1982) Intermediate filaments. Cold Spring Harbour Symp Quant Biol 42:413–429

18. Traub P, Nelson WJ, Kuhn S, Vorgias CE (1983) Interaction in vitro of the intermediate filament protein vimentin with naturally occurring RNAs and DNAs. J Biol Chem 258: 1456–1466

19. Jones JCR, Goldman AE, Steinert PM, Yuspa S, Goldman RD (1982) Dynamic aspects of the supramolecular organization of intermediate filament networks in cultured epidermal cells. Cell Motil 2:197–213

20. Cartwright J, Goldstein MA (1985) Microtubules in the heart muscle of the postnatal and adult rat. J Mol Cell Cardiol 17:1–7

21. Herdson PB, Sommers HM, Jennings RB (1965) Comparative study of the fine structure of normal and ischemic dog myocardium with special reference to early changes following temporary occlusion of a coronary artery. Am J Pathol 46:367–386

22. Jennings RB, Ganote CE (1974) Structural changes in myocardium during acute ischemia. Circ Res 34/35(suppl III):156–172

23. Jennings RB, Hawkins HK, Lowe JE, Hill ML, Klotman S, Reimer KA (1978) Relationship between high energy phosphate and lethal injury in myocardial ischemia in the dog. Am J Pathol 92:187–214

24. Steenbergen C, Hill ML, Jennings RB (1985) Volume regulation and plasma membrane injury in aerobic and ischemic myocardium in vitro: effects of osmotic cell swelling on plasma membrane integrity. Circ Res 57:864–875

25. Steenbergen C, Hill ML, Jennings RB (1987) Cytoskeletal damage during myocardial ischemia: changes in vinculin immunofluorescence staining during total in vitro ischemia in canine heart. Circ Res 60:478–486

26. Iwai K, Hori M, Kitabatake A, Kurihara H, Uchida K, Inoue M, Kamada T (1990) Disruption of microtubules as an early sign of irreversible ischemic injury: immunohistochemical study of in situ canine hearts. Circ Res 67:694–706

27. Bennet V (1992) Ankyrins: adaptor between diverse plasma membrane proteins and the cytoplasm. J Biol Chem 267:8703–8706

28. Vybiral T, Winkelmann JC, Roberts R, Joe E, Casey DL, Williams JK, Epstein HF (1992) Human cardiac and skeletal mucscle spectrins: differential express and localization. Cell Motil Cytoskeleton 21:293–304

29. Carlier MF, Simon C, Cassoly R, Pradel LA (1984) Interaction between microtubule-associ-ated protein tau and spectrin. Biochimie 66:305–311

30. Braunwald E, Kloner RA (1982) The stunned myocardium: prolonged postischemic ventricular dysfunction. Circulation 66:1146–1149

31. Gross JG, Farber NE, Hardman HF, Warltier DC (1986) Beneficial actions of superoxide dismutase and catalase in the stunned myocardium of dogs. Am J Physiol 250: H372–H377

32. Krause SM, Jacobus WE, Becker LC (1989) Alterations in cardiac sarcoplasmic reticulum transport in the postischemic "stunned" myocardium. Circ Res 65:526–530

33. Kusuoka H, Porterfield JK, Weisman HF, Weisfeldt ML, Marban E (1987) Pathophysiology and pathogenesis of stunned myocardium: depressed Ca^{2+} activation and contraction as a consequences of reperfusion-induced cellular overload in ferret hearts. J Clin Invest 79:950–961

34. Kitakaze M, Weisman HF, Marban E (1988) Contractile dysfunction and ATP depletion after transient calcium overload in perfused ferret hearts. Circulation 77:685–695

35. Deboer FWV, Ingwall JS, Kloner RA, Braunwald E (1980) Prolonged derangements of canine myocardial purine metabolism after a brief coronary artery occlusion not associated with anatomic evidence of necrosis. Proc Natl Acad Sci USA 77:5471–5475

36. Greenfield RA, Sawain JL (1987) Disruption of myofibrillar energy use: dual mechanisms that may contribute to postischemic dysfunction in stunned myocardium. Circ Res 60: 283–289

37. Hori M, Kitakaze M, Sato H, Takashima S, Iwakura K, Inoue M, Kitabatake A, Kamada T (1991) Staged reperfusion attenuates myocardial stunning in dogs; role of transient acidosis during early reperfusion. Circulation 84:2135–2145

38. Pike MM, Kitakaze M, Marban E (1990) Sodium-23 NMR measurements of intracellular sodium in intact perfused ferret hearts during ischemia and reperfusion. Am J Physiol 259:H1767–1773

39. Philipson ED, Bersohn MM, Nishimoto AY (1982) Effects of pH on Na^+-Ca^{2+} exchange in canine cardiac sarcolemmal vesicles. Circ Res 50:287–293

40. Kusuoka H, Jacobus WE, Marban E (1988) Calcium oscillation in digitalis-induced ventricular fibrillation: pathogenetic role and metabolic consequences in isolated ferret hearts. Circ Res 62:609–619

41. Sato H, Hori M, Kitakaze M, Iwai K, Takashima S, Kurihara H, Inoue M, Kamda T (1993) Reperfusion after brief ischemia disrupts the microtubule network in canine hearts. Circ Res 72:361–375

42. Kitakaze M, Weisman HF, Marban E (1987) Contractile dysfunction and ATP depletion after transient calcium overload in perfused ferret heart. Circulation 77:685–695

43. Porterfield JK, Kusuoka H, Weisman HF, Weisfeldt ML, Marban E (1987) Ryanodine prevents the changes in myocardial function and morphology induced by reperfusion after brief periods of ischemia [abstract]. Clin Res 35:315

44. Kitakaze M, Weisfeldt ML, Marban E (1988) Acidosis during reperfusion prevents myocardial stunning in ferret heart. J Clin Invest 82:920–927

45. Zhao M, Zhang H, Robinson TF, Factor SM, Sonnenblick EH, Eng C (1987) Profound structural alterations of the extracellular matrix in postischemic dysfuntion ("stunned") but viable myocardium. J Am Coll Cardiol 10:1322–1334

46. Marcum JM, Dedman JR, Brinkley BR, Means AR (1978) Control of microtubule assembly-disassembly by calcium-dependent regulator protein. Proc Natl Acad Sci USA 75:3771–3775
47. Yamamoto H, Fukunaga K, Goto S, Tanaka E, Miyamoto E (1985) Ca^{2+} calmodulin-dependent regulation of microtubule formation via phosphorylation of microtubule-associated protein 2, tau factor, and tubulin, and comparison with the cyclic AMP-dependent phosphorylation. J Neurochem 44:759–768
48. Matsumura Y, Kusuoka H, Inoue M, Hori M, Kamada T (1993) Protective effect of the protease inhibitor leupeptin against myocardial stunning. J Cardiovasc Pharmacol 22:135–142
49. Reddy MK, Etlinger JD, Rabinowitz M, Fischman DA, Zak R (1975) Removal of Z-lines and alpha-actinin from isolated myofibrils by a calcium-activated neural protease. J Biol Chem 250:4278–4284
50. Dayton WR, Goll DE, Zeece MG, Robinson RM, Reville WJ (1976) A Ca^{2+}-activated protease possible involved in myofibrillar protein turnover: purification from porcine muscle. Biochemistry 15:2150–2158
51. Carlier MF, Pantaloni D (1981) Kinetic analysis of guanosine 5'-triphosphate hydrolysis associated with tubulin polymerization. Biochemistry 20:1918–1924
52. Klein I (1983) Colchicine stimulates the rate of contraction of heart cells in culture. Cardiovasc Res 17:459–465
53. Tsutsui H, Ishihara K, Cooper G IV (1993) Cytoskeletal role in the contractile dysfunction of hypertrophied myocardium. Science 260:682–687
54. Goldstein MA, Entman ML (1979) Microtubules in mammalian heart muscle. J Cell Biol 80:183–195
55. Kelly RB (1990) Microtubules, membrane traffic, and cell organization. Cell 61:5–7
56. Chidsey CA, Harrison DC, Braunwald E (1962) Augmentation of plasma norepinephrine response to exercise in patients with congestive heart failure. N Engl J Med 267:650–654
57. Thomas JA, Marks BH (1978) Plasma norepinephrine in congestive heart failure. Am J Cardiol 41:233–243
58. Francis GS, Goldsmith SR, Ziesche S, Cohn JN (1982) Response of plasma norepinephrine and epinephrine to dynamic exercise in patients with congestive heart failure. Am J Cardiol 49:1152–1156
59. Hasking GJ, Esler MD, Jennings GL, Burton D, Korner PI (1986) Norepinephrine spillover to plasma in patients with congestive heart failure: evidence of increased overall and cardiorenal sympathetic nervous activity. Circulation 73:615–621
60. Leimbach WN, Wallin BG, Victor RG, Aylward PE, Sundlof G, Mark AL (1986) Direct evidence from intraneural recordings for increased central sympathetic outflow in patients with heart failure. Circulation 73:913–919
61. Golstein DS, McCarty R, Polinsky RJ, Kopin IJ (1983) Relationship between plasma norepinephrine and sympathetic neural activity. Hypertension 5:552–559
62. Hirsch AT, Dzau VJ, Creager MA (1987) Baroreceptor function in congestive heart failure: effect on neurohumoral activation and regional vascular resistance. Circulation 75(suppl IV):36–48
63. Wang W, Chen JS, Zucker IH (1990) Carotid sinus baroreceptor sensitivity in experimental heart failure. Circulation 81:1959–1966
64. Abboud FM, Thames MD, Mark AL (1981) Role of cardiac afferent nerves in the regulation of the circulation during coronary occlusion and heart failure. In: Abboud FM, Fozzard HA, Gilmore JP, Reis DJ (eds) Disturbances in neurogenic control of the circulation. American Physiological, Society, Bethesda, pp 65–86
65. Christensen NJ, Galbo H (1983) Sympathetic nervous activity during exercise. Annu Rev Physiol 45:139–153
66. Freud PR, Rowell LB, Murphy TM, Hobbs SF, Butler SH (1979) Blockade of the pressor response to muscle ischemia by sensory nerve block in man. Am J Physiol 237:H433–H439
67. Stebbins CL, Maruoka Y, Longhurst JC (1986) Prostaglandins contribute to cardiovascular reflexes evoked by static muscle contraction. Circ Res 59:645–654

68. Sato H, Hori M, Kitabatake A, Inoue M (1989) Adrenergic regulation during exercise in patients with heart failure. In: Hori M, Suga H, Baan J, Yellin EL (eds) Cardiac mechanics and function in the normal and diseased heart. Springer, Berlin Heidelberg New York Tokyo, pp 325–334

69. Waagstein F, Hjalmarson A, Varnauskas E, Wallentin I (1975) Effect of chronic beta-adrenergic receptor blockade in congestive cardiomyopathy. Br Heart J 37:1022–1036

70. Waagstein F, Caidahl K, Wallentin I, Bergh CH, Hjalmarson A (1989) Long-term beta-blockade in dilated cardiomyopathy: effects of short- and long-term metoprolol treatment followed by withdrawal and readministration of metoprolol. Circulation 80: 551–563

71. Yamada T, Fukunami M, Ohmori M, Iwakura K, Kumagai K, Kondoh N, Minamino T, Tsujimura E, Nagareda T, Kotoh K, Hoki N (1993) Which subpopulation of patients with dilated cardiomyopathy would benefit from long term beta-blocker therapy? A histological viewpoint. J Am Coll Cardiol 21:628–633

72. Bloom S, Davis DL (1972) Calcium as mediator of isoproterenol induced myocardial necrosis. Am J Pathol 69:459–470

73. Wheatley AM, Thandroyen FT, Opie LH (1985) Catecholamine-induced myocardial cell damage: catecholamines or adrenochrome. J Mol Cell Cardiol 17:349–359

74. Buja LM (1991) Lipid abnormalities in myocardial cell injury. Trends Cardiovasc Med 1:40–44

75. Ganote C, Armstrong S (1993) Ischemia and the myocyte cytoskeleton: review and speculation. Cardiovasc Res 27:1387–1403

76. Hori M, Sato H, Iwai K, Sato H, Inoue M, Kitabatake A, Kamada T (1992) Norepinephrine disrupts cytoskeletal framework of microtubules in rat hearts. Jpn Circ J 56:462–468

77. Hori M, Sato H, Kitakaze M, Iwai K, Takeda H, Inoue M, Kamada T (1994) Beta-adrenergic stimulation disassembles microtubules in neonatal rat cultured cardiomyocytes through intracellular Ca^{2+} overload. Circ Res 75:324–334

78. Kieth C, Dipaola M, Maxfield FR, Shelanski ML (1983) Microinjection of Ca^{2+}-calmodulin causes a localized depolymerization of microtubules. J Cell Biol 97:1918–1924

79. Schliwa M, Euteneuer U, Bulinski JC, Izant JG (1981) Calcium lability of cytoplasmic microtubules and its modulation by microtubules-associated proteins. Proc Natl Acad Sci USA 78:1037–1041

80. Badalamente MA, Hurst LC, Stracher A (1986) Calcium-induced degradation of the cytoskeleton in monkey and human peripheral nerves. J Hand Surg [Br] 11:337–340

81. Geffen LB, Ursh RA, Louis WJ, Doyle AE (1973) Plasma catecholamine and dopamine beta-hydroxylase amounts in pheochromocytoma. Clin Sci 44:421–424

82. Samuel JL, Marotte F, Delcayre C, Rappaport L (1986) Microtubule organization is related to rate of heart myocyte hypertrophy in rat. Am J Physiol 251:H1118–H1125

83. Shimo-oka T, Hayashi M, Satanabe Y (1980) Tubulin-myosin interaction: some properties of biding beween tubulin and myosin. Biochemistry 21:4921–4926

84. Warren RH (1968) The effect of colchicine on myogenesis in vivo in Rana pipiens and Rhodnius prolixus (Hemiptera). J Cell Biol 39:544–555

85. Croop JM, Holtzer H (1975) Response of fibrogenic and myogenic cells to cytochalasin B and to colcemid. I. Light microscopic observations. J Cell Biol 65:271–285

86. Hayashi M, Ohnishi K, Hayashi K (1980) Dense precipitate of brain tubulin with skeletal muscle myosine. J Biochem (Tokyo) 87:1347–1355

87. Antin PB, Forry-Scaudies S, Friedman TM, Tapscott SJ, Holtzer H (1981) Taxol induces postmitotic myoblasts to assemble interdigitating microtubules-myosin arrays that exclude actin filaments. J Cell Biol 90:300–308

88. Samuel JL, Bertier B, Bugaisky L, Marotte F, Swynghedauw B, Schwartz K, Rappaport L (1984) Different distributions of microtubules, desmin filaments and isomyosins during the onset of cardiac hypertrophy in the rat. Eur J Cell Biol 34:300–306

89. Schaper J, Froede R, Hein ST, Buck A, Hashizume H, Speiser B, Friedl A, Bleese N (1991) Impairment of the myocardial ultrastructure and changes of the cytoskeleton in dilated cardiomyopathy. Circulation 83:504–514

90. Hori M, Sato H, Iwai K, Takashima S, Hoki N, Fukunami M, Naka M, Kurihara H, Kitabatake A, Inoue M, Kamada T (1992) Disrupted microtubule structure in the ischemic and failing myocardium. The role of calcium overload. In: Yasuda H, Kawaguchi H (eds) New aspects in the treatment of failing heart. Springer, Berlin Heidelberg New York Tokyo, pp 46–50

Part 2
Mechanics of Contraction
of the Failing Heart

Cardiac Utilization of the Momentum of Blood

Motoaki Sugawara[1], Keisuke Uchida[2], Yukiyoshi Kondoh[1], and Christopher J.H. Jones[3]

Abstract. It is possible that the momentum of blood flowing out of the ventricle near end-systole plays an important role in the initiation of the decline and formation of the maximum rate of decline in left ventricular pressure. We hypothesize that a healthy heart utilizes this momentum of blood effectively.

Key words. Momentum—Inertia—Diastolic function—Maximum $(-dP/dt)$—Time constant

Introduction

It has been generally assumed that left ventricular pressure starts to decline near end-systole because the myocardium loses its tension and cannot maintain the high pressure. We earlier proposed the idea that the inertia force of the blood flowing out of the left ventricle toward the aorta plays an important role in the initiation of decay and formation of the maximum rate of decay in left ventricular pressure [1]. Here we describe the importance of the inertia force of blood in relation to cardiac function.

Time Course of Left Ventricular Pressure Decline

Figure 1 shows simultaneous recordings of left ventricular pressure, aortic pressure, and aortic flow velocity obtained from a dog. The aortic flow velocity signal is electrically delayed about 30 ms. The notch (*b*) in the aortic pressure waveform indicates the time of aortic valve closure. Left ventricular pressure starts to decline before aortic valve closure. The period between the beginning of left ventricular pressure decay and aortic valve closure (*a–b*) may be called "protodiastole," a term coined by Wiggers [2].

---

[1]Department of Cardiovascular Sciences, Tokyo Women's Medical College, 8-1 Kawada-cho, Shinjuku-ku, Tokyo 162, Japan
[2] Nihon Kohden Corporation, 1-31-4 Nishiochiai, Shinjuku-ku, Tokyo 161, Japan
[3] Princess of Wales Hospital, Coity Road, Bridgend, Mid Glamorgan CF31 1RQ, UK

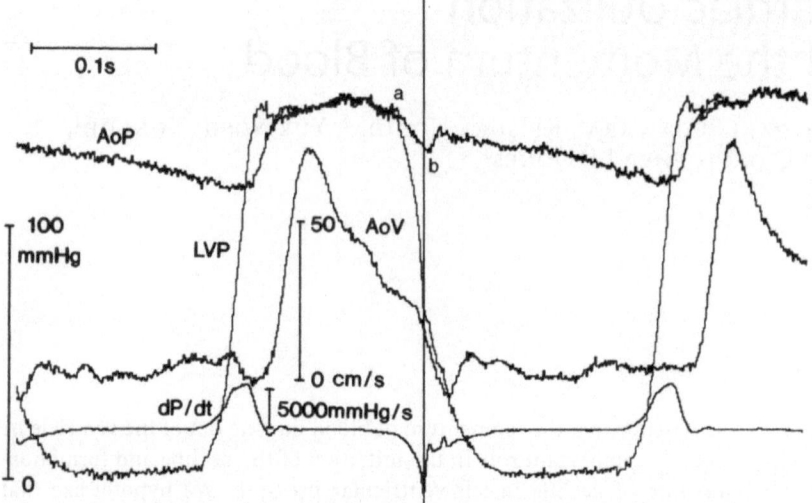

FIG. 1. Simultaneous recordings of left ventricular pressure (*LVP*), aortic pressure (*AoP*), and aortic flow velocity (*AoV*) with a multisensor catheter from a dog. Aortic flow velocity signal was delayed about 30 ms. The data were digitized at a sampling interval of 2 ms. dP/dt was obtained by differentiating digitally the left ventricular pressure with respect to time. *Vertical line* indicates the time of the maximum ($-$dP/dt)

The time course of the decay in left ventricular pressure during protodiastole is different from that during the period of isovolumic relaxation after aortic valve closure. The rate of the fall in left ventricular pressure ($-$dP/dt) increases with time during protodiastole so it reaches its maximum immediately before aortic valve closure. The timing of the maximum ($-$dP/dt) is indicated by the vertical line in Fig. 1. On the other hand, $-$dP/dt decreases exponentially with time during isovolumic relaxation. The exponential pressure decay during isovolumic relaxation is characterized by a time constant, τ. On high-fidelity left ventricular pressure recordings, there is often such a point of inflection, when $-$dP/dt changes discontinuously, at the time of aortic valve closure.

If the decline in left ventricular pressure during protodiastole is caused purely by myocardial relaxation, as must be the case during isovolumic relaxation, the time courses of pressure decline during the two periods should be similar. However, in the case illustrated in Fig. 1, there is a discontinuous change in dP/dt, and the time courses do not seem to be similar.

Effects of the Momentum of Blood

The decline in left ventricular pressure during protodiastole may also be determined by the deceleration of blood flowing out of the ventricle. In isolated cardiac muscle, the shortening ability decreases to zero before the tension-bearing ability declines (Fig. 2) [3]. If this were the case in the intact heart in vivo, the left ventricle would stop actively ejecting blood at the onset of protodiastole before its tension-bearing ability

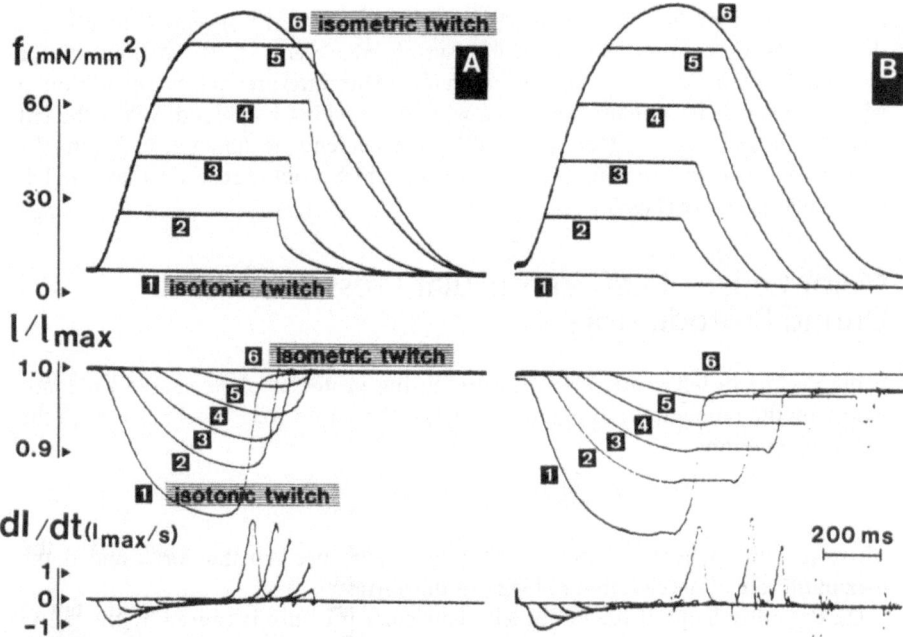

FIG. 2. Traces of force (f), length (l/lmax), and rate of length change (dl/dt) of a series of afterloaded twitches in an isolated cardiac muscle. The panels on the *left* (**A**) illustrate the familiar isotonic-isometric relaxation sequence; those on the *right* (**B**) illustrate the more physiological isometric-isotonic relaxation sequence. In the physiological sequence, shortening velocity decreases to zero before the force starts to decay. (From [3], with permission)

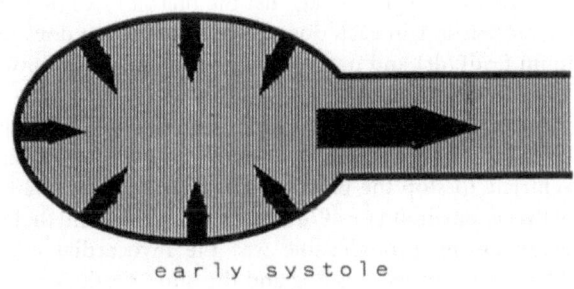

early systole

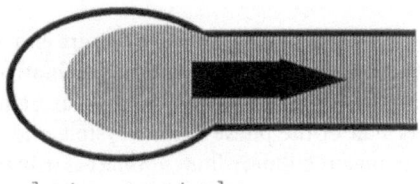

late systole

FIG. 3. Blood tends to flow out of the ventricle under its own momentum near end-ejection

is diminished by relaxation. In fact, Patterson et al. [4] and Wiggers [2] mentioned that the latter portion of ventricular systole represents a *Verharrungszeit* or *rückständige Kontraction*, an early German idea. They interpreted it as a condition in which the ventricles remain contracted without expelling any blood. When the left ventricle stops ejecting, blood may still have a tendency to flow out of it into the aorta under its own momentum (inertia force), which would cause a decrease in left ventricular pressure (Fig. 3).

Major Cause of Left Ventricular Pressure Decline During Protodiastole

If the decline in left ventricular pressure during protodiastole is caused predominantly by the momentum of blood, an analysis based on wave mechanics gives the following relation:

$$\text{Maximum} \left(-dP/dt\right) = \varrho c \alpha$$

where ϱ is the density of blood, c the pulse wave speed in the aorta, and α the maximum rate of deceleration of blood in the aorta.

On the other hand, if the fall in left ventricular pressure is caused by the fall in tension-bearing ability of the left ventricle, there must be a good negative correlation between maximum $(-dP/dt)$ and the time constant of exponential fall in left ventricular pressure during isovolumic relaxation.

To confirm which of these factors determines the maximum $(-dP/dt)$, we performed experiments in seven dogs. We measured (1) aortic flow velocity with an electromagnetic flowmeter, and (2) left ventricular pressure and pulse wave velocity in the aorta with three catheter-tipped micromanometers under conditions of pressure loading, volume loading, and changing cardiac contractility.

Multiple regression analysis was applied to the experimental data. The maximum $(-dP/dt)$ was regressed against the inertia force $\varrho c \alpha$ and the myocardial relaxation characteristic τ in each dog. In six of the seven dogs the correlation between maximum $(-dP/dt)$ and $\varrho c \alpha$ was significant, and that between maximum $(-dP/dt)$ and τ was not signigicant.

Therefore in most cases in our experiments the major determinant of maximum $(-dP/dt)$ was not the time constant of isovolumic relaxation but the ability of the left ventricle to stop the blood flowing out of it. In one dog, however, the correlation between maximum $(-dP/dt)$ and τ was significant; that is, the major cause of pressure decay during protodiastole was the myocardial relaxation. Let us consider the difference between this dog and the other six dogs.

Characteristics of the Phase Loop

Figure 4 shows left ventricular pressure and its derivative with respect to time (dP/dt), aortic flow, and the phase loop representative of the group of six dogs. The abscissa of the phase loop is left ventricular pressure, and the ordinate is its derivative, dP/dt. The upper half of the phase loop is systole and the lower half diastole. If the data point moves on a rectilinear line (not necessarily passing through the origin), left ventricular pressure decays exponentially. It seems that this is the case during the isovolumic

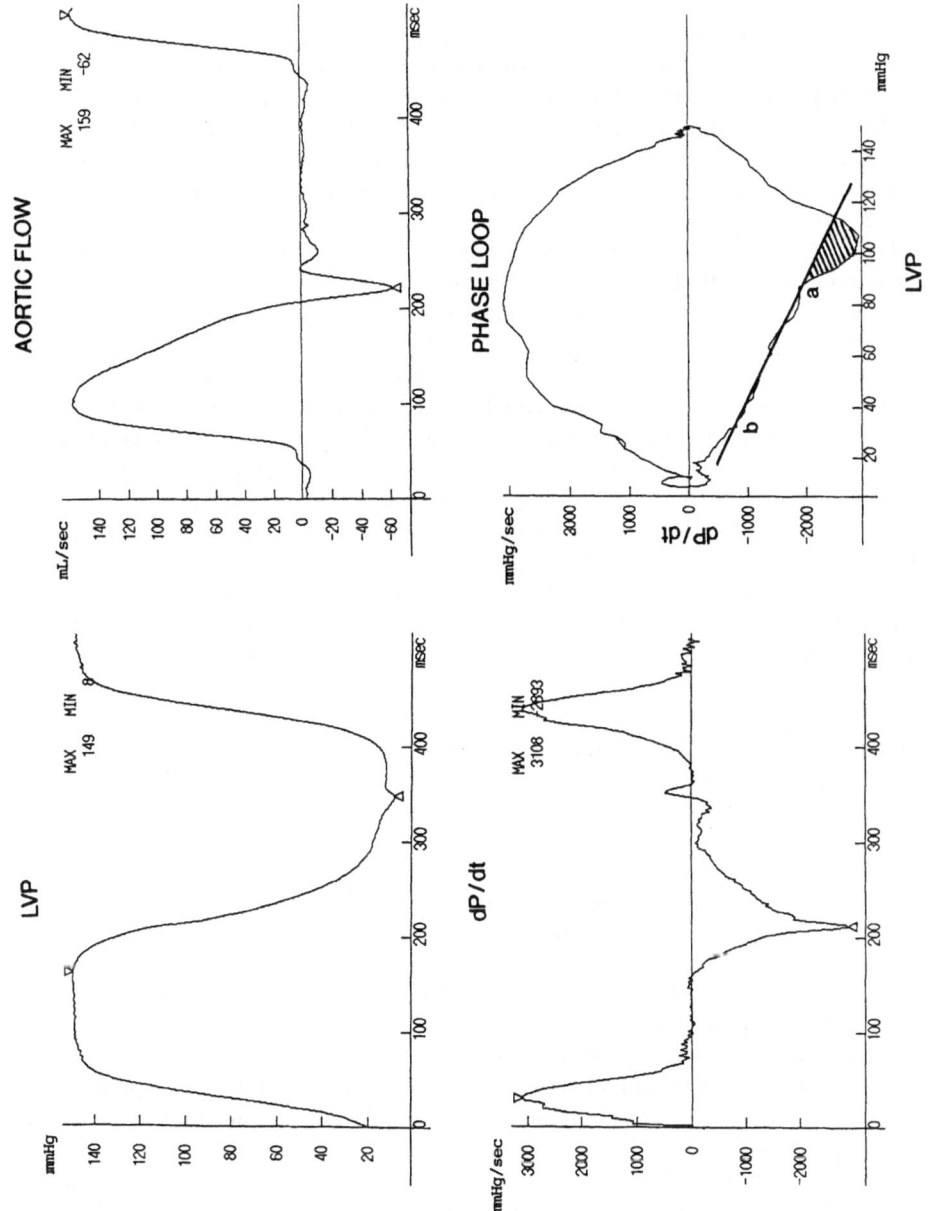

FIG. 4. Traces of left ventricular pressure (*LVP*), its time derivative (*dP/dt*), aortic flow rate, and phase loop obtained from a representative dog with significant effects of the momentum of blood

relaxation phase (*a–b* in lower right panel). However, the phase loop has a downward hump before the isovolumic relaxation phase (*hatched area*), and the data point goes below the imaginary straight line expected if the pressure declines in the same exponential manner as during the isovolumic relaxation phase. Thus peak ($-dP/dt$) becomes considerably large than expected from the exponential pressure decay. We believe that this difference is caused by the momentum of blood.

Figure 5 shows the data from the other dog. The phase loop has no downward hump, and $-dP/dt$ reached its maximum on the line expected from the exponential pressure decay. We believe that in such a case the momentum of blood is not effective.

The aortic flow waveform in Fig. 4 has a round contour with rapid deceleration near end-ejection, which seems suitable for obtaining a large cardiac output. The high deceleration rate near end-ejection generates a large effect of the momentum of the blood flowing out of the ventricle, which causes a rapid decay in left ventricular pressure. On the other hand, the aortic flow waveform in Fig. 5 has a lean triangular contour with a relatively low deceleration rate near end-ejection, which does not seem suitable for obtaining a large cardiac output. Empirically, we believe that the former heart is in better condition than the latter heart. Thus we hypothesize that a good heart mobilizes the momentum of blood to improve its cardiac function.

Effects of the Momentum of Blood on Cardiac Function

The momentum of blood decreases left ventricular pressure rapidly near end-ejection, which is late-systolic unloading for the heart. Gillebert et al. [5] analyzed the effects of systolic load clamps on relaxation in isolated cat papillary muscles. They reported that late-systolic unloading increased the peak rate of tension decline, made muscle lengthening occur earlier, and increased the peak rate of lengthening. All these effects enhance diastolic function.

We hypothesized that a good heart utilizes the momentum of blood. Having analyzed a considerable amount of clinical data, we are convinced that the hypothesis works well. Here we present examples of a normal and a diseased heart taken from a report by Katayama et al. [6].

Figure 6 shows recordings of left ventricular pressure obtained from a normal subject and a patient with congestive cardiomyopathy. Figure 7 shows the phase loops obtained from the left ventricular pressure waveforms in Fig. 6. For the normal patient the phase loop has a large downward hump, and $-dP/dt$ reaches a value much higher than expected from the exponential pressure decline during isovolumic relaxation (*straight line*). This case is typical of patients with normal hearts, with the momentum of blood having a large effect. On the other hand, in the patient with a diseased heart, the phase loop has no downward hump, and $-dP/dt$ barely reaches the same value expected from the exponential pressure decline during isovolumic relaxation. In this case the momentum of the blood has no effect.

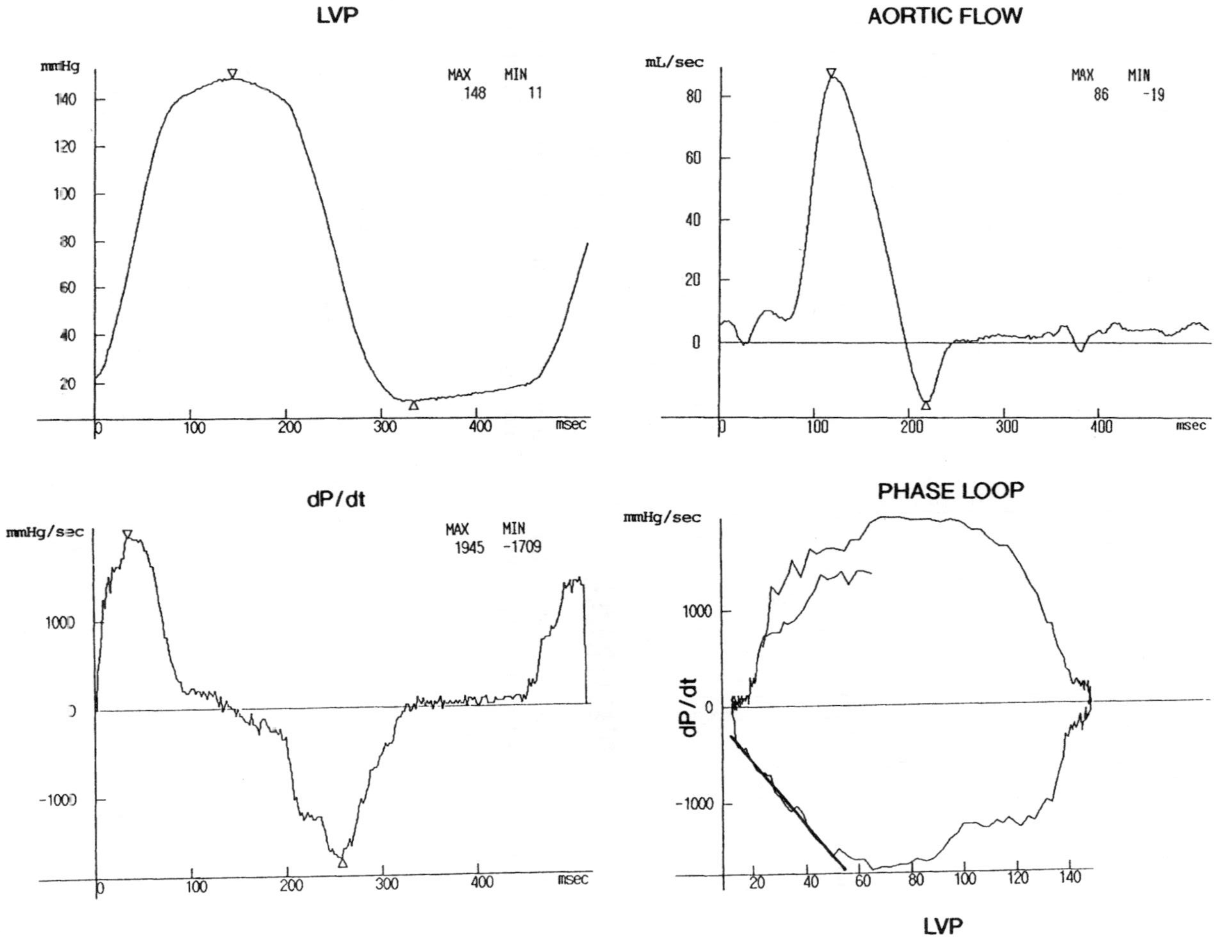

Fig. 5. Traces of left ventricular pressure (*LVP*), its time derivative (*dP/dt*), aortic flow rate, and phase loop obtained from a dog with no effect of the momentum of blood

75

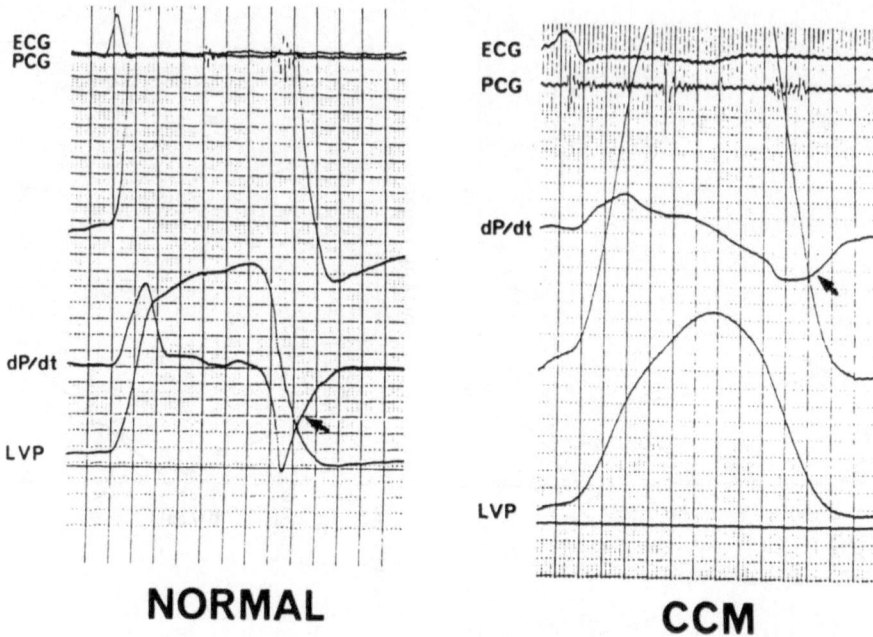

FIG. 6. Representative examples of left ventricular pressure (*LVP*) and its time-derivative (*dP/dt*) tracings from a normal subject and a patient with congestive cardiomyopathy (*CCM*). (From [6], with permission)

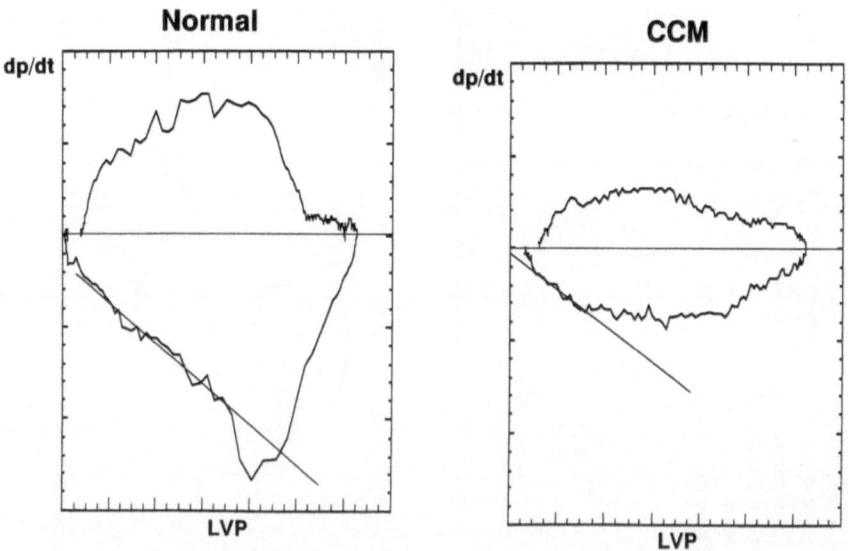

FIG. 7. Phase loops obtained from the data in Fig. 6. The phase loop obtained from a normal subject has a large downward hump, which is formed by the effects of the momentum of blood. In contrast, the phase loop obtained from a patient with congestive cardiomyopathy (*CCM*) has no downward hump, and the −dP/dt barely reaches the maximum value expected from the exponential pressure decline during isovolumic relaxation (*straight line*)

References

1. Jones CJH, Sugawara M (1993) "Wavefronts" in the aorta—implications for the mechanism of left ventricular ejection and aortic valve closure. Cardiovasc Res 27:1902–1905
2. Wiggers CJ (1921) Studies on the consecutive phases of the cardiac cycle. I. The duration of the consecutive phases of the cardiac cycle and the criteria for their precise determination. Am J Physiol 56:415–438
3. Brutsaert DL, Sys SU (1989) Relaxation and diastole of the heart. Physiol Rev 69:1228–1314
4. Patterson SW, Piper H, Starling EH (1914) The regulation of the heart beat. J Physiol (Lond) 48:465–513
5. Gillebert TC, Sys SU, Brutsaert DL (1989) Influence of loading patterns on peak length-tension relation and on relaxation in cardiac muscle. J Am Coll Cardiol 13:483–490
6. Katayama K, Kumada T, Fujii T, et al (1984) Clinical characteristics of left ventricular pressure decline during isovolumic relaxation in normal and diseased hearts. Am Heart J 107:332–338

Two Major Pumps of the Heart: Difference and Interdependence of the Right and Left Ventricles

Hitonobu Tomoike, Yoshitoshi Urabe*, Keizaburo Ohzono†, and Seiji Yamaguchi

Abstract. The right and left ventricles are the two major pumps of the heart that deliver blood to the pulmonary and systemic circulations, respectively. Both ventricles propel the same amount of blood but are different with regard to intracavitary pressure, wall thickness, and shape. Coronary perfusion pressure and regional wall motion are closely linked to myocardial metabolic states and regional myocardial blood flow. When coronary perfusion pressure is decreased below the level of coronary flow autoregulation, regional wall motion deteriorates. However, the mechanism of a reduced level of autoregulation in the right coronary artery remains unclear. The transmural distribution of myocardial necrosis was also different between right and left coronary artery ligations. The interdependence of the right and left ventricles is clearly seen. The resetting of regional diastolic lengths may affect systolic and diastolic functions. Thus the structural and hemodynamic differences of these two pumping chambers determine the perfusion pressure–flow function integrity of the regional myocardium and the distribution of myocardial necrosis. Understanding the interdependence of these chambers will allow us to develop a better assist mechanism for depressed pump performance.

Key words. Autoregulation—Regional wall motion—Ischemia—Infarction—Ventricle

Introduction

The heart propels blood throughout the body so as to deliver nutrients to and remove wastes from the organs, thereby maintaining homeostasis and adjusting the body's performance to alterations of the environment [1]. The heart is divided into four chambers. The right and left ventricles are the two major pumps of the heart. The ventricles are different in shape, wall thickness, and intracavitary pressure, although they eject the same amount of blood per minute. Such coordination as is shown by the right and left ventricles depends partly on the Frank-Starling law. Differences in

First Department of Internal Medicine, Yamagata University School of Medicine, 2-2-2 Iida-Nishi, Yamagata 990-23, Japan
* Present address: Kitakyushu Medical Center, Kitakyushu 802, Japan
† Present address: Kyushu Medical Center, Fukuoka 812, Japan

morphology and loading condition between the right and left ventricles determine the hemodynamics and clinical manifestations in the presence of stress and disease states.

Characteristics of Perfusion Pressure: Function Relation in Right Ventricle

Coronary flow remains relatively constant over a wide range of perfusion pressures. When the mean coronary driving pressure decreases below 50–70 mm Hg, left coronary flow begins to fall sharply. The level of perfusion pressiure required for maintaining normal regional wall motion in the left ventricle is above 40–60 mm Hg [2–4]. Thus autoregulation adjusts coronary vascular resistance to maintain relatively constant myocardial perfusion and performance. Although extravascular compressive forces are markedly different in the right and left ventricles, the pressure–function relation of the right ventricle has not been extensively investigated. We examined the effects of graded reductions in regional coronary perfusion pressure on regional segment shortening in the right ventricular (RV) free wall [5]. As the level of afterload alters the extent of systolic wall motion and myocardial oxygen consumption, segment shortening was measured with and without an increased level of RV pressure. The level of afterload to the right ventricle can easily be elevated by constricting the pulmonary artery without altering right coronary perfusion pressure. Thus the right ventricle seems to be a naturally designed model for elucidating the relations among perfusion pressure, coronary flow, pump performance, and afterload.

Experimental Setup

Thirteen mongrel dogs (19–23 kg) were sedated with intramuscular morphine sulfate (10 mg) and then anesthetized with intravenous α-chloralose (45 mg/kg) and urethane (450 mg/kg). After endotracheal intubation, a left thoracotomy at the third intercostal space was performed under positive-pressure respiration, and the pericardium was opened. A hydraulic vascular occluder (diameter = 16 mm) was placed around the main pulmonary artery. The pericardium was loosely closed, and the chest was closed. A right thoracotomy then was performed through the fourth intercostal space, and the heart was supported in a pericardial cradle. The autoperfusion system from the right carotid artery to the proximal portion of the right coronary artery was established using a large-bore cannula. Right coronary blood flow and pressure were monitored using a cannulating type electromagnetic flow probe (diameter = 3 mm, Statham, SP7517, Oxford, CA, USA) and a Statham P23Db transducer, respectively. Systemic arterial pressure was monitored continuously at the ascending aorta with a P23Db pressure transducer through an 8F catheter, and both left (LV) and right ventricular pressures were measured by catheter-tip pressure transducers (PC350; Millar Houston, TX, USA). For pressure measurements, zero level was taken at the middle of the chest. For assessment of regional wall motion in the right ventricle, two pairs of miniature (1.5–1.7 mm in diameter) piezoelectric crystals (5 MHz; Murata, Kyoto, Japan) were positioned approximately midway between the endocardium and the epicardium in the RV free wall. One pair was implanted 0.8–1.2 cm apart, parallel to the atrioventricular groove, and the other pair was oriented perpendicular to the first pair. The correct location of these crystals relative to the vascular bed of the right coronary artery was verified by postmortem soft radiographic examination.

Regional shortening was calculated by the formula

$$\left[(\text{End-diastolic length} - \text{end-systolic length})/\text{end-diastolic length}\right] \times 100$$

and was termed percent shortening. We recorded the aortic pressure, RV pressure, coronary flow, and regional segmental lengths along with the LV pressure and its first derivative (dP/dt) on a direct-writing pen recorder, eight-channel rectigraph (Sanei Sokuki, Tokyo, Japan).

Experimental Design

After 20 min of control recordings, the perfusion pressure was reduced abruptly using a stopcock. A reduced level of coronary perfusion pressure was maintained for 60 s, after which the constriction was released. This procedure was repeated at several levels of coronary perfusion pressure. Graded reductions of the right coronary perfusion pressure were repeated with or without banding the pulmonary artery. The cuff around the pulmonary artery was gradually inflated by infusing saline until the systolic RV pressure was elevated 10–30 mm Hg without producing changes in peak systolic LV pressure. For each experiment the order of the two conditions— banding or not banding the pulmonary artery (PA)—was random. The anatomical perfusion area of the right coronary artery was measured angiographically postmortem in order to calculate coronary blood flow (in milliliters per minute per gram).

Critical Coronary Perfusion Pressure for Maintaining Wall Motion

Figure 1 shows representative tracings of regional wall motion at various levels of right coronary perfusion pressure before (top panel) and after (bottom panel) PA banding. Before PA banding the regional wall motion remained almost constant at a perfusion pressure of 48 mm Hg and then decreased progressively depending on the level of perfusion pressure. When the RV systolic pressure was increased by 25 mm Hg without affecting the mean arterial and LV peak systolic pressures, regional hypokinesis was first noted at a perfusion pressure of 60 mm Hg, which means that the perfusion pressure critical for maintaining regional wall motion depends on the level of afterload.

The relation between right coronary perfusion pressure and regional shortening is plotted in Figure 2. Regional shortening was insensitive to changes in right coronary perfusion pressure when the pressure was higher than a critical level. Below this perfusion pressure, the regional shortening of both base to apex and circumferential segments were directly dependent on the right coronary perfusion pressure.

In Figure 3, all data points for each dog are replotted to demonstrate the pressure-shortening relation (Fig. 3A) and flow-shortening relation (Fig. 3B) in the right ventricle. The inflection points, below which the regional shortening was dependent on perfusion pressure, were estimated by visual inspection (arrows in Fig. 2). The

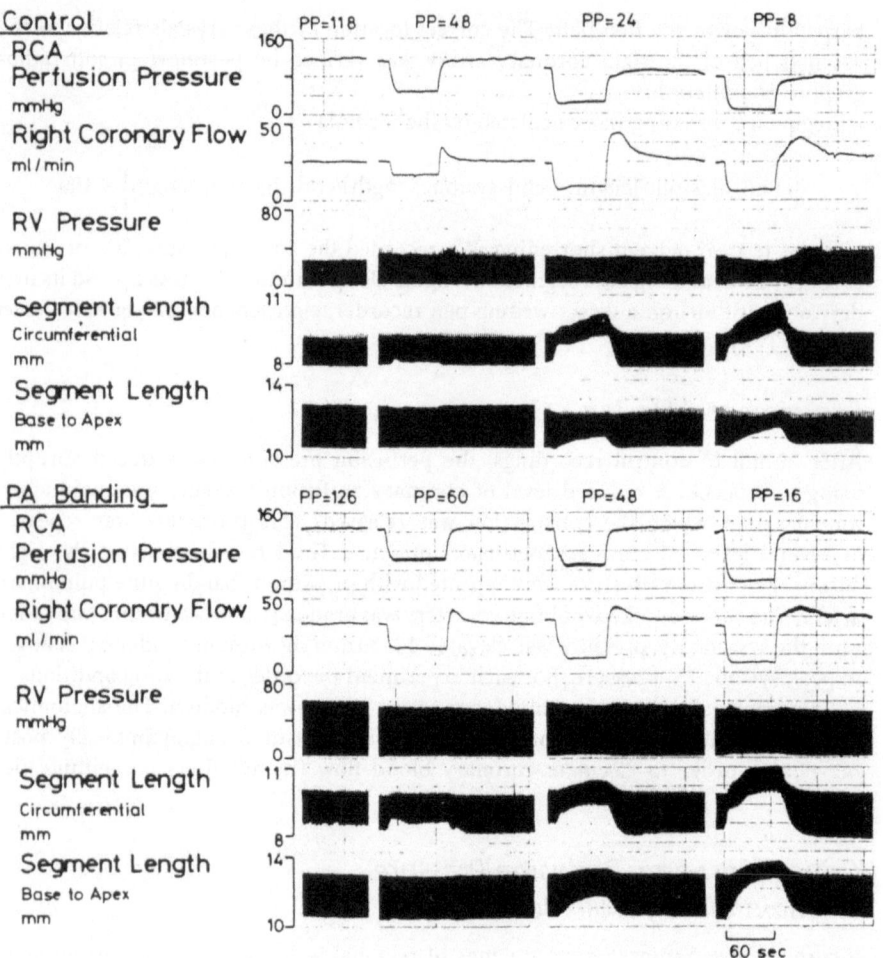

FIG. 1. Effects of various perfusion pressures on right ventricular (RV) pressure and segment length from a representative experiment. At *top*, tracings obtained at normal RV pressure (control); *bottom*, tracings obtained during pulmonary artery (PA) banding. After abrupt changes in coronary perfusion pressure, coronary blood flow changed, depending on the pressure level, and was maintained constant during the procedure; this phenomenon indicates the absence of autoregulation in the right coronary vasculature. RV pressure was increased by constricting the PA with a cuff occluder. Reactive hyperemia was always noted, and its degree depended on the reduced level of coronary perfusion pressure. *RCA*, right coronary artery; *PP*, perfusion pressure (in millimeters of mercury); *RV*, right ventricle. (From [5], with permission)

average inflection pressures were 30 ± 9 and 45 ± 16 mm Hg before and after PA banding, respectively ($P < 0.01$), in the base-to-apex segment and 32 ± 6 and 42 ± 11 mm Hg before and after PA banding, respectively ($P < 0.01$), in the circumferential segment. Accordingly: (1) the critical perfusion pressure was lower in the right than in the left ventricle [2]; and (2) an increase in RV afterload elevated the critical perfusion pressure below which regional function was deteriorated.

The difference in the critical perfusion pressure between the right and left ventricles may be explained by (1) a marked difference in afterload for performing systolic

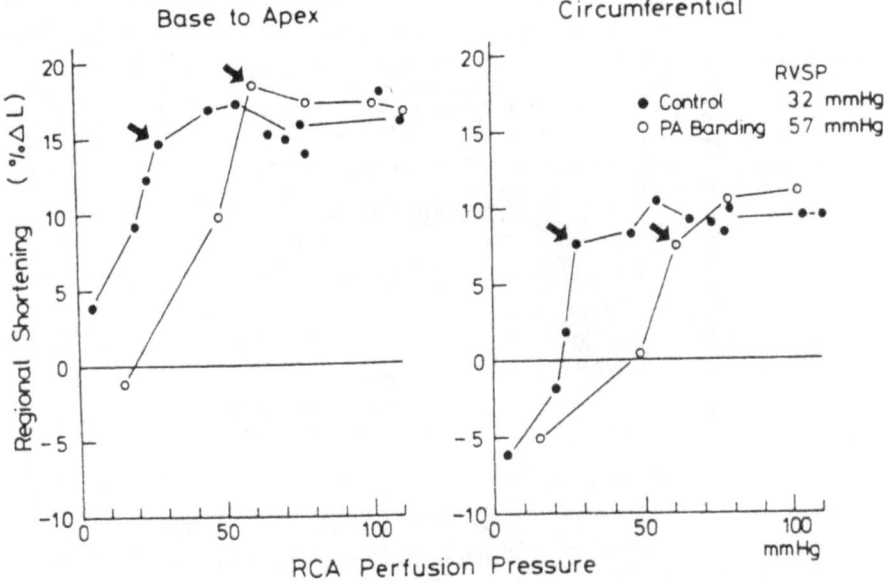

FIG. 2. Right coronary artery (RCA) perfusion pressure—regional shortening data from a representative dog before (*closed circles*) and after (*open circles*) PA banding. *Left* and *right* panels show data obtained at the base-to-apex and circumferential planes, respectively. Curve falls off steeply below the perfusion pressure at the inflection point (*arrow*), indicating the presence of critical perfusion pressure unique to the regional RV free wall, after which regional wall motion became highly dependent on the perfusion pressure. PA banding obviously shifts this relation toward the right. (From [5], with permission)

wall motion; (2) lower oxygen consumption of the right than the left ventricle due to lower RV pressure and work [6, 7] and (3) thinner wall thickness; and (4) lower extravascular compressive force of the right than the left ventricle.

Homogeneous Deterioration of Wall Motion

In Figure 4 the relation between coronary perfusion pressure or flow and systolic shortening in the circumferential direction is replotted by normalizing the perfusion pressure, flow, and regional shortening data as decimal fractions of the data observed at the inflection point. A highly significant correlation coefficient was obtained when normalized pressure (x) and shortening (y) were fitted to a monoexponential curve after transforming the ordinate to $y' = y + 1.5$. The equations derived for data from all 13 open-chest dogs were as follows: $y' = 70x^{0.24}$ ($r = 0.67, n = 126, P < 0.001$) in the base-to-apex direction at normal RV pressure; $y' = 25x^{0.44}$ ($r = 0.72, n = 118, P < 0.001$) in the circumferential direction at normal RV pressure; $y' = 42x^{0.35}$ ($r = 0.79, n = 85, P = 0.001$) in the base-to-apex direction during RV hypertension: and $y' = 15x^{0.54}$ ($r = 0.68, n = 74, P < 0.001$) in the circumferential direction during RV hypertension. There was no significant difference in the level of critical perfusion pressures between the base-to-apex and circumferential segments. Thus the wall motion abnormalities appeared at the same perfusion pressure, irrespective of the direction of segment length measurements.

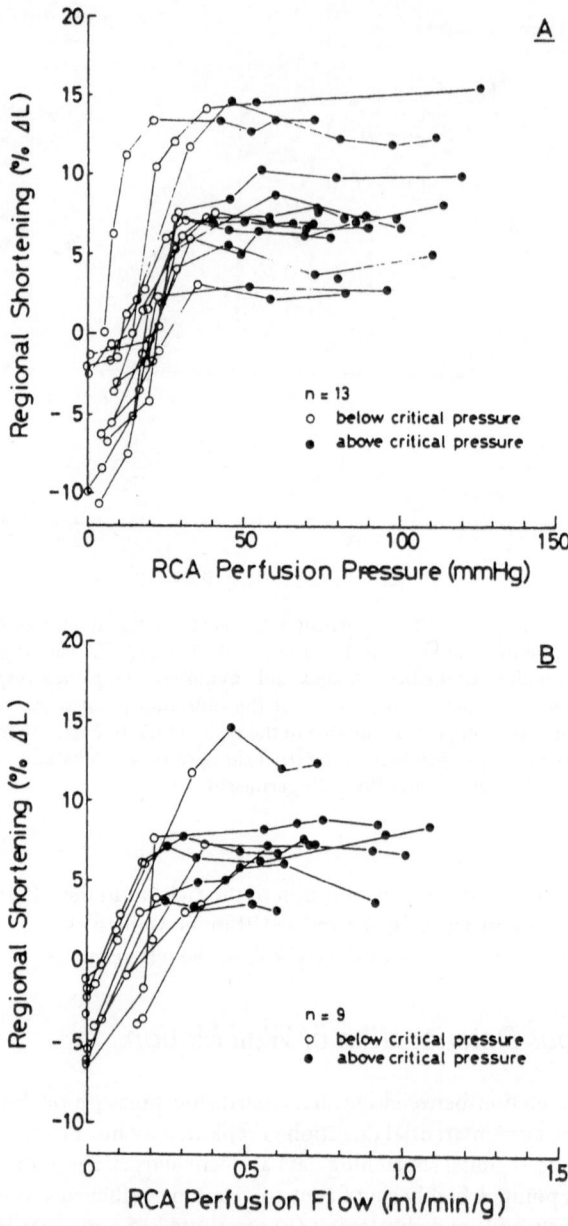

FIG. 3. Relation between right coronary perfusion pressure (**A**) or perfusion flow (**B**) and regional shortening in circumferential direction. *Open* and *closed circles* represent the relation below and above the critical perfusion pressure in 13 dogs (**A**) or the critical perfusion flow in nine dogs (**B**), respectively. Similar relations also were obtained in the base-to-apex direction and in both directions during PA banding (not shown). (From [5], with permission)

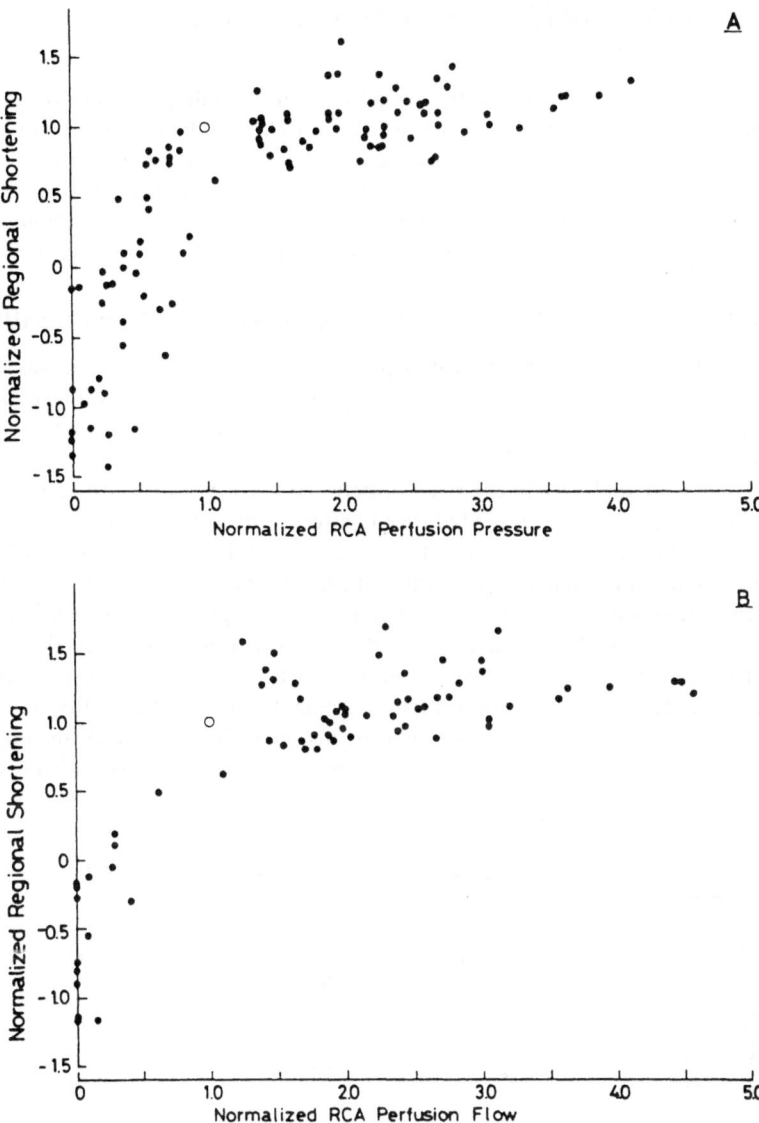

FIG. 4. Relation between normalized right coronary perfusion pressure (A) or perfusion flow (B) and regional shortening in circumferential direction of the data in Fig. 3. Shortening was normalized by expressing it with a unity fraction of shortening at the inflection point, as shown by the arrows in Fig. 2. This normalization procedure for perfusion pressure or flow and regional shortening accounts for individual variations in cardiac metabolism and shape among animals. Dependence of regional shortening on perfusion pressure below the critical perfusion pressure is clearly demonstrated. Above the critical level of coronary perfusion, regional shortening tends toward an asymptotic value. (From [5], with permission)

Hemodynamic Stability During Right Coronary Underperfusion

Changes in RV and LV pressures during right coronary underperfusion were minimal. Statistically significant reductions in RV and LV systolic pressures and some increases in RV end-diastolic pressure were noted during PA banding below the critical perfusion pressure. Because these changes were too small to consider as physiologically significant alterations, a marked reduction of regional function in the RV free wall did not affect global performance of either the right or left ventricle.

Systolic Pressure-Dependent Shift in Critical Perfusion Pressure

Independent control of ventricular cavity pressure and perfusion pressure was feasible in the present in situ right ventricle. This point was an unique advantage of this experimental set-up and facilitated detailed analysis of pressure–wall motion–flow relations.

A monoexponential curvilinear relation between perfusion pressure or flow rate and percent shortening was noted before and after PA banding. In addition, a direct linear relation between normalized perfusion pressure and regional shortening below the inflection point was noted with or without PA banding ($r = 0.71–0.89$, $n = 21–56$, $P < 0.001$). It is noteworthy that the relations shifted rightward after PA banding (Fig. 2). Increases in RV systolic pressure during PA banding were directly related to the level of critical perfusion pressure, as shown in Fig. 5. The higher level of critical perfusion pressure during PA banding may be attributable to the elevation of RV pressure, which presumably reflects increases in wall stress during PA banding. Correlation coefficients and slopes between changes in systolic RV pressure

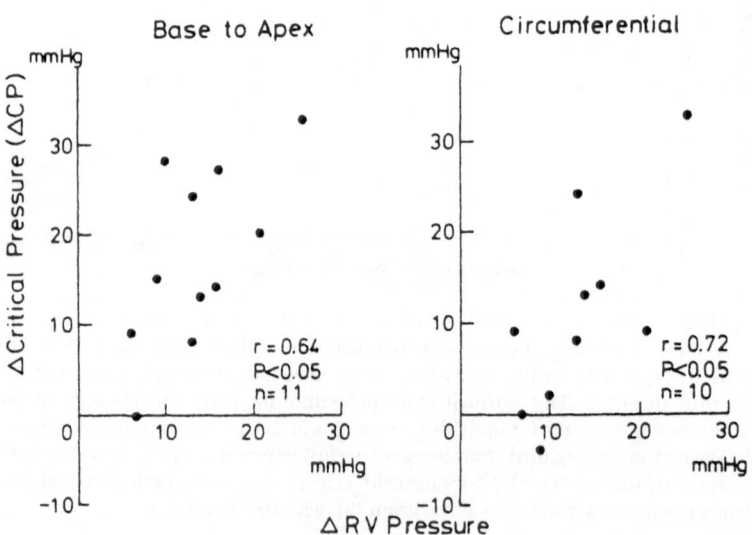

FIG. 5. Relative changes in critical perfusion pressure versus changes in the increase of RV systolic pressure. A statistically significant correlation was noted between them, suggesting that the RV systolic pressure determines the degree of critical perfusion pressure. (From [5], with permission)

and critical perfusion pressure were practically the same between the base-to-apex and the circumferential planes (Fig. 5). An increase of afterload surely increases myocardial oxygen consumption [8, 9]. An area of the RV free wall, calculated from end-diastolic lengths of the base-to-apex and circumferential segments, increased after PA banding. The wall tension, calculated from a pressure and an area at end-diastole by Laplace's law, increased significantly, suggesting an augmentation of preload during PA banding. Ellis and Klocke described a rightward shift of the pressure–flow relation of the left coronary artery during diastole when the preload was increased [10]; similarly, the rightward shift of the pressure–wall motion relation during PA banding may be explained in part by the increases in preload and oxygen consumption.

Autoregulation

The inflection point of the curvilinear relation between perfusion pressure and contractile force was considered to be the limit of autoregulatory reserve [11]. Although the inflection point of the curvilinear relation between right coronary perfusion pressure and regional wall motion was easy to detect, it was difficult to determine the inflection between perfusion pressure and coronary flow, especially during RV hypertension. Thus autoregulation is a different category of flow and wall motion with regard to perfusion pressure. These data also suggest that the effectiveness of autoregulation in vessels that perfuse the right and left ventricles is strikingly different. Mechanisms of the reduced level of autoregulation in the right coronary artery remain unclear.

Determinants of Infarct Size

In experimental studies, the evolution of myocardial infarction after ligating a branch of the coronary artery is determined by the time after flow cessation, the oxygen consumption of the heart, the level of collateral blood flow, and the size of the area at risk. A consistent linear relation between infarct area and the area at risk or the perfusion size of the ligated coronary artery has been repeatedly noted in the left ventricle [12, 13]. The ratio of infarct size to the area at risk has been used for normalizing the infarct size.

We attempted to determine if there is any topological difference in the distribution of myocardial necrosis through different transmural layers between the right and left ventricles, with reference to risk area and regional myocardial blood flow [14]. Fifty-one adult mongrel dogs of either sex (weight 16–29 kg) were anesthetized with sodium pentobarbital (25 mg/kg IV) and ventilated by room air and supplemental oxygen. The chest was opened at the left fourth intercostal space. The largest obtuse marginal branch of the left circumflex coronary artery and the main trunk of the right coronary artery were ligated to produce myocardial infarction.

Measurements of Regional Myocardial Flow and Infarct Size

A tracer microsphere technique was used to determine regional myocardial blood flow before, 5 min after, and 24 h after coronary occlusion. We used carbonized tracer microspheres, 8–11 μm in diameter, labeled with γ-emitting nuclides: [141]Ce, [113]Sn, [46]Sc (New England Nuclear, Boston, MA, USA), and [85]Sr (3M, St. Paul, MN, USA) [15].

Postmortem coronary angiography was used to determine the risk areas. At 24 h after coronary ligation the dog was anesthetized with sodium pentobarbital (15–20 mg/kg IV), 5000 units of heparin was infused, and the animal was killed by intravenously administering 20 ml of saturated KCl. The heart was excised, and the left main coronary artery and right coronary artery proximal to its ligated portion were then cannulated and flushed with buffered saline. A barium–gelatin mixture (BaSO$_4$ 42 g, gelatin 17 g, and water 53 ml) was perfused simultaneously at a perfusion pressure of 120–140 mm Hg for 5 min at 37°C. The heart was then immersed in crushed ice for 5 min to harden the barium–gelatin mixture. The right and left ventricles were sliced parallel to the atrioventricular groove into four and five slices, respectively, of equal thickness (0.8–1.2 cm). Each slice was immediately incubated in 1% solution of triphenyl tetrazolium chloride (TTC), buffered in Tris buffer (0.2 mol/L) to pH 7.8 at 20°C for 30 min, and fixed in 20% formalin to define the infarct area. The area at risk was determined by stereoscopic radiograms (SRO-M40S; Sofron, Osaka, Japan) [16–18].

Regional Flow After Coronary Occlusion

At 5 min after coronary occlusion, regional myocardial blood flow to the purely necrotic area decreased from 0.67 ± 0.03 to 0.06 ± 0.03 ml/min per gram in the right ventricle and from 1.47 ± 0.09 to 0.19 ± 0.03 ml/min per gram in the left ventricle. Blood flow to the total risk or central risk areas was also decreased but was greater ($P < 0.05$) than that at the purely necrotic site in either the right or left ventricle. Between 5 min and 24 h after coronary occlusion, transmural myocardial blood flow toward the total or central risk area did not change significantly in either the right or left ventricle, whereas that to the purely necrotic area of the left ventricle decreased significantly from 0.19 ± 0.03 to 0.01 ± 0.01 ml/min per gram ($P < 0.01$). This phenomenon is explained by (1) disruption of the microvasculature in the region of severe ischemia [19, 20], (2) redistribution of collateral blood flow from the necrotic to the salvaged myocardium [21], and (3) ischemia-induced vasoconstriction along the border of the ischemic zone [22].

The physiological appropriateness of our risk determination was examined by changes in regional flow across the boundary of the risk region after administration of dipyridamole. Regional myocardial blood flow of the area 5 mm outside the risk area increased from 0.87 ± 0.10 to 2.99 ± 0.38 ml/min per gram ($P < 0.01$) and from 1.09 ± 0.13 to 2.55 ± 0.34 ml/min per gram ($P < 0.01$) after dipyridamole in the right and left ventricles, respectively, which were larger ($P < 0.01$) than the increases in regional flow of the area 5 mm inside the risk area, that is, from 0.52 ± 0.08 to 0.96 ± 0.15 ml/min per gram ($P < 0.05$) and from 0.70 ± 0.10 to 1.04 ± 0.12 ml/min per gram ($P < 0.05$) in the right and left ventricles, respectively. Regional myocardial blood flow was unchanged in both the purely necrotic and central risk areas. Accordingly, a sharp change in regional myocardial blood flow across the border after dipyridamole suggested that demarcation of the risk area by a postmortem angiogram was appropriate physiologically. A collateral flow in the risk area was defined as regional flow toward the central risk area in the following analysis.

Transmural distribution of myocardial blood flow inside the risk area differed between the right and left ventricles at 5 min and 24 h after coronary occlusion. The subendocardial to subepicardial flow ratio in the central risk area of the right ventricle was reduced slightly from 1.19 ± 0.06 before coronary occlusion to 0.85 ± 0.05 at 5 min and, significantly, to 0.69 ± 0.06 at 24 h ($P < 0.01$). This ratio in the left ventricle decreased remarkably from 1.29 ± 0.08 before occlusion to 0.51 ± 0.09 at 5 min ($P <$ 0.01 versus before occlusion) and 0.09 ± 0.02 at 24 h of coronary occlusion ($P < 0.01$ versus 5 min). Hence the transmural flow distribution after coronary ligation was more homogeneous in the right ventricle than in the left ventricle.

Infarct Size and Collateral Flow in the Right and Left Ventricles

We determined risk areas by postmortem stereoscopic coronary arteriography [16, 23]. This procedure provides an anatomical risk region supplied by the occluded coronary artery [24, 25]. With TTC staining, the infarcted myocardium was clearly detectable from the surrounding normal tissue. The mean infarct size of the risk area was similar between the right coronary artery (RCA) and the obtuse marginal branch occlusions: 11.3 ± 0.5 g and 10.3 ± 0.9 g, respectively. The size of the risk area was more variable in the case of occlusion of the obtuse marginal branch than for RCA occlusion ($P < 0.05$). The mean infarct size and the ratio of the infarct size to the risk area (IS: RA) were not significantly different between occlusions of these two vessels. There was a linear relation between infarct size and risk area for both vessels (Fig. 6). The infarcted area was always located inside the risk area, in both right and left ventricles. Accordingly, the usefulness and rationale of risk determination were confirmed for both RV and LV infarctions.

The relation between the necrotic area (percent of the risk area size, or y) and transmural collateral flow (x) 24 h after coronary occlusion was inversely related in the left and right ventricles (Fig. 7). The slope of the relation was steeper in the right than the left ventricle and the x-axis intercept was lower in the right than in the left ventricle. The correlation coefficients between necrotic area and collateral flow remained unchanged between 5 min and 24 h of occlusion in the right ventricle (-0.87

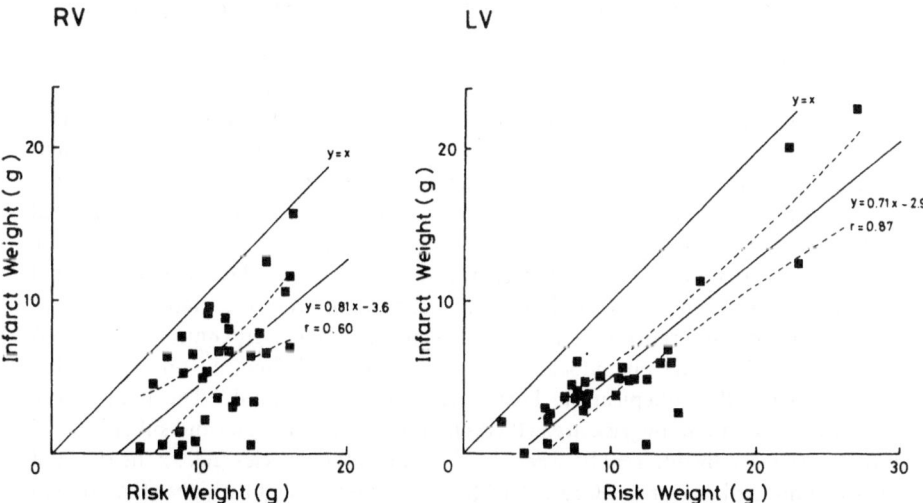

FIG. 6. Relation between the weight of infarcted and risk areas. The line labeled $y = x$ is the line of identity; the other *solid line* is the regression line. The standard error of estimate is shown by *dotted lines*. Two coronary arteries (obtuse marginal branch and right coronary artery) were ligated at a fairly constant anatomical site. *RV*, right ventricle; *LV*, left ventricle. Each point represents data from one dog. (From [14], with permission)

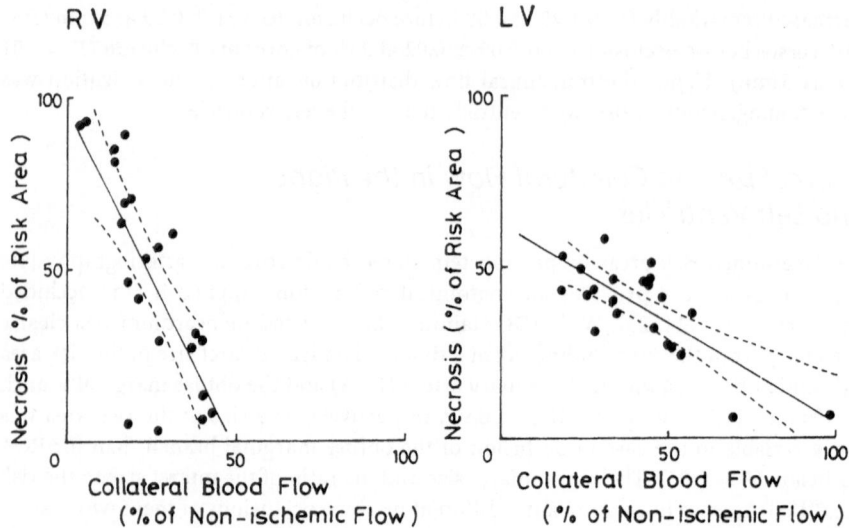

FIG. 7. Relation between percent of necrosis of the risk area and transmural collateral flow in the percent of nonischemic flow 24 h after coronary ligation. Right ventricle (RV): y = −2.1x + 97.8 (r = −0.77). Left ventricle (LV): y = −0.6x + 62.0 (r = −0.77). The standard error of estimate is shown by *dotted lines*. (From [14], with permission)

versus −0.75) but increased from −0.47 to −0.78 over 24 h in the left ventricle. This finding means that flow redistribution was obvious in cases of LV infarction, suggesting the operation of a wave front phenomenon [12]. However, the mechanisms of postocclusive flow redistribution remain unclear.

Regional Differences in Distribution of Myocardial Necrosis

To explain the difference of the risk–infarct relation between the right and left ventricles, the regional relation between infarct size and risk area from subendocardium to the subepicardium, was examined. In the left ventricle the subepicardial layer tended to be salvaged in most dogs. On the other hand, myocardial necrosis in the right ventricle was distributed rather homogeneously from the subendocardium to the subepicardium. The relation between infarct size and risk area for the subendocardial and the subepicardial layers in the right and left ventricles is shown in Fig. 8. In the right ventricle data from the subepicardial and subendocardial layers are distributed between the x-axis and a line of identity (y = x) of an infarct–risk relation, and there is no significant difference in variance between these layers. In contrast, in the left ventricle data from the subendocardial layers are grouped along the line of identity, and data from the subepicardial layers are scattered randomly. The infarct size, expressed as a ratio of the risk area (IS:RA), in the subendocardial and subepicardial layers was markedly different between the right and left ventricles (fig. 9); the IS:RA of the subendocardial layer was 0.53 ± 0.05 (n = 33) and was slightly higher than that of the subepicardial layer(0.40 ± 0.05), (P < 0.01) in the right ventricle, whereas in the left ventricle the IS:RA was markedly higher in the subendocardial layer (0.71 ± 0.04) than in the subepicardial layer (0.21 ± 0.04) (P < 0.01). The ratios of subepicardial IS:RA to subendocardial IS:RA in the right and left ventricles were 0.76 ± 0.06 and

RV   LV

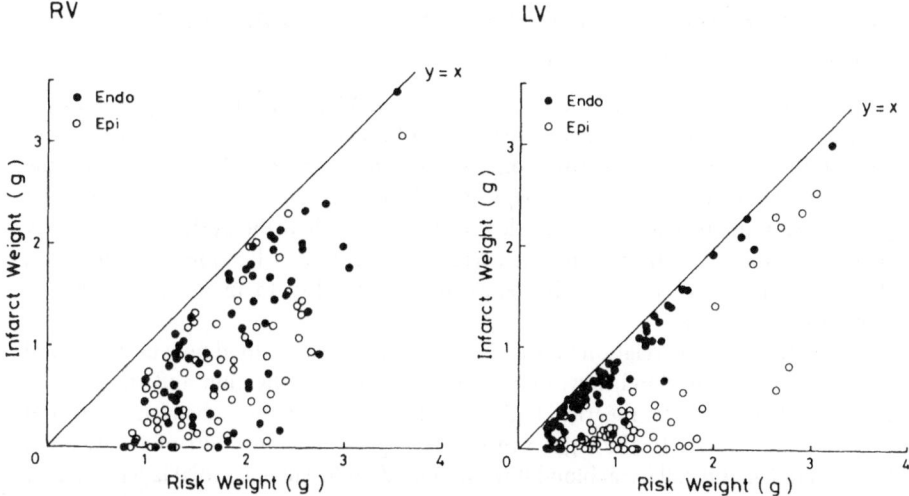

FIG. 8. Relation between the weight of infarcted and risk areas in the subendocardial (*closed circles*) and subepicardial (*open circles*) layers. Note that in the right ventricle the subendocardial and subepicardial samples are plotted in almost the same manner, whereas in the left ventricle the subendocardial samples give a linear line and the subepicardial samples are plotted rather randomly between the line of identity and the x-axis. (From [14], with permission)

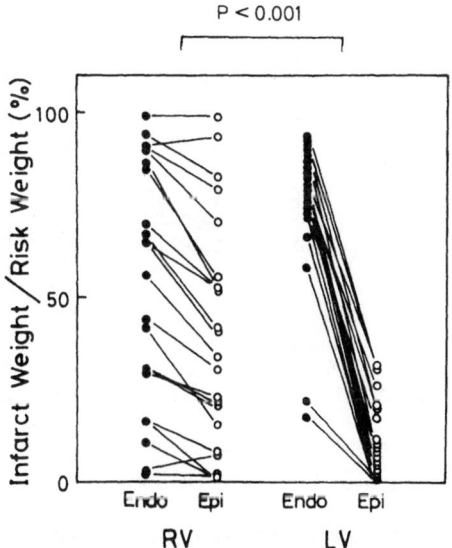

FIG. 9. Infarct size expressed as a percentage of the risk area (IS:RA) transmurally in the right and left ventricles. Each line represents one slice and shows the transmural distribution of IS:RA of each risk area. A marked transmural gradient of infarction was noted in the left ventricle (*LV*) and is negligible in the right ventricle (*RV*). (From [14], with permission)

0.28 ± 0.05, respectively ($n = 31$) ($P < 0.01$ between ventricles). Such a marked difference in the regional distribution of myocardial necrosis between the right and left ventricles suggests that the risk area per se is not a sole determinant of infarct size. Differences in hemodynamic burden and wall thickness between the two ventricles may affect the distribution of coronary flow and then determine the extent of necrosis.

Regional Difference in the Relation Between Infarct Size and Collateral Blood Flow

A transmural difference in flow level in the normal left ventricle is explained by a difference in myocardial oxygen consumption between layers. Weiss et al. demonstrated that regional myocardial oxygen consumption was 20% higher in the subendocardial layer than in the subepicardial layer [26]. The tissue pressure gradient is also a dominant determinant of flow distribution when the peripheral coronary pressure of the collateral channels is decreased by coronary ligation [27]. However, the question of the regional difference in susceptibility to myocardial ischemia remained unanswered.

Figure 10 shows the relation between regional myocardial blood flow in the central risk area (collateral blood flow, or x) 24h after coronary ligation and the ratio of myocardial necrosis to the risk region (IS:RA, or y) in the subendocardial and subepicardial layers. In the right ventricle a slight rightward shift of the relation between IS:RA and collateral blood flow was noted in the subepicardial layer, whereas in the left ventricle the infarcted area was always larger in the subendocaridal than in the subepicardial layer, along with a markedly reduced slope of this relation in the subepicardial layer. An inverse relation between regional collateral flow and infarct size inside the risk area was evident in the case of both ventricles. Relative sub-

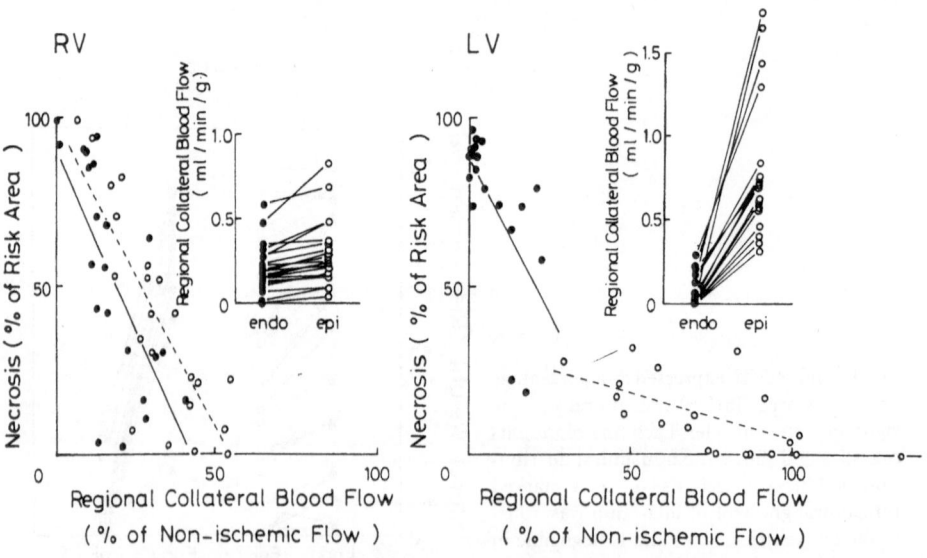

FIG. 10. Relation between collateral blood flow (percent of control flow at 24h of coronary ligation) and percent of infarct to risk size in subendocardial (*closed circles*) and subepicardial (*open circles*) layers in the right (*RV*) and left (*LV*) ventricles. Note that the slope of the relation is steeper for the subendocardium than for the subepicardium in the left, but not the right, ventricle. RV subendocardial layer: $y = -2.19x + 93.2$; $r = -0.708$; $n = 20$. RV subepicardial layer: $y = -1.89x + 101.4$; $r = -0.829$; $n = 20$. LV subendocardial layer: $y = -1.92x + 89.4$; $r = -0.668$; $n = 19$. LV subepicardial layer: $y = -0.83x + 32.5$; $r = -0.631$; $n = 19$. Insets show regional myocardial blood flow in milliliters per minute per gram in the subendocardial (*endo*) and subepicardial (*epi*) layers examined 24h after coronary ligation. (From [14], with permission)

endocardial underperfusion was noted in the right ventricle (Fig. 10), which was clearly demonstrated in cases of RV systolic hypertension [28, 29] and RV hypertrophy [30, 31]. In general, the subendocardial region of the right ventricle is also prone to be underperfused, as is the left ventricle. However, a transmural difference in flow in the necrotic area was not as prominent in the right ventricle as in the left ventricle. Accordingly, transmural flow distribution after abrupt coronary ligation may explain the variations in infarct size. The relation between collateral flow and infarct size was similar in the subendocardial and subepicardial halves of the right ventricle and the subendocardial layer in the left ventricle. Salvage of the subepicardial layer in the left ventricle suggests a tissue-sparing effect in the case of left coronary artery occlusion. Thus sacrificing the injured myocardium may be appropriate for maintaining viable epicardium in better condition.

In summary, the regional distribution of myocardial necrosis was determined by the level of regional myocardial blood flow inside the risk area. The slopes of the necrosis–area at risk relation were similar for the subendocardium and subepicardium in the right ventricle, whereas in the left ventricle it was larger in the subendocardium than in the subepicardium. Thus in the dog the inherent characteristics of regional distribution of coronary collateral blood flow, thickness of the wall, intracavitary pressure, and level of oxygen consumption [32] are important modifiers in the evolution of myocardial infarction, especially in the left ventricle.

Interdependence of Right and Left Ventricles

The interdependence of the right and left ventricles has been qualitatively and quantitatively demonstrated by the pressure–volume relation in the respective ventricles [33–35]. For example, acute increases in RV volume or pressure (or both) can elevate LV diastolic and systolic pressures, and increasing the LV volume or pressure (or both) can elevate the RV diastolic and systolic pressures. Such circumstances are exaggerated by the presence of pericardium, which surrounds the heart and determines the limits of acute diastolic expansion—and therefore the extent to which the Frank-Starling mechanism is utilized [36].

A shape change, including a change in surface area, of either ventricle can be elicited by a volume change of the opposite ventricle, although the volume of the ventricular chamber is unchanged [37]. The goal of this study was to test whether shifts in the ventricular pressure–volume relation during changes in the volume of the opposite ventricle is explained by resetting the regional length related to the ventricular shape change [38]. The study was designed in an isolated heart preparation after removal of the pericardium to demonstrate ventricular interaction resulting solely from the anatomical arrangements of the right and left ventricles.

Experimental Preparations

In 15 experiments, two dogs, a small dog (13.6 ± 0.3 kg) and a large dog (19.9 ± 1.0 kg) were anesthetized with pentobarbital sodium (30 mg/kg IV), intubated, and ventilated with a respirator (model SN-480-3; Shinano, Tokyo, Japan). The chest of the small dog was opened bilaterally at the fourth intercostal space. Sodium heparin (2000 IU) was injected via the femoral vein. The thoracic cavity was filled with ice for cooling the heart. About 500 ml of blood was withdrawn, and 10% dextran in saline was infused.

We used the withdrawn blood to prime the perfusion system. After 5–15 min of cooling, asystole occurred. The pericardium was removed, and the heart was isolated from the systemic and pulmonary circulations and removed from the chest.

The aortic valve cusps were sewn up, and a patch was sutured below the aortic valve through the mitral valve orifice. The chordae tendineae of the left ventricle were cut, and a thin latex balloon (condom, 0.03 mm thick) attached to a rigid cannula was inserted into the LV cavity through the mitral orifice. The chordae tendineae of the right ventricle were cut through the tricuspid orifice. A pacing wire was sewn to the upper portion of the interventricular septum and the midpoint of the septum. The pulmonary valve was sutured. Another latex balloon attached to a rigid cannula was inserted into the RV cavity through the tricuspid orifice. The tricuspid orifice was fixed to a plastic ring that was attached to the cannula. The maximum balloon capacity was 20–30 ml, at which volume there was no pressure because of balloon distension and the balloon capacity was greater than the chamber volume used in the experiment. The tips of 6F micromanometer catheters (Millar Instruments, Houston, TX, USA) were positioned in the LV and RV balloons through the cannulas. The total volume of the balloon, pressure transducer, and adapter for mounting was about 2.0 ml. The balloons were filled with saline. Vents were placed in the apex of the left and right ventricles to decompress these chambers from any thebesian drainage. To ensure proper positioning of the balloons, strings were attached to the apical portion of each balloon and withdrawn through the drainage ports. The ascending aorta was cannulated with the perfusion line. The isolated heart was suspended by a clamp at the tops of the three cannulas. The femoral arteries and veins of the larger (support) dog were cannulated and connected to a perfusion line.

Placement of Ultrasonic Crystals

To measure regional changes in the geometry of the LV free wall, the interventricular septum, and the RV free wall, pairs of piezoelectric crystals (5 MHz, 2 mm diameter) were implanted circumferentially as well as longitudinally. The long axis of the left ventricle and interventricular septum was defined as the line connecting the bifurcation of the left main coronary artery and the apical dimple. A circumferential pair of crystals was placed perpendicular to the midpoint of the LV long axis. The segment measured in longitudinal direction crossed the circumferential segment crystals at their midpoints. The RV circumferential plane was determined from the axis connecting the tricuspid valve and the pulmonary valve. LV free wall crystals were placed at approximately the one-third depth of the myocardium from LV epicardium for 12 of the 15 isolated hearts. In 11 of the 15 hearts, two pairs of crystals were inserted through the tricuspid orifice before insertion of the balloon-cannula assembly into the right ventricle. The septal crystals were placed at approximately one-third the depth of the myocardium from the RV side endocardium, and the slit for the septal crystal insertion was sutured with fine suture material (ophthalmological use). In 6 of the 15 hearts, two pairs of crystals were implanted in the midwall of the RV free wall. These segments were about 1 cm in length.

Experimental Protocol

About 5 min after the perfusion line was opened, the isolated heart was defibrillated. The heart was paced at 130 or 140 beats per minute with bipolar electrodes on the upper interventricular septum and atrium. After the heart began to contract isovolumically, LV, RV, and perfusion pressures (measured with a P23 Db strain gauge manometer; Statham) were checked for stability. The data were then collected according to the following protocols. The order of increasing RV and LV volume was random. Large and small volumes of both ventricles were set according to the following definition. When large volumes were found in both ventricles the LV and RV volumes were increased up to about 100 mm Hg of pressure in the left ventricle and up to about 45 mm Hg in the right ventricle. The LV and RV volumes were then slightly readjusted so that the LV volume was similar to the RV volume. When determining small volumes, we increased the volumes up to about 50 mm Hg of pressure in the left ventricle and up to about 15 mm Hg in the right ventricle. A small LV volume was similar to the RV volume. A middle volume was midway between large and small volumes. Large and small LV (RV) volumes (mean ± SE) were 18.6 ± 1.5 and 7.4 ± 0.7 ml, respectively.

Extent of Interdependence

Changes in Chamber Pressures

Figure 11 shows the pressure changes of one ventricle elicited by the opposite ventricle. At a large RV volume the RV diastolic pressure increased from 14 ± 2 to 17 ± 2 mm Hg ($P < 0.01$) after increasing the LV volume from small to large. The RV diastolic pressure at small RV volume also increased from 3 ± 1 to 4 ± 1 mm Hg ($P < 0.01$). A similar increase in LV pressure can be seen with increasing RV volume (Fig. 11B, D). At large LV volume the LV diastolic pressure increased from 14 ± 2 to 16 ± 2 mm Hg ($P < 0.01$) when the RV volume was increased from small to large. The LV diastolic pressure at small LV volume increased from 3 ± 1 to 4 ± 1 mm Hg ($P < 0.01$). The extent of diastolic interaction was 1 to 3 mm Hg within the range of the volume used and depended on the end-diastolic volume of the opposite ventricle. Janicki and Weber reported the maximum diastolic interaction for either ventricle to be 1–6 mm Hg in the absence of pericardium [39]. In previous studies the basis for diastolic interaction was explained by the interventricular septum from the ventricle that is being distended shifting toward the other ventricle [40].

The RV systolic pressure increased from 44 ± 2 to 49 ± 2 mm Hg ($P < 0.01$) at a large RV volume and from 17 ± 1 to 19 ± 1 mm Hg ($P < 0.01$) at a small RV volume when the LV volume was increased from small to large. The LV systolic pressure increased from 97 ± 6 to 105 ± 6 mm Hg ($P < 0.01$) at a large LV volume and from 49 ± 5 to 54 ± 5 mm Hg ($P < 0.01$) at a small LV volume when the RV volume was increased from small to large. The extent of systolic interaction was similar to that in previous studies [39].

Changes in Segmental Lengths in RV Free Wall
and Interventricular Septum with the Alteration of LV Volume

With the RV volume held constant, we increased the LV volume and measured the changes in diastolic circumferential and longitudinal segment lengths in the RV free wall and interventricular septum. Figure 12 shows the graded increases in RV circumferential and longitudinal lengths with increasing LV volume (from 6 ml to 18 ml) at a fixed RV volume (18 ml). The systolic bulging in longitudinal RV length was due to an isovolumically beating heart used in the present study. Thus shortening in one direction was accompanied by bulging in the other direction in most experiments.

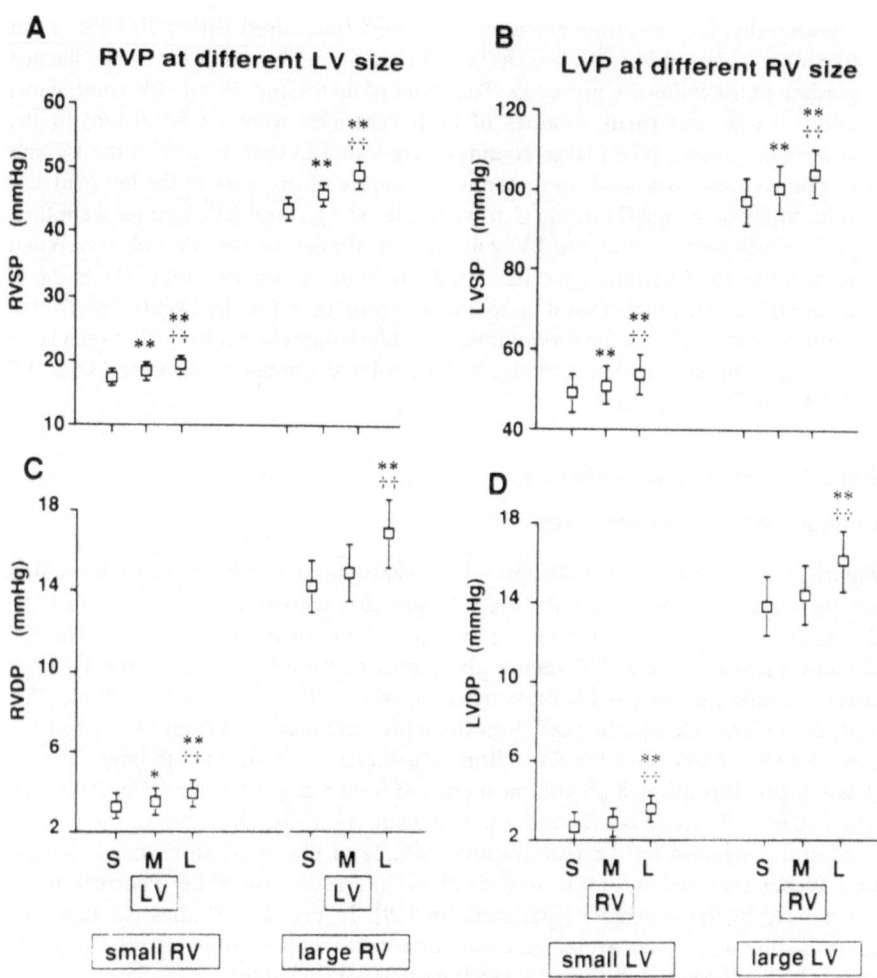

FIG. 11. **A, C** Effects of the left ventricular (*LV*) volume on right ventricular (*RV*) systolic pressure (*RVSP*) and RV diastolic pressure (*RVDP*), respectively. **B, D** Effect of RV volume on LV systolic pressure (*LVSP*) and LV diastolic pressure (*LVDP*), respectively. The left ventricle was altered at different sizes [small (*S*), middle (*M*), and large (*L*)], whereas the right ventricle was held constant at a small or large size (*left*). The right ventricle was altered at different size, with the LV volume held constant (*right*). Results are means ± SE. *P < 0.05 versus S. **P < 0.01 versus S. ††P < 0.01 versus M. (From [38], with permission)

Figure 13 shows RV free wall diastolic lengths at different LV sizes (*n* = 6). When the LV volume was increased from small (9.3 ± 1.6 ml) to middle (14.2 ± 1.7 ml) size and further increased to a large (19.0 ± 1.8 ml) size, the circumferential diastolic length in RV free wall at large RV volume increased from 108 ± 2% to 109 ± 2% and further to 110 ± 2% (*P* < 0.01) (Fig. 13, top). At a small RV volume increasing the LV volume from small to large increased the RV free wall circumferential diastolic length (100 to 102 ± 1%; *P* < 0.01). In longitudinal direction, increasing the LV volume increased the diastolic length in the RV free wall at a large RV volume (112 ± 3% to 113 ± 3%; *P* < 0.01) (Fig. 13, middle). When increasing the LV volume from small

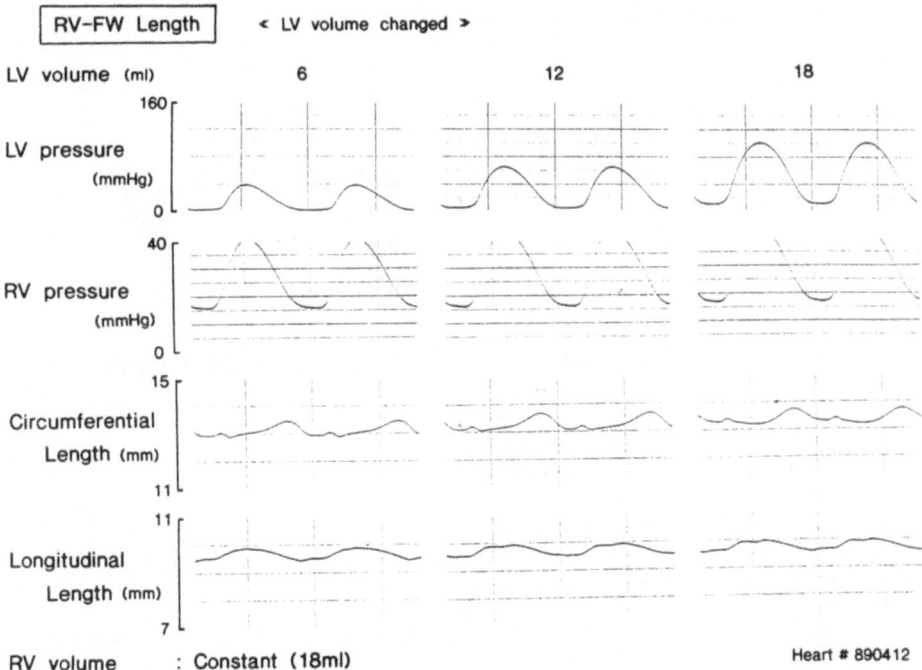

FIG. 12. Recordings from a representative heart showing the effect of LV volume on RV free wall (FW) lengths. RV volume was held constant (18 ml), and LV volume was increased from 6 ml to 18 ml. RV circumferential and longitudinal diastolic lengths increased with the increment of LV volume. Model used in this study was an isovolumically contracting heart. Note in the tracings of these lengths that there was no atrial contribution, and a constant ventricular volume was maintained even during systole. (From [38], with permission)

to large (or middle) volume, the RV free wall area, calculated by multiplying the circumferential and longitudinal diastolic lengths, increased from 121 ± 4% to 125 ± 5% (middle, 122 ± 4%) at a large RV volume ($P < 0.01$). The RV free wall area at a small RV volume also increased from 100 to 103 ± 1% (Fig. 13, bottom) ($P < 0.01$).

Figure 14 illustrates interventricular septal diastolic lengths and the calculated regional wall area ($n = 11$). The circumferential septal length at two RV volumes was significantly increased with increasing LV volume (100 ± 1% to 105 ± 2% at a large RV volume and 100 ± 1% to 106 ± 1% at small RV volume) ($P < 0.01$). In the longitudinal direction, the septal length showed no significant difference by altering LV volume. The regional area of the interventricular septum increased from 103 ± 2% to 109 ± 2% at a large RV volume ($P < 0.01$) and increased from 100 to 107 ± 2% at a small RV volume ($P < 0.01$).

Changes in Segment Lengths in Interventricular Septum and LV Free Wall with the Alteration of RV Volume

Figure 15 shows a slight increase in LV free wall lengths with increasing RV volume but a constant LV volume. With a large LV volume the circumferential LV free wall diastolic length increased from 105 ± 1% to 106 ± 1% ($P < 0.01$) with an increasing

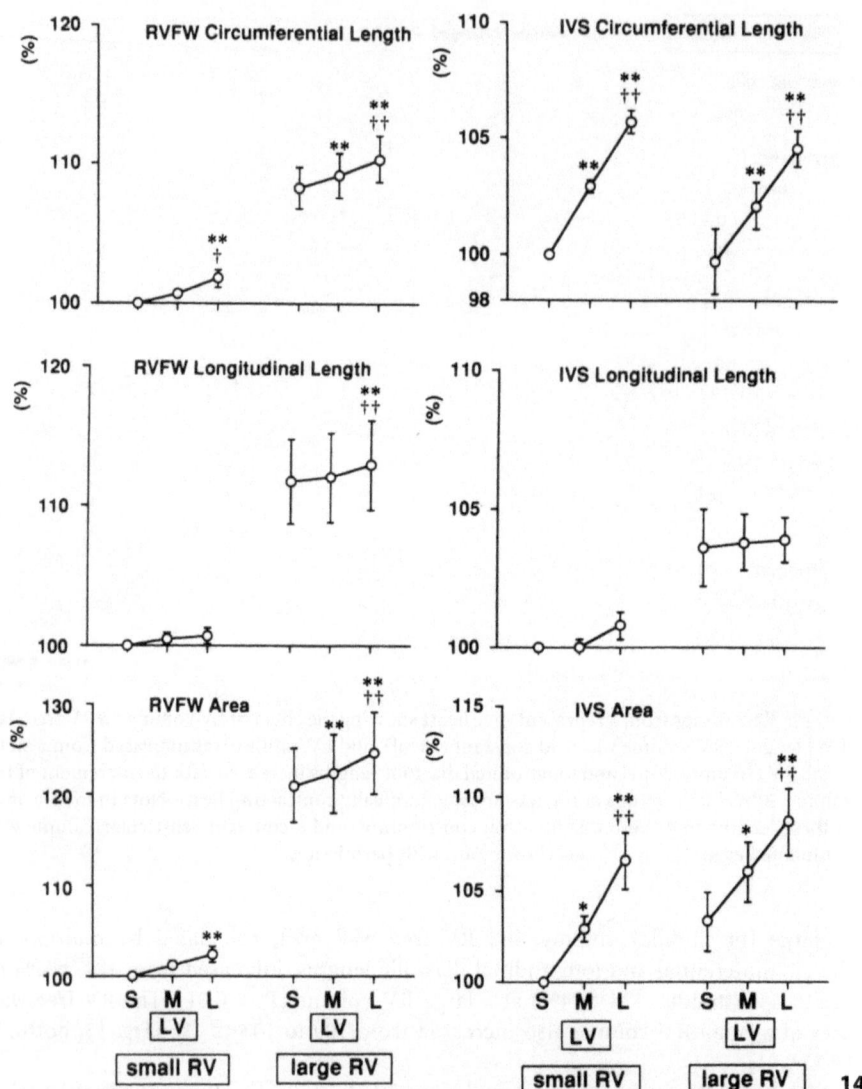

FIG. 13. Effects of altering the LV at small (S), medium (M), and large (L) volumes on circumferential and longitudinal diastolic lengths (*top, middle*) and calculated regional area (*bottom*) in the right ventricular free wall (*RVFW*). The right ventricle was held constant at a small or large volume. Results are means ± SE. **$P < 0.01$ versus S. †$P < 0.05$ versus M. ††$P < 0.01$ versus M. (From [38], with permission)

FIG. 14. Altering LV volumes to small (S), medium (M), and large (L): effects on circumferential and longitudinal diastolic length (*top, middle*) and calculated regional area (*bottom*) in interventricular septum (*IVS*). The RV volume was held constant at small or large. Results are means ± SE. *$P < 0.05$ versus S. **$P < 0.01$ versus S. ††$P < 0.01$ versus M. (From [38], with permission)

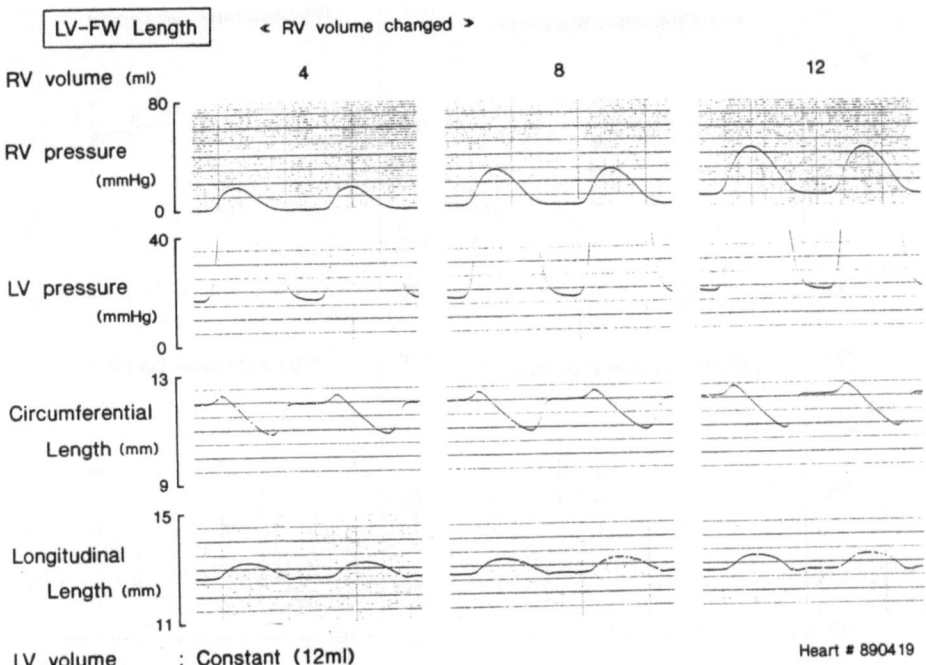

FIG. 15. Recordings from a representative heart showing the effect of RV volume on LV-FW lengths. LV volume was held constant (12 ml), and RV volume was increased from 4 ml to 12 ml. LV-FW circumferential and longitudinal lengths slightly increased with the increment of RV volume. (From [38], with permission)

RV volume (from small to large) (Fig. 16, top). The longitudinal LV free wall diastolic length increased from $105 \pm 1\%$ to $106 \pm 1\%$ at a large LV volume ($P < 0.01$) (Fig. 16, middle). With increasing RV size, the calculated regional area increased from $110 \pm 2\%$ to $112 \pm 2\%$ ($P < 0.01$) at a large LV volume and from 100% to 101% ($P < 0.05$) at a small LV volume (Fig. 16, bottom).

Circumferentially, there was no significant difference in the interventricular septal diastolic length with increasing RV volume (Fig. 17). On the other hand, the interventricular septal longitudinal length was significantly increased with increasing RV volume (from small to large) [$101 \pm 1\%$ to $104 \pm 1\%$ at a large LV volume ($P < 0.01$) and 100 to $103 \pm 2\%$ at a small LV, volume ($P < 0.05$)]. The calculated regional wall area at a large LV volume increased from $107 \pm 1\%$ to $109 \pm 2\%$ ($P < 0.05$) with increasing RV volume (from small to large).

The findings of the above study are as follows. (1) Under fixed RV volume, increasing the LV volume increased the circumferential and longitudinal RV free wall diastolic lengths. Increasing the LV volume increased the circumferential interventricular septal diastolic lengths without significantly increasing the septal longitudinal length. Within the range of LV volume change examined in the present study, the calculated regional area of RV free wall and interventricular septum increased by about 3% and 7%, respectively. (2) Under a fixed LV volume, increasing the RV volume increased the longitudinal diastolic length in interventricular septum without significantly changing the circumferential length. At a relatively large LV

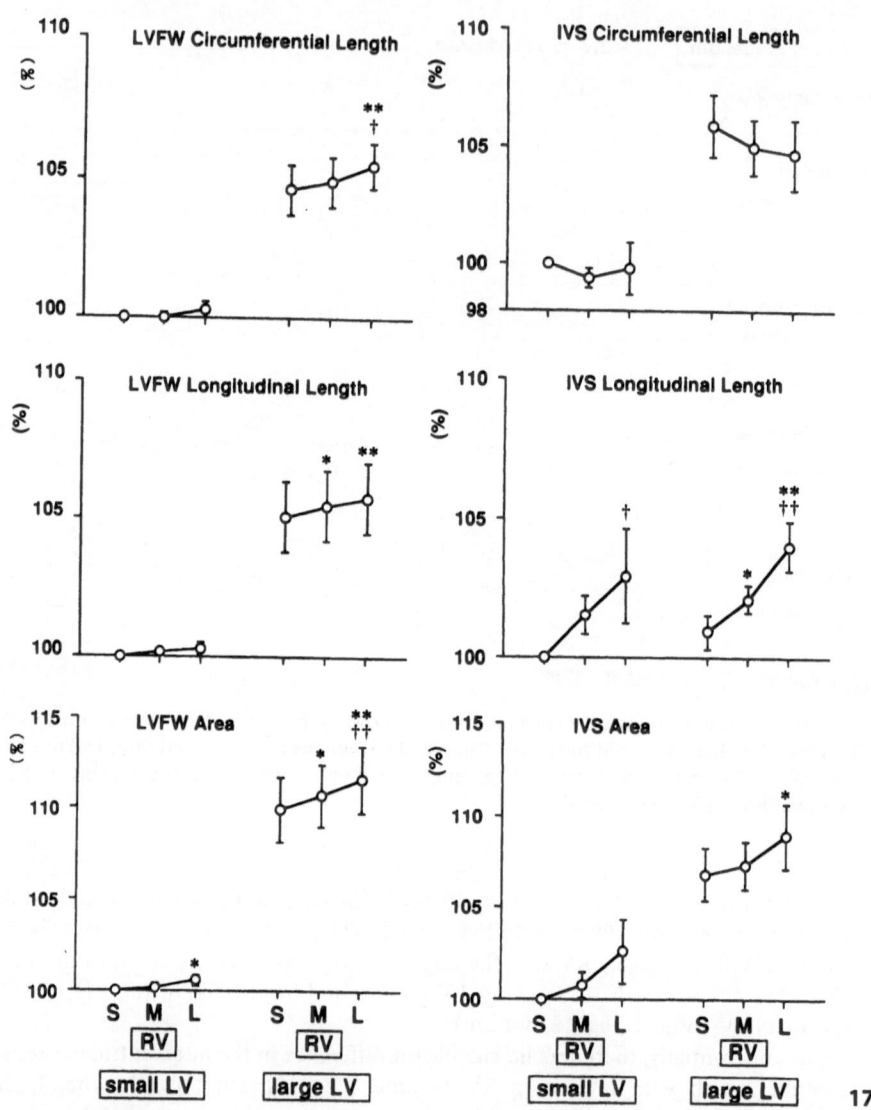

FIG. 16. Altering the RV volume from small (S), to medium (M), to large (L): effects on circumferential and longitudinal diastolic length (*top, middle*) and calculated regional area (*bottom*) in LVFW. The LV volume was held constant (small or large). Results are means ± SE. *P < 0.05 versus S. **P < 0.01 versus S. †P < 0.05 versus M. ††P < 0.01 versus M. (From [38], with permission)

FIG. 17. Altering the RV volume from small (S), to medium (M), to large (L): effects on circumferential and longitudinal diastolic lengths (*top, middle*) and the calculated regional area (*bottom*) in the IVS. The RV volume was held constant (small or large). *P < 0.05 versus S. **P < 0.01 versus S. †P < 0.05 versus M. ††P < 0.01 versus M. (From [38], with permission)

volume, it increased the LV free wall circumferential and longitudinal diastolic lengths. The calculated regional areas in LV free wall and interventricular septum increased by 0.6%–1.5% and 2.0%, respectively. Thus a volume overload of one ventricle can increase the regional lengths of the septum and the free wall in the other ventricle, even when its volume is held constant. This finding implies that ventricular interaction may alter the mean fiber diastolic length of either ventricle (resetting of the regional preload), probably owing to a global shape change of the ventricle.

The observed changes in regional diastolic dimensions probably alter the myocardial length–tension relation. The length–tension relation represents the mechanical characteristics of the myocardium. When the regional length of the tissue is increased, a working point on the resting length–tension relation moves rightward and the resting tension of the tissue increases. Because the ventricular volume was held constant, this increase in resting tension probably causes the observed increase in ventricular chamber diastolic pressure. Because an increase in ventricular pressure may occur at any value of the ventricular volume, the diastolic pressure–volume relation may shift upward.

The resetting of regional diastolic lengths may also affect systolic function. The increase in resting tension should be accompanied by an increase in active tension. Because the tension increases with the chamber being constant, a point of the systolic pressure moves upward on the systolic pressure–volume relation. The increase in active tension with movement of the working point on the length–tension curve is larger than the increase of the resting tension. As a consequence, the magnitude of the enhancement of ventricular pressure was larger during systole than during diastole (2.0- to 5.5-mm Hg increase in RV systolic pressure and 4.0- to 7.5-mm Hg increase in LV systolic pressure in the present study). The diastolic dimensional alteration may change the working point of the active tension relation of the tissue and thus may enhance the ventricular systolic performance with the ventricular volume being constant.

It is still unclear that the resetting of diastolic dimensions explain our observed phenomenon of ventricular interaction. Other mechanisms, such as interventricular septal shifting [41, 42] and a three-element elastance model [43], have also been proposed. However, there has been no experimental evidence and no solid theoretical background for supporting the concept of septal shifting.

Acknowledgments. The work was partly supported by Grants for Scientific Research from the Ministry of Education, Science, and Culture, Japan. The authors thank Ms. Aiko Funaki for the preparation of this manuscript.

References

1. Katz AM (1992) Physiology of the heart, 2nd edn. Raven, New York, pp 1–7
2. Wyatt HL, Forrester JS, Tyberg JV, Goldner S, Logan SE, Pamley WW, Swan HJC (1975) Effect of graded reductions in regional coronary perfusion on regional and total cardiac function. Am J Cardiol 36:185–192
3. Waters DD, Da Luz P, Wyatt HL, Swan HJC, Forrester JS (1977) Early changes in regional and global left ventricular function induced by graded reductions in regional coronary perfusion. Am J Cardiol 39:537–543
4. Banka VS, Bodenheimer MM, Helfant RH (1977) Relation between progressive decreases in regional coronary perfusion and contractile abnormalities. Am J Cardiol 40:200–205
5. Urabe Y, Tomoike H, Ohzono K, Koyanagi S, Nakamura M (1985) Role of afterload in determining regional right ventricular performance during coronary under perfusion in dogs. Circ Res 57:96–104

6. Amold G, Kosche F, Miessner E, Neitzert A, Lochner W (1968) The importance of the perfusion pressure in the coronary arteries for the contractility and the oxygen consumption of the heart. Pflugers Arch 299:399–356

7. Henquell L, Honig CR (1976) O_2 extraction of right and left ventricles. Proc Soc Exp Biol Med 152:52–53

8. Isoyama S, Maruyama Y, Ashikawa K, Sato S, Suzuki H, Watanabe J, Shimizu Y, Ino-oka E, Takishima T (1983) Effects of afterload reduction on global left ventricular and regional myocardial functions in the isolated canine heart with stenosis of a coronary arterial branch. Circulation 67:139–147

9. Lekven J, Kill F (1975) Myocardial function in general and regional left ventricular ischaemia in dogs at control and high aortic blood pressure. Cardiovasc Res 9:373–383

10. Ellis AK, Klocke FJ (1979) Effects of preload on the transmural distribution of perfusion and pressure-flow relationships in the canine coronary vascular bed. Circ Res 46:68–77

11. Downey JM (1976) Myocardial contractile force as a function of coronary blood flow. Am J Physiol 230:1–6

12. Reimer KA, Jennings RB (1979) The "wavefront phenomena" of myocardial ischemic cell death. II. Transmural progression of necrosis within the framework of ischemic bed size. (myocardium at risk) and collateral flow. Lab Invest 40:633–644

13. Sakai K, Tomoike H, Ootsubo H, et al (1982) Preocclusive perfusion area as a determinant of infarct size in a canine model. Cardiovasc Res 16:408–416

14. Ohzono K, Koyanagi S, Urabe Y, Harasawa Y, Tomoike H, Nakamura M (1986) Transmural distribution of myocardial infarction: difference between the right and left ventricles in a canine model. Circ Res 59:63–73

15. Tomoike H, Ootsubo H, Sakai K, et al (1979) Tissue edema and loss of tracer microspheres in infarcted myocardium. Basic Res Cardiol 74:46–53

16. Tomoike H, Ogata I, Maruoka Y, et al (1983) Differential registration of two types of radionuclides on macroautoradiograms for studying coronary circulation. J Nucl Med 24:693–699

17. Lie JT, Pairolero PC, Holley KE, et al (1975) Microscopic enzyme-mapping verification of large, homogenous, experimental myocardial infarct of predictable size and location in dogs. J Thorac Cardiovasc Surg 69:599–605

18. Schaper W, Franzel H, Hort W (1979) Experimental coronary artery occlusion. I. Measurement of infarct size. Basic Res Cardiol 74:46–53

19. Kloner RA, Ganote CE, Jennings RB (1974) The "no-reflow" phenomenon after temporary coronary occlusion in the dog. J Clin Invest 54:1496–1508

20. Leaf A (1973) Cell swelling; a factor in ischemic injury. Circulation 48:455–458

21. Hirzel HO, Nelson GR Sonnenblick EH, et al (1976) Redistribution of collateral blood flow from necrotic to surviving myocardium following coronary occlusion in the dog. Circ Res 39:214–222

22. Grayson J, Irvine M, Parrat JR, et al (1968) Vasospastic elements in myocardial infarction following coronary occlusion in the dog. Cardiovasc Res 2:54–62

23. Becker LC, Schester EH, Jugdutt BI, et al (1983) Relationship between myocardial infarct size and occluded bed size in the dog: difference between left anterior descending and circumflex coronary artery occlusions. Circulation 67:549–557

24. Schaper W, Sass S (1981) Right ventricular infarct size and collateral blood flow following occlusion of the right coronary artery in the dog [abstract]. Circulation 64(suppl IV):118

25. Shaper W, Remijse P, Xhonnneux R (1969) The size of myocardial infarction after experimental coronary artery ligation. Z Kreislaufforsch 58:904–909

26. Weiss HR, Neubauer JA, Lipp JA, et al (1978) Quantitative determination of regional oxygen consumption in the dog heart. Circ Res 42:394–401

27. Downey JB, Kirk ES (1975) Inhibition of coronary blood flow by a vascular waterfall mechanism. Circ Res 36:753–760

28. Fixler DE, Archie JP, Ullyot DJ, et al (1973) Effects of acute right ventricular systolic hypertension on regional myocardial blood flow in anesthetized dogs. Am Heart J 85:491–500

29. Gold FL, Bache RJ (1982) Transmural right ventricular blood flow during acute pulmonary artery hypertension in the sedated dog: evidence for subendocardial ischemia despite residual vasodilator reserve. Circ Res 51:196–204
30. Murray PA, Vatner SF (1980) Fractional contribution of the right and left coronary arteries to perfusion of normal and hypertrophied right ventricle of conscious dogs. Circ Res 47:190–200
31. Manohar M, Bisgard GE, Bullard V, et al (1981) Blood flow in the hypertrophied right ventricular myocardium of unnanesthetized ponies. Am J Physiol 240:H881–H888
32. Kusachi S, Nishiyama O, Yasuhara K, et al (1982) Right and left ventricular oxygen metabolism in open-chest dogs. Am J Physiol 243:H761–H766
33. Janicki, JS, Weber KT (1979) The pericardium and ventricular interaction, distensibility, and function. Am J Physiol 237:H494–H503
34. Little WC, Badke FR, O'Rourke RA (1984) Effect of right ventricular pressure volume relationship on the end-diastolic left ventricular pressure volume relationship before and after chronic right ventricular pressure overload in dogs without pericardia. Circ Res 54:719–730
35. Maughan WL, Sugawara K, Sagawa K (1987) Ventricular systolic interdependence: volume elastance model in isolated canine hearts. Am J Physiol 253:H1381–H1390
36. Maruyama Y, Ashikawa K, Isoyama S, Kanatsuka H, Inooka E, Takishima T (1982) Mechanical intereactions between four heart chambers and without the pericardium in canine hearts. Circ Res 50:86–100
37. Yamaguchi S, Tsuiki H, Miyawaki Y, Tamada I, Ohta H, Sukekawa M, Watanabe M, Kobayashi T, Yasui S (1989) Effect of left ventricular volume on right ventricular end-systolic pressure-volume relation: resetting of regional preload in right ventricular free wall. Circ Res 65:623–631
38. Yamaguchi S, Tamada Y, Miyawaki H, Niida Y, Fukui A, Shirakabe M, Ohta I, Tsuiki K, Tomoike H (1993) Resetting of regional preload due to ventricular shape change alters diastolic and systolic performance. Am J Physiol 265:H1629–H1637
39. Janicki JS, Weber KT (1980) The pericardium and ventricular interaction, distensibility and function. Am J Physiol 238:H494–H503
40. Santamore WP, Lynch PR, Heckman JL, Bove AA, Meier GO (1976) Myocardial interaction between the ventricles. J Appl Physiol 41:362–368
41. King ME, Braun H, Goldblatt A, Liberthson R, Weyman AE (1983) Interventricular septal configuration as a predictor of right ventricular systolic hypertension in children. Circulation 68:68–75
42. Kingma I, Tyberg JV, Smith ER (1983) Effects of diastolic transseptal pressure gradient on ventricular septal position and motion. Circulation 68:1304–1314
43. Santamore WP, Burkhoff D (1991) Hemodynamic consequences of ventricular interaction as assessed by model analysis. Am J Physiol 260:H146–H157

Dahl Salt-Sensitive Rats: Model to Study Transitions from Compensatory Hypertrophy to Left Ventricular Failure

Yasuki Kihara, Moriaki Inoko, and Shigetake Sasayama

Abstract. To establish an experimental model for studying a transitional stage from compensatory hypertrophy to heart failure, we studied the pathophysiology of the left ventricle in Dahl salt-sensitive (DS) rats fed a high-salt diet. DS rats fed an 8% NaCl diet after the age of 6 weeks developed concentric left ventricular (LV) hypertrophy at 11 weeks, followed by marked LV dilatation at 15–20 weeks. During the latter stage, the DS rats showed labored respiration with LV global hypokinesis. All of these DS rats died within a week owing to massive pulmonary congestion. The dissected left ventricles revealed chamber dilatation and a marked increase in mass without myocardial necrosis. In contrast, corresponding Dahl salt-resistant (DR) rats fed the same diet showed neither mortality nor any of these pathological changes. The in vivo LV end-systolic pressure–volume relation (ESPVR) shifted to the right with a slope that was less steep in the failing DS rats than in age–matched DR rats. Therefore the DS rat is a useful model for demonstrating rapidly developing congestive heart failure, in which the transition from compensatory hypertrophy to decompensatory dilatation of the left ventricle is consistently manifested.

Key words. Left ventricular hypertrophy—Congestive heart failure—Animal model—Dahl salt-sensitive rats—Myocardial contraction

Introduction

Despite numerous studies on cardiac hypertrophy and heart failure, the precise mechanisms by which a well-compensated hypertrophied heart eventually decompensates are not fully understood [1]. A major shortcoming of previous experimental models is that progression from compensated left ventricular (LV) hypertrophy to overt, clinically relevant congestive heart failure could not be clearly demonstrated in an individual animal.

The Dahl salt-sensitive (DS) rat is a model animal that develops systemic hypertension depending on the amount of sodium supplied in the diet [2–4]. As a contrasting model, there is the Dahl salt-resistant (DR) rat, which is derived from the same colony as the DS rat [5] and is genetically distinguishable only by a polymorphism in the renin gene [6]. Previous studies have shown that most DS rats fed a high-salt diet after

Third Division, Department of Internal Medicine, Kyoto University School of Medicine, 54 Shogoin Kawahara-cho, Sakyo-ku, Kyoto, 606 Japan

weaning die by the age of 20 weeks [2, 4]. Lethality was shown not to correlate with the level of blood pressure [2], and the major cause of death in these animals remains unknown. When the timing of initiating a high-salt diet is properly selected, DS rats have a life expectancy of 4–5 months. During this limited life-span we consistently found the occurrence of compensation with concentric LV hypertrophy and subsequent decompensation with a dilated hypokinetic left ventricle without significant myocardial loss [7]. The cause of death was massive pulmonary congestion. Therefore the DS rats may provide a unique opportunity to elucidate the transition and the underlying mechanisms.

Methods

Experimental Animals

Inbred DS and DR rats were obtained from Brookhaven National Laboratories, were further inbred for three or four generations by Eisai Co. (Tokyo, Japan), and were then supplied to us [8]. The rats were fed a 0.3% NaCl (low-salt) diet after weaning [8] until the age of 6 weeks, after which they were fed an 8% NaCl (high-salt) diet [2, 3, 8].

The systemic blood pressure and body weight of each animal were measured every 2 weeks. The peak systolic pressure was recorded by a photoelectric pulse device (model PS-100; Riken Kaihatsu Yokohama, Japan) placed on the tail of unanesthetized rats.

To evaluate LV dimensions and the contractile state in vivo, transthoracic echocardiography [9] (model SSD-280 with a 5.0 MHz sector scan probe, Aloka, Tokyo, Japan; and model HP77010, with a 7.5 MHz sector scan probe, Hewlett–Packard, Palo Alto, CA, USA) was performed at ages 6, 11, 15, and 18 weeks. M-mode echocardiograms at the papillary muscle level were determined, guided by two-dimensional long-axis images. We determined the LV end-diastolic diameter (EDD) as the widest and the end-systolic diameter (ESD) as the narrowest dimensions in the M-mode recordings, respectively. The LV posterior wall thickness (PWT) was measured at the time of EDD measurement. From these measurements, the LV fractional shortening (FS) and LV mass [10] were calculated according to the following formulas:

$$\text{LV FS}\,(\%)\ = \left[(\text{EDD} - \text{ESD})/\text{EDD}\right] \times 100$$

$$\text{LV mass}\,(\text{g}) = 1.05 \times \left[(\text{EDD} + 2 \times \text{PWT})^{3} - \text{EDD}^{3}\right]$$

General Protocols and Study Objects

The rats were divided into three groups according to the study protocol. The *first group* (DS, $n = 20$; DR, $n = 17$) was used for determining the natural survival time and for postmortem pathological study. Rats that were continuously fed with a 0.3% NaCl diet after the age of 6 weeks (DS/DR: $n = 7$, respectively) were included in this group. The general conditions of animals were inspected every 24 h; when animals were found dead, they were immediately subjected to postmortem pathological examination. As noted in the Results section, all DS rats fed the high-salt diet in this group developed rapid, labored respiration during the period of 15–20 weeks (failing DS rats) and died within 7 days thereafter. Therefore in the second and third groups, failing DS rats with labored respiration were subjected to experiments before their natural death.

In the *second group* (6-week DS/DR: $n = 7$, respectively; 11-week DS/DR: $n = 7$, respectively; failing DS: $n = 13$; and age-matched DR: $n = 10$), the rats were anesthetized with sodium pentobarbital 30 mg/kg IP, and the chest was quickly opened. The heart was forced to arrest by intraaortic injection of 3 ml of 1 M KCl solution, removed, and retrogradely perfused with a formalin fixative solution under a constant perfusion pressure for subsequent histological study.

The *third group* (11-week DS/DR: $n = 6$, respectively; failing DS and age-matched DR: $n = 6$, respectively) was used for an in vivo study to examine the LV end-systolic pressure–volume relation (ESPVR) [11] under light anesthesia. A 22-gauge angiocath cannula was inserted into the ascending aorta through an arteriotomy of the right carotid artery. The pressure was measured by a 0.018-inch guidewire-mounted optical pressure sensor (Pressure Guide 0.018-inch; RADI Medical Systems, Uppsala, Sweden) [12], which was advanced to the ascending aorta through the cannula. The tip sensor was calibrated using a Statham pressure transducer connected to the side arm of the cannula. The ESPVR was assessed by simultaneous measurements of the end-systolic LV volume (the cube of ESD) [13] using echocardiography and the end-systolic aortic pressure, which was measured at the time of ESD measurement. In each animal the ESPVR were recorded at five points during changes in aortic pressure induced by intraluminal bolus infusion of methoxamine (0.25 μg/g body weight) or phentolamine (0.25 μg/g body weight).

Results

Development of Heart Failure

Figure 1 (A, B) shows the effects of dietary salt intake on the systolic blood pressure and body weight of Dahl rats between the age of 6 and 18 weeks. In DS rats fed the 8% NaCl (high-salt) diet from the 6th week (8% DS), blood pressure gradually rose, reached 230 mm Hg by the 12th week, and remained elevated above 200 mm Hg thereafter (Fig. 1A). In contrast, in DR rats on the same high-salt diet (8% DR), blood pressure did not change significantly during this period. When these animals (both DS and DR) were kept on the 0.3% NaCl (low-salt) diet beyond the age of 6 weeks (0.3% DS, 0.3% DR), neither group developed hypertension. The left ventricle/body weight ratio in DS rats with hypertension was markedly increased and reached the level of 0.45 at the 18th week. This value was twofold higher than that of the age-matched DR rats (Fig. 1C).

At the age of 15–22 weeks, all DS rats with hypertension displayed characteristic rapid, labored respiration associated with loss of activity. At this stage, although remaining at a level higher than 200 mm Hg, the blood pressure also tended to decrease. When these DS rats were continuously fed the high-salt diet, the general condition became progressively worse and they died within a week after the onset of respiratory distress. In contrast, during the same period all DR and DS rats fed the low-salt diet survived; and none of these animals showed any signs of labored respiration or loss of activity (Fig. 1D). Thus the DS rats on the high-salt diet survived only about 5 months, in contrast with other experimental groups examined.

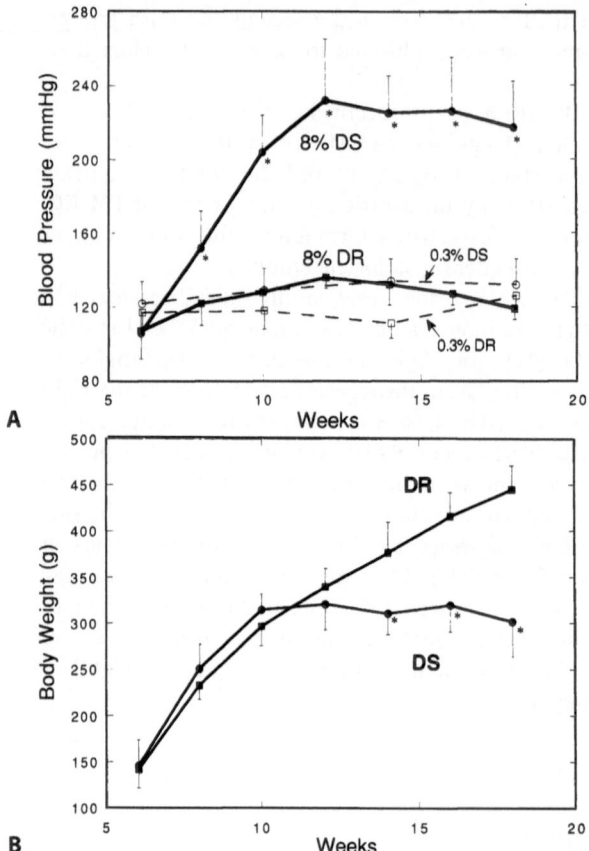

A

B

FIG. 1. **A** Time course of blood pressure changes in Dahl salt-sensitive (*DS*) and Dahl salt-resistant (*DR*) rats. The 8%DS (*n* = 13) and 8%DR (*n* = 10) represent DS and DR rats, respectively, fed an 8% NaCl diet after the age of 6 weeks; 0.3%DS (*n* = 7) and 0.3%DR (*n* = 7) represent DS and DR rats, respectively fed a 0.3% NaCl diet for 18 weeks. *P < 0.01 versus 8%DR. **B** Time course of body weight gain in DS and DR rats fed an 8% NaCl diet. *P < 0.01 versus DR. **C** Left ventricular weight normalized for body weight (LV/BW) taken at the ages of 6, 11, and 18 weeks in DS (*n* = 13) and DR (*n* = 10) rats fed an 8% NaCl diet. *P < 0.01 versus DR. **D** Survival curves of DS (*n* = 13) and DR (*n* = 10) rats fed an 8% NaCl diet. These two curves were statistically different (*P* < 0.0001) by the generalized wilcoxon test. (From [7], with permission)

Transthoracic Echocardiography and Left Ventricle

Figure 2A shows the M-mode echocardiograms of the left ventricle at the papillary muscle level at three stages in both DS and DR rats. Figure 2B shows the corresponding transverse tissue slices of the left ventricle from rats taken at the same stages as for the echocardiograms. At 6 weeks echocardiograms and tissue slices of the DS rats did not differ from those of the DR rats. At 11 weeks, the LV posterior wall thickness (PWT) increased and the LV end-diastolic diameter (EDD) decreased in the DS rats compared with the values for the DR rats, indicating the establishment of LV concentric hypertrophy in DS rats (LVH DS). In contrast, at 18 weeks the EDD was markedly increased and PWT was decreased with reduced LV motion (increase in ESD and decrease in FS) in DS rats (failing DS), whereas the wall and the cavity of the left ventricle of the DR rats developed proportionally. There was no significant difference in the LV fractional shortening (FS) between these two strains until age 15 weeks. However, at the failing stage, reductions in FS became greater in the DS rats than in the DR rats (Table 1).

Histological Characteristics

Histological observations of the lung of the failing DS rats revealed that the alveolar spaces were filled owing to massive transudate and capillary hemorrhaging (Fig. 3A).

FIG.1 *Continued*

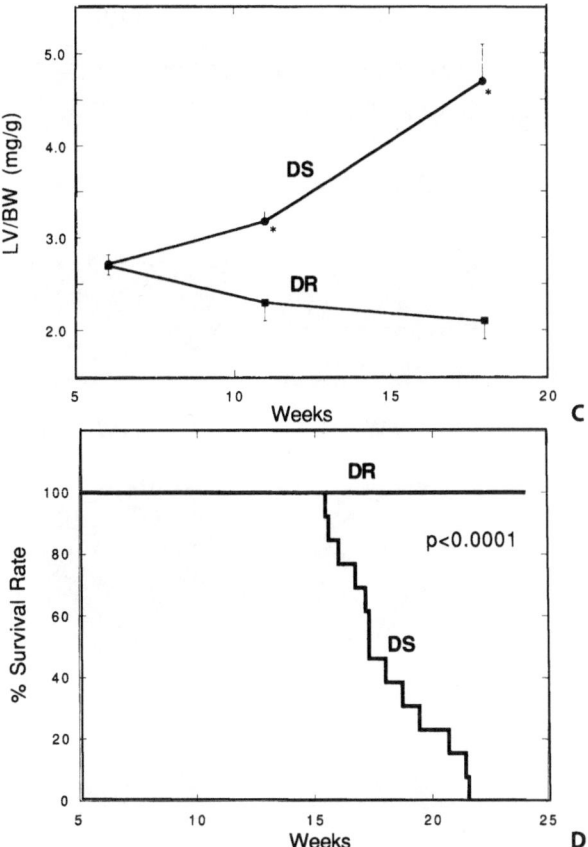

Hemosiderosis was also observed in the alveolar wall. These serious conditions well matched the rats' labored respiration and indicated that massive pulmonary congestion as the outcome of elevated left atrial and LV diastolic pressure was the primary cause of death.

In the LV myocardium, the short-axis diameter of myocytes was $18.1 \pm 0.9\,\mu m$ in the 11-week-old DS rats (LVH DS) and $21.2 \pm 1.5\,\mu m$ in the failing DS rats ($P < 0.01$ versus LVH DS). These values were significantly greater than the corresponding values for the DR rats ($15.6 \pm 0.2\,\mu m$ in 11-week-old DRs, $P < 0.01$ versus LVH DSs;

TABLE 1. Echocardiographic data

Age (weeks)	DS ($n = 13$)				DR ($n = 10$)			
	EDD (mm)	FS (%)	PWT (mm)	LVmass (g)	EDD (mm)	FS (%)	PWT (mm)	LVmass (g)
6	4.9 ± 0.4	50 ± 6	1.4 ± 0.1	0.38 ± 0.06	5.0 ± 0.4	49 ± 4	1.5 ± 0.1	0.40 ± 0.05
11	5.8 ± 0.4	44 ± 4	$2.2 \pm 0.1^*$	$0.93 \pm 0.12^*$	6.1 ± 0.5	45 ± 4	1.6 ± 0.1	0.64 ± 0.12
15	7.0 ± 0.8	40 ± 7	$2.0 \pm 0.2^*$	$1.07 \pm 0.14^*$	7.1 ± 0.5	41 ± 6	1.6 ± 0.2	0.73 ± 0.08
Failing	$9.8 \pm 0.3^*$	$25 \pm 5^*$	1.6 ± 0.1	$1.29 \pm 0.12^*$	7.4 ± 0.4	41 ± 3	1.7 ± 0.1	0.90 ± 0.10

DS, Dahl salt-sensitive rat; *DR*, Dahl salt-resistant rat; *EDD*, left ventricular end-diastolic diameter; *FS*, left ventricular fractional shortening; *PWT*, left ventricular posterior wall thickness; *LVmass*, left ventricular mass calculated from echocardiogram; *Failing*, data at the failing stage in DS rats and at the age of 18 weeks in DR rats.
Values are means $\pm$ SD.
* $P < 0.01$ *vs* DR.

110   Y. Kihara et al.

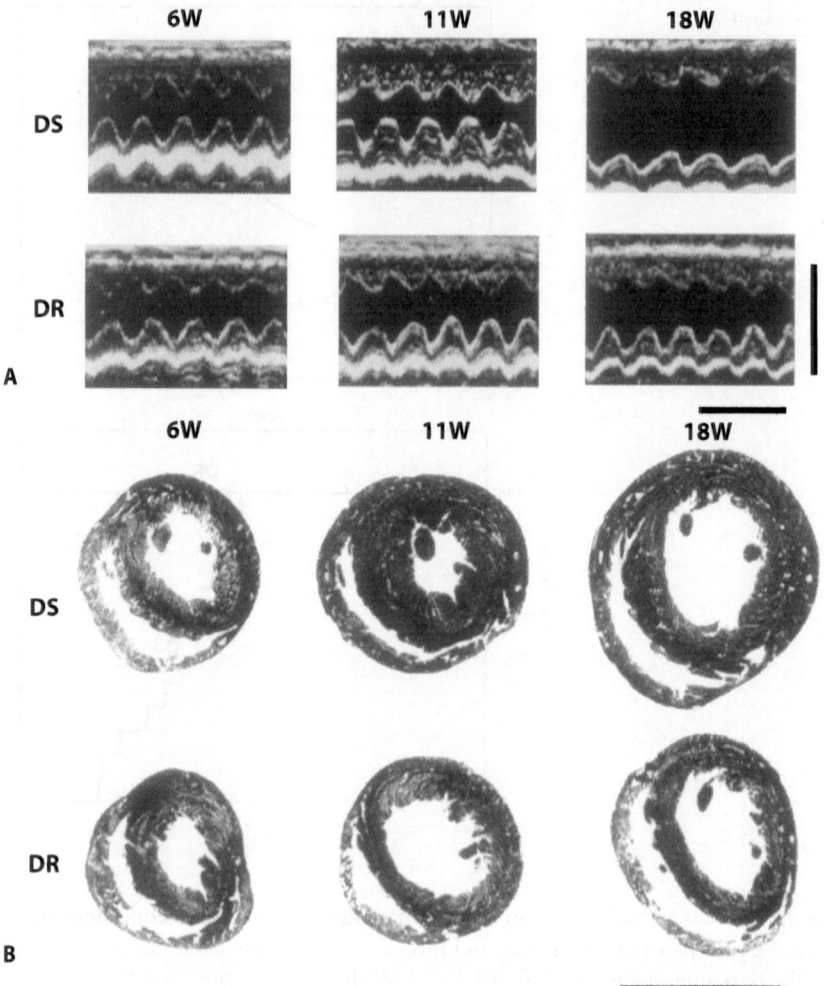

FIG. 2. **A** Serial M-mode echocardiography obtained from representative Dahl salt-sensitive (*DS*) and Dahl salt-resistant (*DR*) rats. The echocardiograms were recorded at the level of the papillary muscles guided by two-dimensional long-axis images. For group data, see Table 1. **B** Cross-sectional tissue slices of the left ventricle from rats sacrificed at stages corresponding to the echocardiograms shown in **A**. (From [7], with permission)

→

FIG. 3. **A** Sections of lungs from a Dahl salt-sensitive rat in the failing stage (*failing DS*) and an age-matched Dahl salt-resistant rat (*DR*). Hematoxylin-eosin staining; original magnification ×100. **B** Sections of the left ventricle from a failing DS rat and an age-matched DR rat Masson's trichrome staining, ×100. **C** Low magnification (×40) of the LV sections shown in **B**. (From [7], with permission)

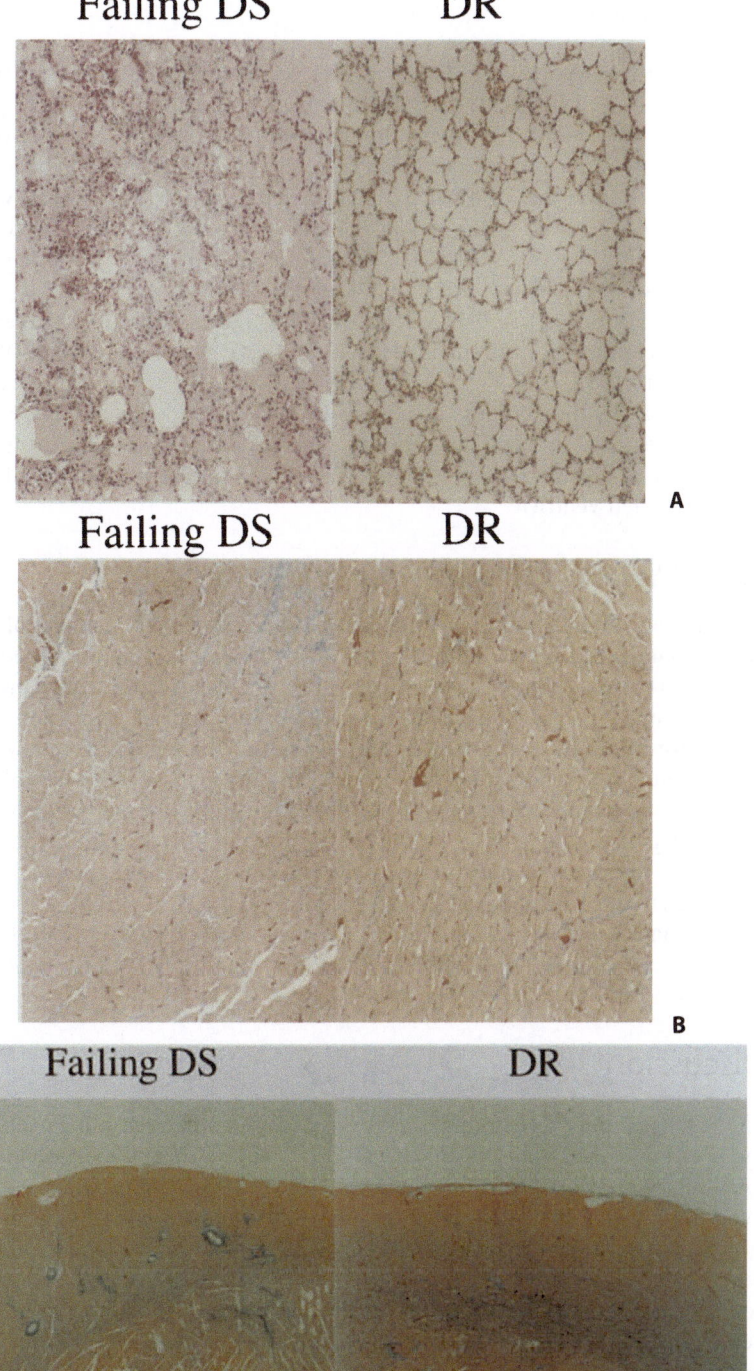

Failing DS   DR

Failing DS   DR

Failing DS   DR

A

B

C

16.2 ± 1.0 μm in 18-week-old DRs, $P < 0.01$ versus failing DSs). Myocardial fibrosis was also increased in the DS rats, which appeared focally and tended to precipitate around the subendocardial layer. The focal fibrosis, however, was not distributed along with specific coronary perfusion (Fig. 3B), and its extent in papillary muscles did not differ from that of other parts of the left ventricle. The fibrosis was mainly localized to the perivascular regions of the arterioles and partly extended into the intermyofibrillar spaces (Fig. 3C). The amount of the area of fibrosis in slices at the papillary muscle level was 1.3 ± 0.4% in the LVH DS rats and 2.0 ± 0.5% in the failing DS rats ($P < 0.05$ versus LVH DS). In contrast, the percent fibrosis in the 18-week-old DR rats remained at 0.5 ± 0.1% ($P < 0.01$ versus LVH DS; $P < 0.01$ versus failing DS). Thus despite the significant increase when compared with the control animals, the amounts of fibrosis in the DS rats were modest. No massive regional necrosis or significant broad replacement of the contractile elements occurred with fibrosis. The pattern of fibrosis was similar in both apical and basal slices of the left ventricle.

LV End-Systolic Pressure–Volume Relation

In the failing DS and age-matched DR rats, the relation of the LV end-systolic pressure versus volume (estimated as the cube of ESD in the echocardiogram) fitted a narrow, linear correlation (DS: $r = 0.96 ± 0.02$; DR: $r = 0.92 ± 0.08$) within the observed pressure range. Figure 4 shows all measured points and the regression line of the ESPVR for the individual rats. The ESPVR lines of the failing DS rats were shifted to the right and were less steep than those of the age-matched (18-week-old) DR rats (the slope in failing DS rats was 0.46 ± 0.15 mmHg/μl; in DR rats it was 1.50 ± 0.51 mm Hg/μl; $P < 0.01$) (Fig. 4A). In contrast, in the 11-week-old DS rats (LVH DS) the ESPVR lines were located farther to the left and were steeper than those of the 11-week-old DR rats (the slope in LVH DS rats was 7.66 ± 3.93 mm Hg/μl, $r = 0.95 ± 0.02$; the slope in DR rats was 1.74 ± 0.80 mm Hg/μl, $r = 0.93 ± 0.03$, $P < 0.01$; $P < 0.01$ for LVH DS versus failing DS; the difference was not significant for 11-week-old DR rats versus 18-week-old DR rats) (Fig. 4B).

Discussion

The results of the present study demonstrated that when fed a high-salt diet after the age of 6 weeks Dahl salt-sensitive (DS) rats have a short life expectancy, limited to about 20 weeks. During this period the compensated stage with concentric LV hypertrophy and the subsequent decompensated stage with LV dilatation and systolic dysfunction are clearly distinguishable. All these rats died within a short period after developing clinically relevant pulmonary congestion, which was confirmed by postmortem pathological examination. These findings not only demonstrated the pathophysiology of heart failure in DS rats but also indicated the usefulness of this experimental model for studying the mechanisms and treatments of heart failure.

Serial echocardiographic examinations in each animal in the present study showed that a decrease in LV systolic function coincided with the transition from the concentric hypertrophy to the dilated failing left ventricle. This decrease in LV systolic function was not due to an acute maladaptation of the heart to its loading condition ("afterload mismatch") [14] because abrupt afterload reduction with phentolamine

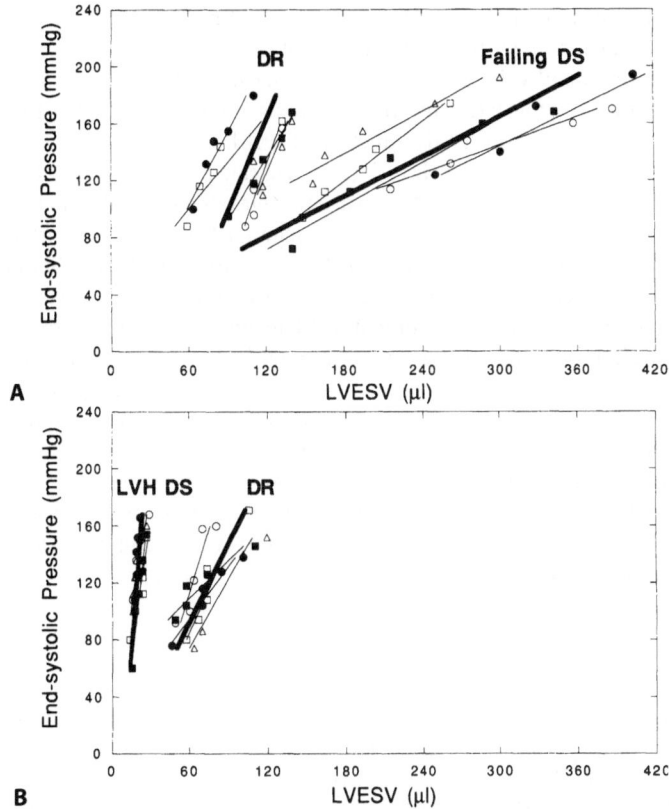

FIG. 4. **A** End-systolic pressure–volume relations (ESPVR) of Dahl salt-sensitive rats in the failing stage (*failing DS*) ($n = 6$) and age-matched Dahl salt-resistant rats (*DR*) ($n = 6$). **B** ESPVR of Dahl salt-sensitive rats in the hypertrophic stage (*LVH DS*) ($n = 6$) and age-matched Dahl salt-resistant rats (*DR*) ($n = 6$). **A, B.** *Thin regression lines* were calculated from five measuring points obtained for each animal. *Thick regression lines* represent the mean for each group. (From [7], with permission)

did not recover the LV functional state. The estimation of ESPVR by this pharmacological intervention confirmed that the LV contractile state was reduced during the transition. The developed tension of isolated myocardium from failing DS rats showed a significant decrease relative to that of age-matched DR rats (data not shown). A reduced force production per unit of myocardium occurred during the transition and caused the observed LV contractile dysfunction during the subsequent heart failure state.

As shown in Fig. 3 (B, C), the reduction of force development in the failing myocardium was not primarily due to massive loss of contractile elements. The percent area of fibrosis increased as the stage progressed. However, it remained at about 2% in the entire myocardial tissue of the failing heart. The fibrosis tended to precipitate around small arteries, in which medial thickening and decreases in cavity size were observed. These changes were also found in small arteries in other organs including the kidneys and were consistent with the known pathological findings of hypertensive vascular disease [15]. Although the possible roles of a limited coronary reserve or of latent tissue ischemia [16] in this animal model should be excluded by future studies, our histological findings were not consistent with those reported for ischemic cardiomyopathy in patients or in experimental animals with coronary microembolization, in the latter of which fibrosis ranging from 11% to 32% was required to induce significant LV dysfunction [17, 18].

The following conclusions were drawn: (1) In DS rats put on an 8% NaCl diet from the age of 6 weeks, the systolic blood pressure was elevated over 200 mm Hg, whereas that of DR rats on the same diet remained unchanged. (2) The DS rats presented concentric LV hypertrophy at around 11 weeks of age, followed by LV dilatation with reduced myocardial contraction at 16–22 weeks. In contrast, the hearts of DR rats showed normal proportional development. (3) During the stage of LV dilatation, DS rats developed signs of pulmonary congestion that mimicked symptoms in the clinical setting. They then died within a week. (4) In DS rats the contractility of LV myocardium decreased in vivo during the transition from the compensated LV hypertrophy stage to the failing stage. These observations indicate that this animal model is useful for investigating mechanisms of and therapeutic strategies for heart failure. Furthermore, the present study demonstrated that decompensation was due to a decrease in myocardial contractility rather than to irreversible myocardial cell damage or loss in the left ventricle.

References

1. Katz AM (1990) Cardiomyopathy of overload: a major determinant of prognosis in congestive heart failure. N Egnl J Med 322:100–110
2. Dahl LK, Knudsen KD, Heine MA, Leitl GJ (1968) Effects of chronic excess salt ingestion: modification of experimental hypertension in the rat by variations in the diet. Circ Res 22:11–18
3. Iwai J, Heine M (1986) Dahl salt-sensitive rats and human essential hypertension. J Hypertens Suppl 4:S29–S31
4. Pfeffer MA, Pfeffer J, Mirsky I, Iwai J (1984) Cardiac hypertrophy and performance of Dahl hypertensive rats on graded salt diets. Hypertension 6:475–481
5. Dahl LK, Heine M, Tassinari L (1962) Role of genetic factors in susceptibility to experimental hypertension due to chronic excess salt ingestion. Nature 194:480–482
6. Rapp JP, Wang SM, Dene H (1989) A genetic polymorphism in the renin gene of Dahl rats cosegregates with blood pressure. Science 243:542–544
7. Inoko M, Kihara Y, Morii I, Fujiwara H, Sasayama S (1994) Transition from compensatory hypertrophy to dilated, failing left ventricles in Dahl salt-sensitive rats. Am J Physiol 267:H2471–H2482
8. Ashida T, Kawano Y, Yoshimi H, Kuramochi M, Omae T (1992) Effects of dietary salt on sodium-calcium exchange and ATP-driven calcium pump in arterial smooth muscle of Dahl rats. J Hypertens 10:1335–1341
9. Litwin SE, Katz SE, Morgan JP, Douglas PS (1992) Transthoracic echocardiographic evaluation of post-infarction ventricular remodeling in the rat [abstract]. J Am Coll Cardiol 19:362A
10. Troy BL, Pombo J, Rackley CE (1972) Measurement of left ventricular wall thickness and mass by echocardiography. Circulation 45:602–611
11. Suga H, Sagawa K, Shoukas AA (1973) Load independence of the instantaneous pressure-volume ratio of the canine left ventricle and effects of epinephrine and heart rate on the ratio. Circ Res 32:314–322
12. Emanuelsson H, Dohnal M, Lamm C, Tenerz L (1991) Initial experiences with a miniaturized pressure transducer during coronary angioplasty. Cathet Cardiovasc Diagn 24:137–143

13. Pombo JF, Troy BL. Russell R Jr (1971) Left ventricular volumes and ejection fraction by echocardiography. Circulation 43:480–490
14. Ross J Jr (1976) Afterload mismatch and preload reserve: a conceptual framework for the analysis of ventricular function. Prog Cardiovasc Dis 18:255–264
15. Hollander W (1976) Role of hypertension in athersaclerosis and cardiovascular disease. Am J Cardiol 38:786–800
16. Marcus ML, Harrison DG, Chilian WM, et al (1987) Alterations in the coronary circulation in hypertrophied ventricles. Circulation 75:I19–I25
17. Lavine SJ, Prcevski P, Held AC, Johnson V (1991) Experimental model of chronic global left ventricular dysfunction secondary to left coronary microembolization. J Am Coll Cardiol 18:1794–1803
18. Smiseth OA, Lindal S, Mjos OD, Vik-mo H, Jorgensen L (1983) Progression of myocardial damage following coronary microembolization in dogs. Acta Patho/Microbiol Immunol Scand 91A:115–124

Precordial or Epicardial Input of Phase-Controlled Minute Vibration: Effect on Coronary Flow Rate in Regional Ischemia

Yoshiro Koiwa, Hideyuki Honda, Taihei Naya, and Kunio Shirato

Abstract. Phase-controlled vibration at diastole (diastolic vibration) induces a millisecond time scale response in in situ heart, and the magnitude of the induced response (the improvement of the ventricular relaxation) is related to the severity of the impairment of relaxation as well as the amplitude of the vibration applied. However, it is still unknown whether diastolic vibration increases the coronary flow rate in the heart with impaired relaxation. We examined in experimental and clinical studies if external diastolic vibration to the heart with impaired relaxation could result in an improvement of the coronary flow rate and, if so, how to interpret the underlying mechanism of the response observed in the heart with regional ischemia. In an experimental study using an open-chest canine preparation with regional ischemia, the diastolic vibration applied to the ventricular surface increased coronary flow rate without increasing the coronary perfusion pressure and simultaneously shortened the time constant of the ventricular pressure decay. The diastolic vibration improved the nonuniformity of the relaxation by accelerating myocardial relaxation in the ischemic region. In clinical studies the response of the coronary flow velocity was measured by the transesophageal Doppler method in 10 healthy volunteers (8 men, 2 women; 50.6 ± 12.8 years old, mean ± SD) and 10 patients with coronary artery disease (8 men, 2 women; 66.4 ± 8.0 years old). The intracoronary Doppler catheter method was used in three patients with coronary artery disease (two men, one woman; 60.3 ± 10.5 years old). Mechanical diastolic vibration on the precordium has been demonstrated to transmit effectively to the ventricle and cause an increase in coronary flow velocity with no change in the coronary arterial diameter, blood pressure, or heart rate. We concluded that diastolic vibration increased the coronary flow rate in the clinical situation as well as in an experimental preparation. This increase mainly resulted from an acceleration of the ventricular relaxation rate caused by crossbridge detachment, normalization of the nonuniformity of the relaxation, or both.

Key words. Diastolic mechanical vibration—Ischemic heart disease—Dyskinesia—Transesophageal Doppler—Ventricular relaxation

First Department of Internal Medicine, Tohoku University, School of Medicine, 1-1 Seiryo-machi, Aoba-Ku, Sendai 980, Japan

Introduction

Impairment of left ventricular (LV) relaxation has been observed in patients with congestive heart failure, ischemic heart disease, hypertrophic cardiomyopathy, dilated cadiomyopathy, and hypertensive heart disease [1-3]. It is considered to be one of the important factors regulating pathophysiology during congestive heart failure [2]. Serious impairment of LV relaxation could depress subsequent ventricular systolic function through the Frank-Starling mechanism [4] and reduce the coronary blood flow rate of the ventricle [5]. Determinants of ventricular relaxation are the load of the myocardium, the function of sarcoplasmic reticulum, and the temporal and spacial nonuniformity of ventricular relaxation [6].

Palacios et al. [7] reported that myocardial relaxation during acute global ischemia was impaired through a direct effect on the left ventricle and not through changes in load or contractility. A potential mechanism involved in impaired relaxation during ischemia is the slower uptake of cytosolic calcium by the sarcoplasmic reticulum because of an inadequate adenosine triphosphate (ATP) supply [7, 8], which results in a number of crossbridges remaining in the attached position during diastole.

Several investigators have reported that an abrupt change in myofibril length or mechanical oscillation induces a decline of tension development by deactivating or detaching active crossbridges [9-11]. In particular, Brutsaert et al. reported that an abrupt change in muscle length induces more rapid relaxation (load-dependent relaxation) [12]. The characteristic features of its rapidity of induced response, observed in in situ open-chest canine preparations (Fig. 1), to external vibration strongly suggested that the perturbation directly modifies the myocardial crossbridge kinetics [4, 13]. Our study on the effect of a small-amplitude (heart sound level) mechanical vibration during diastole (diastolic vibration) on LV relaxation and ventricular systolic function demonstrated that such diastolic vibration improved the ventricular relaxation rate. The magnitude of the improvement of the relaxation rate of the pressure decay depended on both the input amplitude of the vibration and the magnitude of the relaxation impairment of the ventricle. Therefore when diastolic vibration was applied to the ventricle with severe heart failure, it could result in greater improvement of ventricular relaxation than that reported previously.

These features of the LV response to diastolic vibration have also been observed in clinical studies [14]. During routine cardiac catheterization, diastolic vibration applied to the precordium adjacent to Erb's area transmits effectively to the left ventricle and causes shortening of the ventricular relaxation time constant. The magnitude of change in the time constant is correlated to the input amplitude of the vibration (determined by the measured amplitude of the superposed oscillation on the ventricular pressure from the catheter-tip micromanometer, $P < 0.0001$), the level of impairment of the ventricle (estimated by the time constant of the ventricular relaxation, $P < 0.0001$), and the ventricular end-diastolic volume ($P < 0.05$). These observations indicate that mechanical vibration could be a new clinical tool for modulating ventricular function if we carefully determine the phase of the vibration and input site on the precordium to induce effective transmission through the thorax to the ventricle.

The coronary flow rate has been reported to decrease under the condition of impaired relaxation in an open-chest canine heart model with regional ischemia [5], even though verification in the clinical condition has not been accomplished. We have examined the effect of diastolic vibration on coronary flow rate with the idea

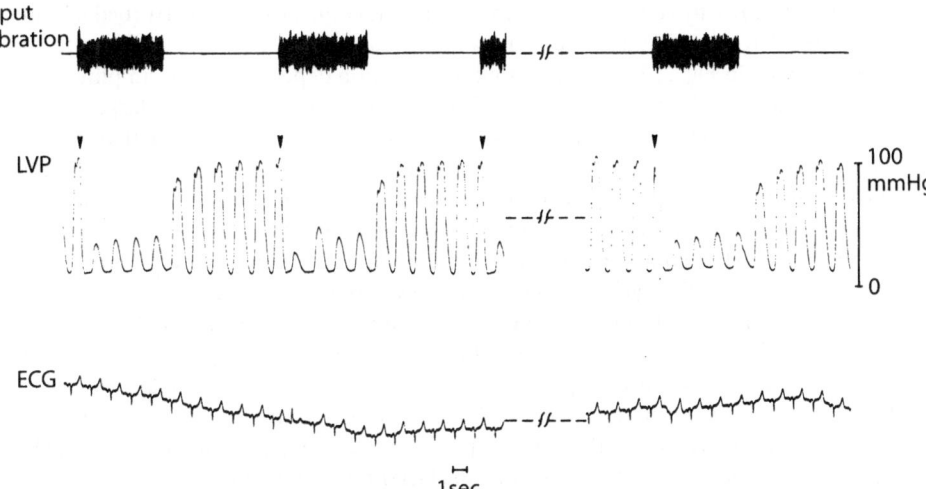

FIG. 1. Note the dramatic onset and termination of the vibration-induced response when vibration is applied and removed. In this open-chest, propranolol-injected canine preparation there was pretreatment with 30 min of tachycardia (>200 bpm) and afterload increment (mean aortic pressure >200 mmHg). These pretreatments were used to reduce ATP, which has been shown to play a dominant role in crossbridge kinetics. This rapid onset was commonly observed in drug-induced failing hearts or in ischemic hearts, but the rate of reversion to the previbration level differed according to the imposed condition that caused the heart failure. That is, in models using negative inotropic drugs recovery was immediate. In the model of coronary ischemia, however, recovery was gradual, taking several beats to return to the previbrational level

that coronary perfusion of the left ventricle with impaired relaxation might be improved by external diastolic vibration mainly through correction of the relaxation impairment. Here we present briefly the results of studies to clarify whether diastolic vibration could exert some influence on coronary flow rate and, if so, to identify the possible underlying mechanisms of the observed response using open-chest canine preparations with regional ischemia and then extrapolating to the clinical situation. We first present the effect of diastolic vibration in a papillary muscle preparation to clarify the muscular response to diastolic vibration, eliminating other complex interventions through metabolic, neural or loading conditions in the in situ ventricle.

Papillary Muscle Preparation

Using the method of Ter Keurs et al. [15, 16], isolated papillary muscle preparations from the right ventricle of male Sprague-Dawley rats were superfused with carbogenated Krebs-Henseleit solution containing 2.5 mM $CaCl_2$ at a constant flow of 3 ml/min. Mechanical sinusoidal vibration was applied at diastole from the point of peak tension to the point after which no active force was observed. In the beginning field stimulation was used, and the vibration was set at 0.25% of Lmax in amplitide and 50 Hz in frequency. The response of muscle function to the vibration was measured with the amplitude and frequency varying between 0.25% and 2.00% Lmax and between 20 and 80 Hz, respectively.

Figure 2 shows three sequential isometric contractions, with the perturbed one in the center. The vibration induced an instantaneous response in the relaxation rate, as demonstrated in Fig. 2. This acceleration of relaxation depended on the amplitude of the input vibration and input frequency. That is, the acceleration became larger as the amplitude of the vibration increased and the frequency was set higher than 40 Hz. These features in the papillary muscle preparation are essentially consistent with those from previous reports [4, 13], suggesting that the response of the entire ventricle is not due to changes in neural or metabolic regulation but to the change imposed on the myocardial contractile element. In cardiac muscle perturbed continuously throughout the cardiac cycle, the active force development decreased remarkable [17, 18] as the frequency or amplitude of the vibration increased [18]. It was speculated that the number of actin–myosin interactions (attached crossbridges) would decrease because of externally forced decoupling; that is, the perturbation detaches cross-bridges during the rising phase of the force in twitch contractions. Eventually, the number of crossbridges at the time of peak force development is decreased. This observation supports the hypothesis that the faster relaxation induced by the diastolic vibration is a result of the mechanical decoupling of crossbridges.

Pilot model calculations using existing crossbridge models in which the length perturbation on cardiac muscle tissue was simulated indicated that diastolic vibration induces an increased net detachment rate; that is, the vibration decouples cross-bridges. The mechanism behind this change was already present in the model, as proposed by Huxley and Simmonds [9] and Julian et al. [19]. The relative influence of a short stretch that led to an increase in the number of crossbridges (by increased attachment) was less than that of release, which led to a decreased number of attached bridges (due to the decreased attachment rate). Vibration can be seen as a repetitive

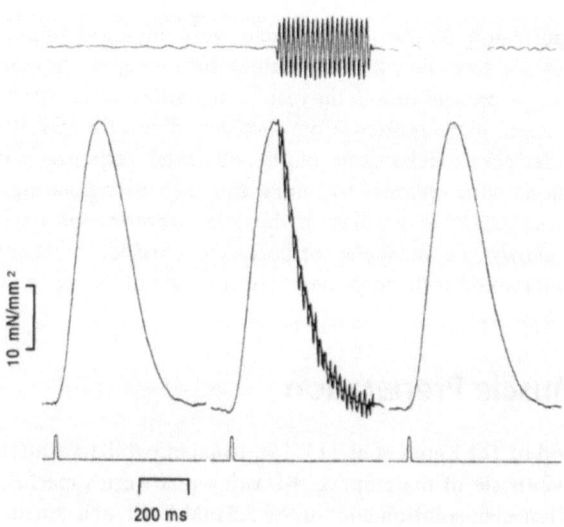

FIG. 2. Three consecutive twitches of a papilary muscle. During relaxation of the second twitch, diastolic vibration was applied. The preparation was stretched to Lmax, and the amplitude of the vibration (middle twitch) was 1.0% of Lmax at a frequency of 50 Hz. The vibration signal is shown at the top of the figure, and at the bottom is the stimulation tracing. Note that the change in relaxation is instantaneous

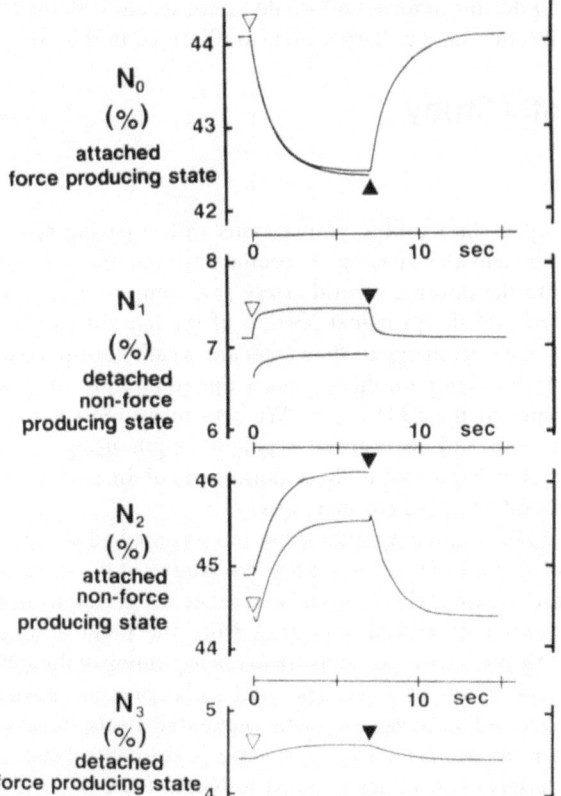

FIG. 3. Results of mathematical simulation [21] of crossbridge kinetics when applying a 50 Hz, 2 mm amplitude mechanical vibration. At application of the vibration (indicated by the *solid line on the top*) the number of attached, strongly binding crossbridges decreased as did the attached non-force-producing crossbridges. *Open triangle*, vibration starts; *closed triangle*, vibration stops. In N_0, N_1, and N_2, the two lines indicate the upper and lower limit of sinusoidal effects induced by vibration

sequence of stretches and releases, and the net result of the mean effect of a release and a stretch would be a decrease in the number of attached, force-producing crossbridges. The effect of sinusoidal vibration on these two models was investigated briefly in a model calculation by Janssen et al. [16]. It was found that both the amplitude and the frequency of the perturbation affected the distribution of the crossbridge states over various states of the model. In general, a decrease in tension was found as continuous sinusoidal perturbations were modeled in an isometric contraction of striated muscle. Honda et al. investigated a four-state crossbridge model of cardiac muscle in which they specifically modeled the effect of sinusoidal perturbations and found similar results [20]. Because the attachment rate is low during relaxation, the effect of a stretch is rather small compared to the effect on detachment by a release (Fig. 3).

According to the above-mentioned model calculations, it is likely that, particularly during relaxation, a sinusoidal perturbation has a much greater effect on the deactivation (detachment) of crossbridges than on their activation (attachment). It results in a faster decline of force and would be consistent with the effect of mechanically applied vibration on papillary muscle as observed in this study.

Experimental Study

Methods

We used nine open-chest canine preparations with a pacing rate at 140 beats per minute (bpm) for right atrial pacing. A coronary arterial line was made by inserting a silicone tube into the internal carotid artery and connecting it to a plastic catheter that was inserted into the proximal portion of the left anterior descending (LAD) coronary artery. A electromagnetic flowmeter and a catheter-tipped micromanometer were set distal to the clamp on this coronary line to monitor the perfusion flow and perfusion pressure of the LAD artery. We also measured LV pressure, right and left atrial pressures, and myocardial segment length using two pairs of 5 MHz piezoelectric crystals implanted in the endocardium of the perfusion area of the LAD and the left circumflex (LCX) coronary artery.

Mechanical, 50 Hz, 2 mm amplitude vibration was applied at the epicardium of the border of the LCX and LAD perfused area. The timing of the vibration was triggered by an electrocardiographic (ECG) signal and set as the period from the beginning of isovolumic relaxation to end-diastole (i.e., from the point at which LV pressure was equal to aortic pressure at the incisura to the beginning of the subsequent systole) by monitoring the trends of aortic and ventricular pressure signals. The diastolic vibration was applied at seven or eight sequential beats. Measurements before, during, and after vibration states were repeated in the control state (no reduction of LAD coronary artery) and under regional ischemia (50% of LAD arterial flow) by manually clamping the coronary line. The value of the relaxation time constant by the method of Weiss et al. [21], coronary vascular resistance, and peripheral vascular resistance were also calculated to estimate the change induced by the diastolic vibration.

Results

At the first beat of vibration input, the LAD coronary blood flow during diastole increased, and the time constant of the ventricular relaxation was reduced. That is, the time constant of the LV pressure fall (T) shortened ($P < 0.0001$), and diastolic coronary flow increased ($P < 0.0001$) immediately (from 105.0 ± 22.6 to 110.5 ± 23.3 ml/min per 100 g of left ventricle in the control and from 46.2 ± 10.5 to 50.0 ± 11.5 ml/min per 100 g in the regional ischemic condition). The coronary vascular resistance decreased at this first beat. In this instance, no significant changes in LV systolic pressure, LV end-diastolic pressure, LAD coronary flow during systole, and coronary perfusion pressure were observed during the application of vibration. The coronary blood flow gradually increased during sequential vibration input of 6 to 10 beats (from 50.0 ± 11.5 ml/min per 100 g for the early phase to 54.2 ± 12.0 ml/min per 100 g for the later phase during the vibration); this increase lasted for the succeeding approximately 10 beats after the cessation of vibration (Fig. 4). Coronary perfusion pressure increased, and coronary vascular resistance remained constant during the sequential vibration input. The percentages of increase in LAD coronary flow and decrease in coronary vascular resistance by vibration input were larger for

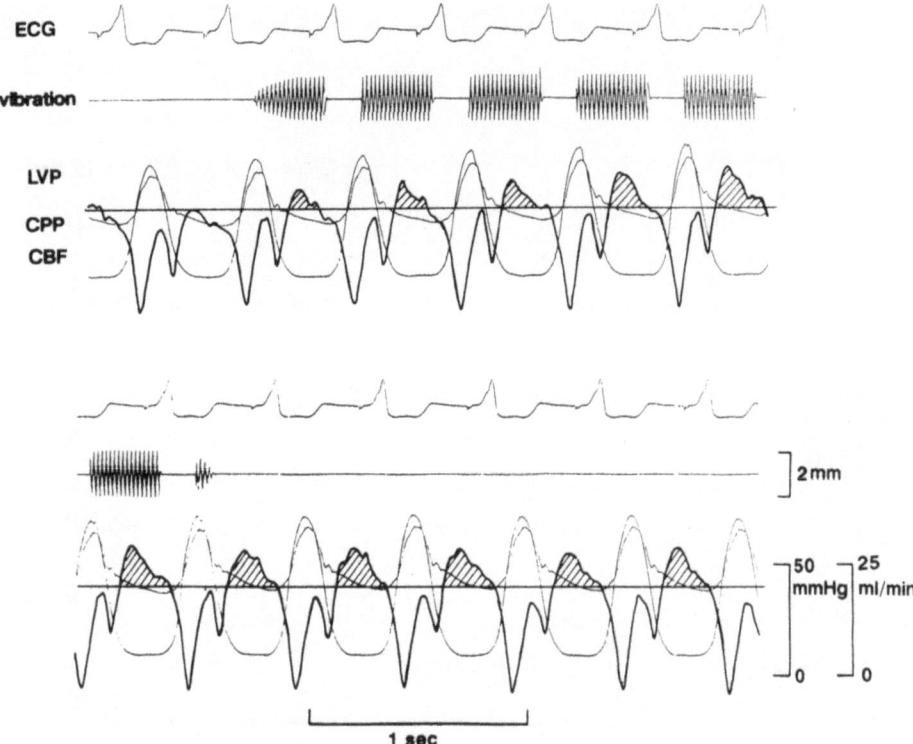

FIG. 4. Sequential trends (from upper to lower panels) show the responses of left ventricular pressure (*LVP*), coronary perfusion pressure (*CPP*), and coronary blood flow (*CBF, thick solid line*) to the mechanical vibration applied to the left ventricle with regional ischemia (50% of control flow). *Horizontal line* is drawn to make clear the change in CBF induced by vibration. The CBF increase due to the vibration input gradually became larger along with the vibration, and this increase lasted for several beats after the cessation of vibration

the ischemic condition than for the control condition ($P < 0.05$ and $P < 0.01$, respectively). Diastolic vibration induced an earlier onset of myocardial relaxation in the ischemic region and reduced nonuniformity of the relaxation sequence between the nonischemic and ischemic regions as shown in trends of myocardial segment length (Fig. 5).

Clinical Study

Methods

We have developed a portable vibrator system for clinical use (Fig. 6). The system includes a mechanical vibration device, monitor, and an electrical, regulatory device. Vibrator tips, which can easily be adapted and changed, were made from pieces of soft silicone rubber attachments of $2 \times 7 \times 2$ cm with three convexities to fit the intercostal space. Before the study we selected the best one to fit the space of the patient to be examined. A 50 Hz, 2 mm amplitude diastolic vibration was applied by placing the tip on Erb's area of the precordium. The phase of the input vibration

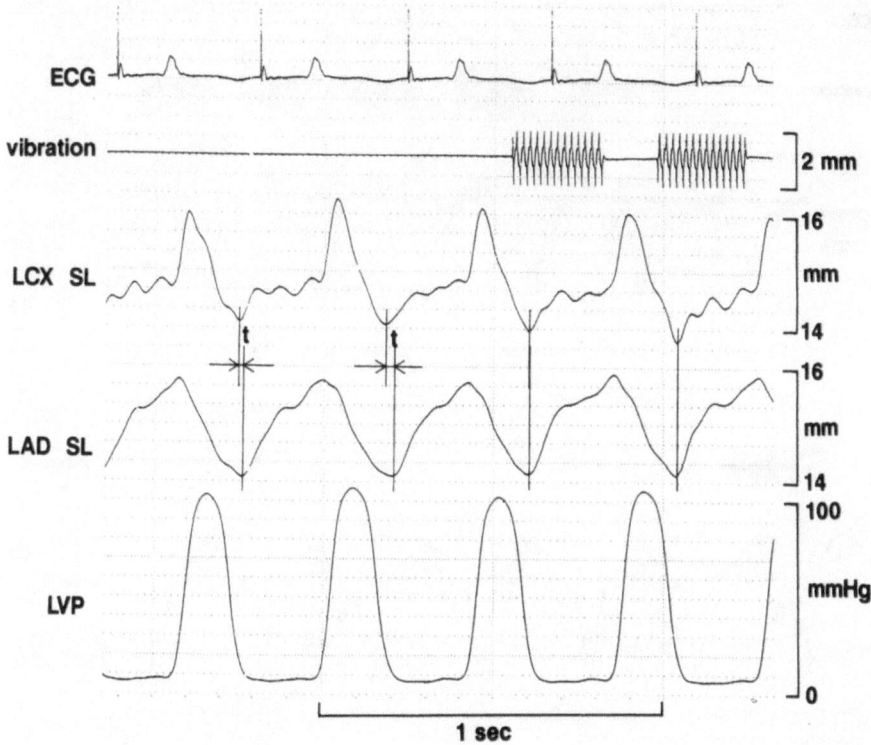

FIG. 5. Change of myocardial segment length at the left anterior descending area under ischemia (*LAD SL*) and nonischemic left circumflex area (*LCX SL*). The interval of time at minimal length between LAD SL and LCX SL (*t*) shortened when diastolic vibration was applied. *LVP*, left ventricular pressure

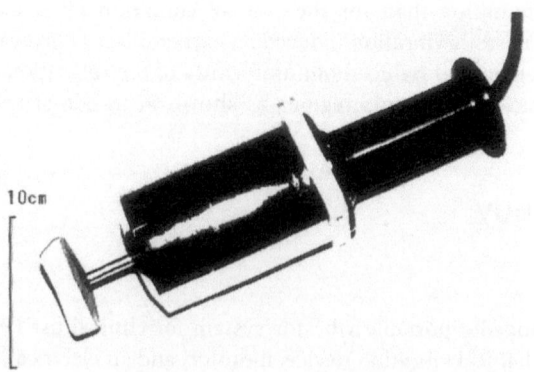

FIG. 6. Prototype of the vibrator used for clinical study. The part of the vibrator that attaches to the chest wall is made of soft silicone rubber. The right upper part of this figure shows the portion that is hand-held

was controlled with an ECG trigger. That is, we manually controlled the input phase from the point of peak contraction of the anterior ventricular wall in the M-mode image of transesophageal echocardiography to the P wave in the ECG, limb lead II.

Changes in coronary arterial flow velocities in the artery (left main or proximal LAD) were measured by two methods. One is a noninvasive method with trans- esophageal Doppler echocardiography (TEE, SSD870; Aloka, Tokyo, Japan) used for ten healthy volunteers (seven men, two women; 50.6 ± 12.8 years old, mean ± SD) and for ten patients with coronary artery disease (CAD) (eight men, two women; 66.4 ± 8.0 years old). The transesophageal echocardiogram was obtained with the subjects under light, local buccal anesthesia and lying in the left lateral position. The other method, which is invasive, calls for inserting a Doppler guidewire (Flowire 1400; Cardiometrics, Mountain View, CA, USA) into the coronary artery. The latter technique was applied to two male and one female CAD patients (60.3 ± 10.5 years old). We analyzed the change in the maximum peak velocity of the coronary artery and the mean arterial blood flow velocity during diastole, as in a previous report [22], while applying diastolic vibration. Special care was taken when estimating the changes of coronary flow velocity to compare those at identical phases of the respiration curve as measured by a nasal thermistor. The variation in peak velocity of coronary blood flow was less than 2.1% in standard deviation under this restriction. In contrast, the variation of the value reached approximately 8% when we measured several succeeding beats throughout the respiration period without the restriction mentioned above. A significant influence of respiration on coronary arterial velocity has been reported [23].

Results

Figure 7 shows the M-mode image of posterior and anterior myocardial wall motions of the left ventricle. The left panel shows the wall movement before applying the vibration; the right panel shows it under vibration. The vibration at the precordium induced myocardial perturbation.

Figure 8 (top to bottom) shows a continuous record of the coronary blood flow velocity measured in the left main trunk of a 52-year-old normal subject. The upper trace was obtained before vibration and the lower trace during vibration. The upper and lower traces are shown so as to compare them at identical respiration phases while measuring the upper and lower beats. When the upper and lower traces of the velocity are compared according to each aspect of the respiration phase, the velocity during diastole increased by precordial vibration input. In contrast, the coronary flow velocity during systole showed no significant difference before and during the vibration input. In all subjects measured by transesophageal echo- cardiography the maximum and mean diastolic velocities of the coronary arterial flow were increased ($P < 0.05$, one-way ANOVA) immediately after application of the diastolic vibration. Moreover, the magnitude of the increase in coronary arterial velocity was significantly larger ($P < 0.05$) in patients (increment of peak velocity 17.7 ± 3.0%; increment of mean velocity 12.7 ± 2.1%) than in normal subjects (increment of peak velocity 9.0 ± 1.4%; increment of mean velocity 6.3 ± 1.7%). Coronary artery diameter, heart rate, and blood pressure showed no change during vibration; and no adverse effects, such as chest pain at the attached portion,

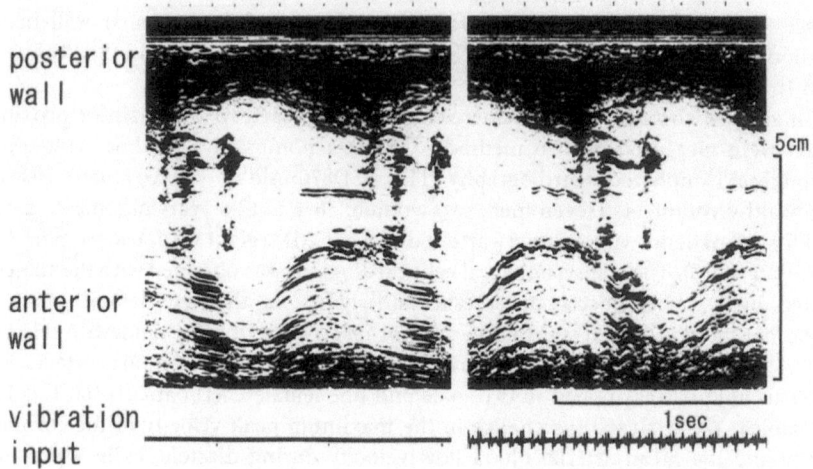

FIG. 7. Short-axis image of the left ventricle as seen by transesophageal echocardiography. Upper portion is an image of the posterior myocardium and the lower portion the anterior myocardium. Vibration of the chest wall by a laboratory-prepared vibrator induced myocardial perturbation, as shown on the right as a zigzag motion of the image compared to the left, previbration state

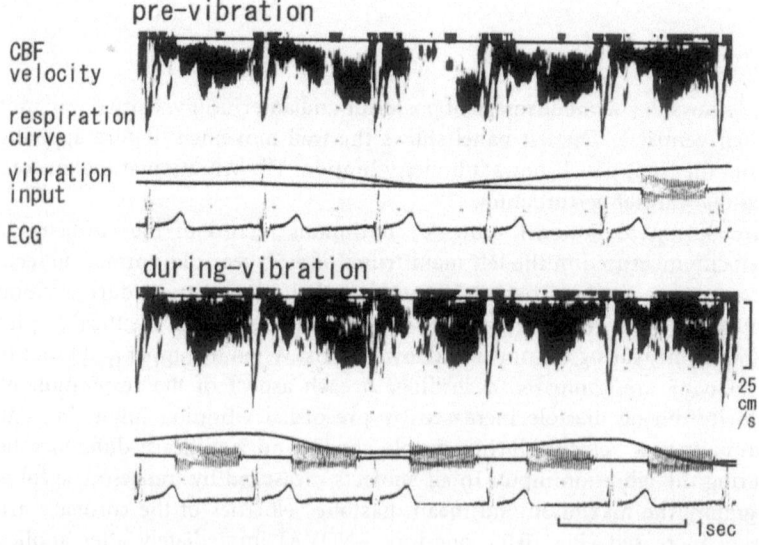

FIG. 8. Coronary blood flow velocity measured by transesophageal Doppler echocardiography in a volunteer. From top to bottom are continuous images of the CBF velocity, respiration curve recorded by nasal thermistor, input vibration monitored at the shaft of the vibrator on the chest wall, and the electrocardiogram. The top traces are those in the previbration state, and the lower traces are those obtained during vibration. Coronary flow velocity, measured by Doppler echocardiography showed an increase in the peak and mean velocities of coronary flow

anginal pain, arrhythmias, or anxiety, were observed during the study. Direct measurements using an intracoronary Doppler guidewire confirmed the increase of coronary flow velocities during vibration.

Discussion

Diastolic vibration increased coronary arterial flow in both normal and ischemic conditions. We believe this improvement likely resulted from acceleration of LV relaxation, which was caused by myocardial crossbridge detachment or normalization of the nonuniformity of relaxation between the ischemic and nonischemic regions, as explained below. We believe that the underlying mechanism responsible for restoration of impaired relaxation is detachment of the residual, force-generating crossbridges during the relaxation period, as discussed in previous reports [4, 13], together with theoretical simulations of crossbridge kinetics [16, 20], though we could not exclude the contribution of intracellular calcium transients [24]. Furthermore, we should be aware of differences in pathological situations imposed on the ventricle when considering the underlying mechanism of the improvement. As for the experimental model, we used a canine preparation with regional ischemia, which differed greatly from previous reports of global ischemia or intravenous injection of negative inotropic drugs characterized by mechanical nonuniformity within the ventricular region. The implication is that a factor of nonuniformity other than the input mode existing between the nonischemic and ischemic areas should be taken into consideration when evaluating the response to external vibration. The nonuniformity has been reported as another major determinant of LV relaxation [6]. Figure 5 demonstrates the effect of diastolic vibration on the nonuniformity of the contraction-relaxation sequence in the regionally ischemic ventricle. Another display of the myocardial segment length at the LAD (horizontal axis) and LCX (vertical axis) is shown in Fig. 9 as a Lissajous loop. In this demonstration it is easy to image the level of the heterogeneous sequence between the different regions; if the relaxation is completely synchronized, the linearly increasing line is displayed. In contrast, when the relaxation sequence is completely inverted in time, that is, when the myocardial lengthening occurred simultaneously with the myocardial shortening of another region, there would be a line from the left upper to the right lower in the graph. Moreover, the concavity implies that the lengthening and shortening occurred simultaneously during the later period of relaxation. In Fig. 9 diastolic vibration reduced the concavity of the loop in the ischemic condition (from right upper at previbration to right lower during vibration) and in the nonischemic condition (left panel). Diastolic vibration applied to the ventricle with regional ischemia therefore should be considered to improve the impaired relaxation by reducing the magnitude of nonuniformity during the relaxation period. This phenomenon might be explained by the synchronizing effect of myocardial relaxation caused by forceful detachment of the residual force generating crossbridges at the ischemic myocardial area by diastolic vibration.

We have demonstrated in this study that external vibration during diastole increases coronary flow rate in the normal and ischemic conditions. This finding can be explained simply by the fact that improvement of the relaxation time constant reduces the compressive force to the intramyocardial coronary vessel in both the ischemic region and the normal area of the ventricular wall. It would be premature to conclude that the method of external perturbation is useful as a therapeutic tool and could be

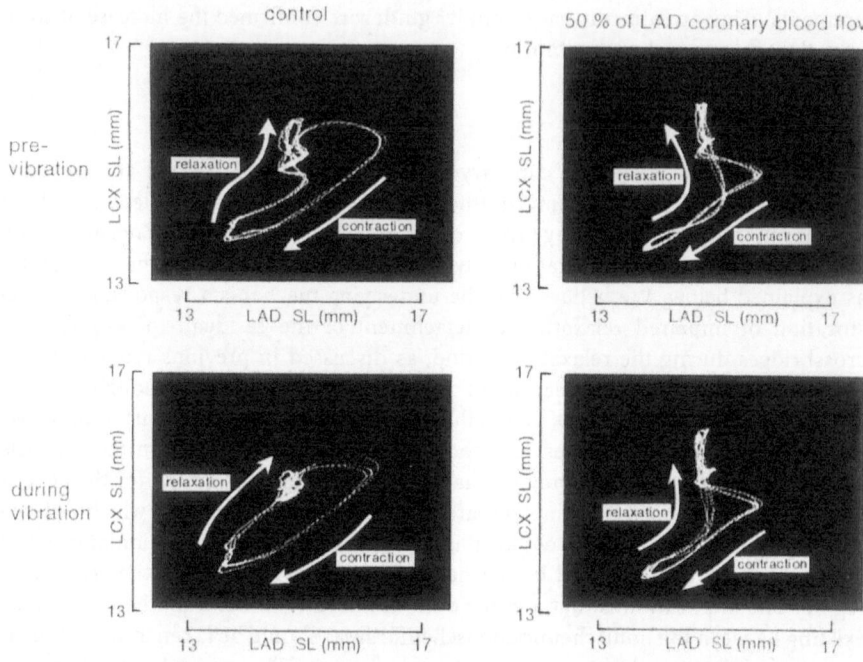

FIG. 9. Change in the Lissajous loop of the myocardial segment length in the nonischemic (*LCX*) and ischemic (*LAD*) areas. When applying vibration, the loop reduced its concavity, suggesting normalization of the nonuniform myocardial contraction and relaxation sequence in the LCX and LAD myocardial areas

used as a probe to investigate the magnitude of the impairment of relaxation. However, we briefly summarize several results that suggest the characteristic features of this vibration method and the possibility of future applicability.

Nishioka et al. discussed the effect of continuous [25] and diastolic [26] 70 Hz, 2 mm amplitude mechanical vibration on ventricular function and myocardial oxygen consumption. They used isolated, isovolumically beating canine LV preparations and applied vibration to the epicardium, measuring Emax, ventricular pressure–volume area (PVA), and myocardial oxygen consumption (Vo_2). Their results showed that (1) the oxygen cost of the contractility is significantly lowered with vibration than that seen with inotropic drugs; (2) PVA-dependent Vo_2 decreased, but Vo_2 for excitation-contraction coupling remained unchanged by this vibration; and (3) myocardial oxygen consumption was reduced during diastolic vibration, whereas the ventricular work remained unchanged. Nishioka et al. concluded that the effect of vibration on ventricular performance is accomplished through a decrease in the number of activated crossbridges, and that mechanical vibration of the failing heart uniquely improves the oxygen cost of contractility by decreasing PVA-related myocardial oxygen consumption. Such an improvement of the oxygen cost of contractility (LV contractility per unit oxygen consumption) was gained only by hypothermia and by external vibration. All of the inotropic drugs examined (catecholamines, digitalis, phosphodiesterase inhibitor [25], Na channel openers [27]) failed to improve the relation of the oxygen consumption and mechanical efficiency in the failing heart model (H. Suga, personal communication).

In previous experiments we confirmed that the magnitude of the response induced by external vibration was related to the input energy of the vibration as well as to the functional severity of the ventricular failure [4, 14, 18]. Therefore we should not accept the magnitude of the ventricular response as maximal using this perturbation method. We did not impose severe hypofunction in the experimental study, nor did we study the response in patients of severe heart failure. The LV relaxation rate during severe heart failure has been reported to be approximately 80 ms [28], but the rates in our study ranged around 40–50 ms [4, 13]. The normal value has been reported to be arround 40–45 ms.

During heart failure impaired relaxation results in myocardial hypoperfusion, which induces further deterioration of ventricular relaxation, resulting in a vicious pathophysiological circle. Therefore selectively breaking the circle by releasing the impaired relaxation and improving the coronary flow rate with external vibration may be a unique, effective way to treat patients with regional ischemia, especially those with impaired relaxation of diastolic heart failure. However, the technology to apply much larger vibration energy to the patient's ventricle from the precordium is still at the prototype level; more importantly, we should continue to examine the possibility of side effects inherent in this perturbation method and consider the benefits of applying it to patients with severe heart failure.

References

1. Carrol DJ, Lang RM, Neumann AL, Bonow KM, Rajfer SI (1986) The differential effects of positive inotropic and vasodilator therapy on diastolic properties in patients with congestive cardiomyopathy. Circulation 74:815–825
2. Grossman W (1990) Diastolic dysfunction and congestive heart failure. Circulation 81 (suppl 3):1–7
3. Hirata Y (1980) A clinical study of left ventricular relaxation. Circulation 62:756–763
4. Takagi T, Koiwa Y, Kikuchi J, Honda H, Hoshi N, Butler JP, Takishima T (1992) Diastolic vibration improves systolic function in case of incomplete relaxation. Circulation 86:1995–1964
5 Domelik-Warzynski LJ, Powell WJ Jr, Guerrero L, Palacios I (1987) Effect of the changes in ventricular relaxation on early diastolic coronary blood flow in canine hearts. Circ Res 62:747–756
6. Brutsaert DL, Radenmaker FE, Sys AU (1984) Triple control relaxation: implications in cardiac disease. Circulation 69:190–196
7. Palacios I, Newell JB, Powell WJ Jr (1978) Effects of acute global ischemia on diastolic relaxation in canine hearts. Am J Physiol 235:H720–H727
8. Gilbert JC, Glantz SA (1989) Determination of left ventricular filling and of the diastolic pressure-volume relation. Circ Res 64:827–857
9. Huxley AF, Simmonds RM (1970) Proposed mechanism of force generation in striated muscle. Nature 233:533–538
10. Kaufmann RL, Bayer RM, Harnasch C (1972) Autoregulation of contractility in the myocardial cell displacement as a controlling parameter. Pflugers Arch 332:96–116
11. Steiger GJ, Brady AJ, Tan ST (1978) Intrinsic regulatory properties of the contractility in the myocardium. Circ Res 42:339–348
12. Brutsaert DL, De Clerck NM, Goethals MA, Housmans PR (1978) Relaxation of ventricular cardiac muscles. J Physiol (Lond) 283:469–480
13. Kikuchi J, Koiwa Y, Takagi T, Honda H, Hoshi N, Butler JP, Takishima T (1992) Effects of mechanical vibration on left ventricular diastolic properties during global ischemia. Am J Physiol 263:H88–H95

14. Koiwa Y, Takagi T, Kikuchi J, Honda H, Hoshi N, Takishima T (1992) Diastolic vibration increases relaxation rate in human left ventricle. Circulation 86(suppl 1):1–380
15. Ter Keurs HEDJ, Rijnsburger WH, Van Heuningen R (1980) Restoring forces and relaxation of rat cardiac muscle. Eur Heart J 1(suppl A):67–80
16. Janssen PML, Van Andel AJ, Sontrop MATA, De Beer EL, Schiereck P (1992) Modelling of the frequency characteristics of striated muscle [abstract]. Pfluegers Arch 420:R94
17. Vukas M, Silvertsson R, Ljung B (1978) Inhibitory effects of vibrations on contractility of isolated rabbit papillary muscle. Scand J Clin Lab Invest 38:415–419
18. Vukas M, Malek I, Hjalmarson AC (1978) Myocardial depressant effect of vibrations in the isolated rabbit heart. Scand J Clin Lab Invest 38:421–424
19. Julian FJ, Sollins KR, Sollins MR (1974) A model for the transient and steady state mechanical behavior of contracting muscle. Biophys J 14:546–563
20. Honda H, Koiwa Y, Takishima T (1994) Mathematical model of the effects of mechanical vibration on crossbridge kinetics in cardiac muscle. Jpn Circ J 58:416–425
21. Weiss JL, Frederiksen JW, Weisfeldt ML (1976) Hemodynamic determinants of time course of fall in canine left ventriclar pressure. J Clin Invest 58:751–760
22. Iliceco S, Malangelli V, Memmola C, Rizzon P (1991) Transesophageal Doppler echocardiography evaluation of coronary blood flow velocity in baseline conditions and during dipyridamol-induced coronary vasodilation. Circulation 83:61–69
23. Erbel R (1991) Transesophageal echocardiography: new window to coronary arteries and coronary blood flow. Circulation 83:339–341
24. Allen DG, Kurihara S (1982) The effects of muscle length on intracellular calcium transients in mammalian cardiac muscle. J Physiol (Lond) 327:79–94
25. Nishioka TY, Goto Y, Hata K, Takasago T, Saeki A, Suga H (1992) Effect of mechanical vibration on myocardial mechanics and energetics in isolated, blood perfused dog heart [abstract]. J Muscle Res Cell Motil 12:485–486
26. Nishioka TY, Goto Y, Hata K, Takasago T, Saeki A, Suga H (1993) Improvement of the ventricular mechanical efficiency by diastolic vibration. Jpn Circ J 57:349 (in Japanese)
27. De Tombe, Burkoff D, Hunter WC (1980) Effects of calcium and EMD-53998 on oxygen consumption in isolated canine hearts. Circulation 86:1945–1954
28. Herrmann HC, Ruddy TD, Dec GW, Strauss HW, Boucher CA, Fifer MA (1987) Diastolic function in patients with severe heart failure: comparison of the effects of enoximone and nitroprusside. Circulation 75:1214–1221

Part 3
Energetics and Exercise

Mechanoenergetics of Acute Failing Hearts Characterized by Oxygen Costs of Mechanical Energy and Contractility

Miyako Takaki, Hiromi Matsubara, Junichi Araki,
Ling Yun Zhao, Haruo Ito, Shingo Yasuhara, Wakako Fujii,
and Hiroyuki Suga

Abstract. We have proposed two key mechanoenergetic concepts: oxygen (O_2) cost of mechanical energy (PVA) and O_2 cost of contractility (Emax). These two O_2 costs proved to be relatively constant under various physiological conditions but have been shown to be altered under pathophysiological conditions such as myocardial stunning and acidosis. In the stunned and acidotic hearts, the O_2 costs of Emax were higher than in the normal hearts without marked changes in O_2 costs of PVA. The energetic changes in these pathological hearts are considered due to decreased Ca^{2+} sensitivity of the contractile machinery, an increased Ca^{2+} handling/ATP ratio, increased Na^+–Ca^{2+} exchange, or all of these factors. However, other types of pathological heart, such as the transient Ca^{2+}-overloaded heart and the negative inotropic agent-treated failing heart, demonstrated similar mechanoenergetics: unchanged O_2 costs of PVA and Emax, different from the above stunned and acidotic hearts. Emax in the second type of pathological heart was depressed comparably to the stunned and acidotic hearts, but its depression is considered due to a decreased total amount of Ca^{2+} handled during excitation-contraction (E-C) coupling. Possible mechanisms responsible for the decreased Ca^{2+} handling include a depression in transsarcolemmal Ca^{2+} influx (channel- or pump-mediated) and a reduction in the amount of Ca^{2+} stored in the sarcoplasmic reticulum. The differences of mechanoenergetics between these two types of pathological heart might derive from the different time courses and degrees of changes in the O_2 cost of Emax. We believe that analyses of these two costs can facilitate better understanding of cardiac mechanoenergetics of both normal and failing hearts.

Key words. Acidosis—Ca^{2+} overload—Contractility—Excitation-contraction coupling—Myocardial oxygen consumption

Introduction

Heart failure is a syndrome caused by heart dysfunction that leads to insufficient cardiac output for metabolic demands of the body. This syndrome remains an obscure clinical entity, and even its definition is controversial. Studies on heart failure have led to new insights into the pathophysiological mechanisms of heart failure, as

Department of Physiology II, Okayama University Medical School, 2-5-1 Shikata-cho, Okayama 700, Japan well as its diagnosis, evaluation, and treatment [1]. The studies have included not only research into gene, molecular, subcellular, and cellular biology of congestive heart failure but also systems physiology in the framework of the pressure–volume relation, enabling assessment of ventricular mechanoenergetics. This conceptual framework is of vital significance, particularly when we consider the failing heart working in the circulatory system.

The heart maintains its pumping action by converting chemical energy contained in metabolic substrates into mechanical energy and work [2]. Adenosine triphosphate (ATP) is the final source of chemical energy for mechanical contraction of muscle [2–5]. Cardiac energy metabolism is normally aerobic (i.e., consuming oxygen); and most ATP is produced by oxidative phosphorylation in mitochondria in the myocardium. Therefore cardiac oxygen consumption (Vo_2) is virtually equivalent to the total energy utilization of the heart ($1 ml O_2 \cong 20 J$) [3–5].

The ATP is utilized in myocardium by three major ATPases: Na^+–K^+ pump ATPase at the sarcolemma, Ca^{2+} pump ATPase at the sarcoplasmic reticulum (SR), and myosin ATPase at the contractile element [6]. The Na^+–K^+ pump ATPase is related to both Na^+ and K^+ handling during electrical activation of the sarcolemma and Na^+ handling coupled with Na^+–Ca^{2+} and Na^+–H^+ exchanges. The Ca^{2+} pump ATPase is related to Ca^{2+} handling during excitation–contraction (E-C) coupling for the activation of contraction and its relaxation. The myosin ATPase is related to crossbridge (CB) cycling for mechanical contraction [6]. The mechanical loading, excitation rate, and inotropic conditions of the heart are known to affect the rate and amount of ATP hydrolysis by these ATPases and hence Vo_2 [3, 4]. However, their quantitative relations in normal and failing hearts remain to be elucidated [7].

In this review, we summarize recent studies, including ours, especially focusing on acute failing hearts, analyzed mainly at the whole-heart level and the mitochondrial level, by applying the two key concepts: O_2 cost of mechanical energy (pressure–volume area, PVA) and O_2 cost of Emax (an index of contractility). These two O_2 costs have been shown to be relatively constant under various physiological conditions but altered under pathophysiological conditions such as myocardial stunning and acidosis [8–11]. We believe that analyses of these two costs can greatly facilitate a better understanding of cardiac mechanoenergetics of normal and failing hearts.

Determinants of Myocardial Oxygen Consumption

Time-Varying Elastance Model

When the Hill two-element model was used to calculate the energy costs of external and internal work, their ratio was $1:3$, leading to the general contention that internal work was three times more costly [12]. However, it was not easily conceivable how the contractile element could discriminate external work from internal work and perform these two types of work with different energy costs and efficiencies. There seems to be no mechanism for CBs to recognize whether the mechanical work performed by CB cycling is conveyed to the outside of the fiber or stored in the series elasticity within the fiber.

Suga developed the idea that the time-varying elastance model of the ventricle could help solve this intriguing problem of cardiac energetics [13]. He proposed this model based on his own ventricular pressure and volume measurements [14–16]. Suga's model of the ventricle is conceptually the same as the time-varying capacitance or elastance models that some cardiovascular modelers had intuitively proposed to simulate cardiac pumping in computer models of the cardiovascular system [14, 17], but he was the first to provide a resolute physiological basis for the time-varying elastance model of the left ventricle [14, 17, 18]. With this model the ventricular contractile state was assessed in terms of a new index, Emax [19, 20]. Emax is the maximal, or end-systolic, value for the ratio $P(t)/[V(t) - V_0]$, where $P(t)$ and $V(t)$ are left ventricular (LV) instantaneous pressure and volume, and V_0 is the ventricular dead volume at which peak isovolumic pressure is zero [14, 21]. The dimensions of Emax are $mm\,Hg\cdot ml^{-1}$. Normalized Emax with respect to LV weight can be expressed in terms of $mm\,Hg\cdot ml^{-1}\cdot100\,g$. The advantages and limitations of the time-varying elastance model and the Emax concept have been well studied and fully reviewed [14, 22–25].

Total Mechanical Energy and Ventricular Pressure–Volume Area

Based on the time-varying elastance model of the ventricle [19, 21–25], Suga [13] proposed a measure of total mechanical energy of ventricular contraction. For this proposal he used the simplest version of the time-varying elastance model, consisting only of an ideal elastance that increases and decreases as a function of time during each contraction [17–19, 26].

The energetic consequences of the time-varying elastance provide a theoretical basis for the definition and measurement of the total mechanical energy. This energy can be quantified as a specific area, the systolic pressure–volume (P-V) area (PVA), in a P-V diagram as shown in Fig. 1A. Mechanical energy is generated with an increase in the time-varying elastance and the counterclockwise rotation of the instantaneous P-V relation curve [13, 21]. The total area swept by the instantaneous P-V curve on the origin side of the working P-V point during a contraction represents the total mechanical energy generated by the contraction. The total area consists of smaller areas: One is the area for external work (EW), surrounded by the P-V loop, and the other is the area for mechanical or elastic potential energy (PE) between the end-systolic and end-diastolic P-V relation curves on the origin side of the P-V loop [13] (Fig. 1A). Thus PVA is a simple sum of EW and PE, as shown in Fig. 1A. The shapes of the instantaneous, end-systolic, and end-diastolic P-V curves do not affect the definition and determination of the total mechanical energy and PVA [13, 27].

Although the amount of EW is independent of the model used, the nature and amount of PE depend on the mechanical model of the heart. PE is a type of internal energy, but it is not equal to the previously defined internal work [28, 29]. Therefore PE was adopted instead of internal work [13, 30].

Although PVA has been determined exclusively on the basis of the ideal time-varying elastance model, more complex time-varying elastance models may be needed to simulate ventricular P-V relations and mechanical energetics under various loading and contractile conditions [31, 32]. An output resistance may be needed to simulate the flow dependence of the elastance [31, 33–35]. This series resistance, if it is a viscous one, consumes energy when ejection flow exists, so EW would be underestimated by the energy loss [13, 32]. Because PVA is determined from measured LV pressure, such a series resistance may make the determined PVA slightly but variably underestimate (by less than 10% in ordinary ejecting contractions) the true total mechanical energy generated inherently in the time-varying elastance [13, 32]. How-

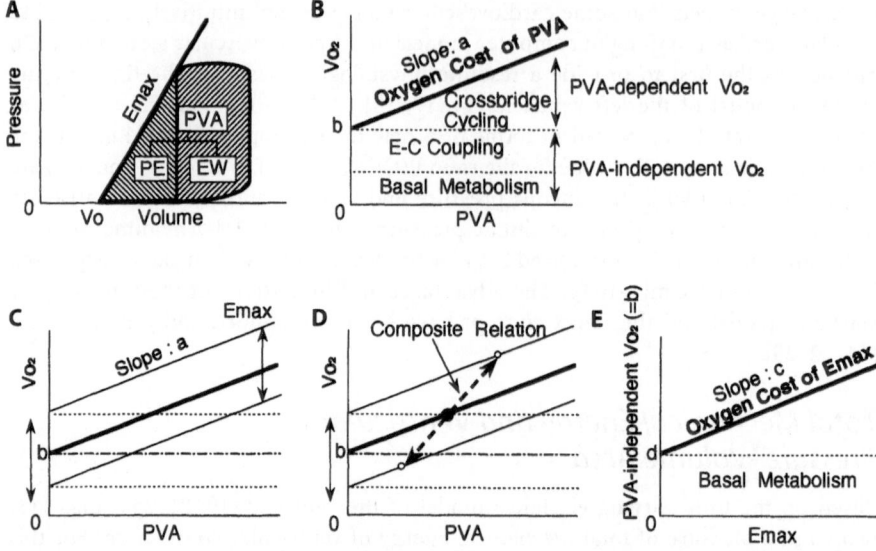

FIG. 1. Framework of the Emax–myocardial oxygen consumption (Vo_2)–left ventricular pressure–volume area (PVA) relation utilized in this review. **A** Emax and left ventricular (LV) systolic pressure (P)–volume (V) area (*PVA*) in the P-V diagram during an ejecting contraction. The slope of the end-systolic P-V relation line is defined as *Emax*. PVA is the area surrounded by the Emax line, the end-diastolic P-V relation curve, and the systolic P-V trajectory. PVA consists of potential energy (*PE*) and external work (*EW*) during an ejecting contraction and of PE alone during an isovolumic contraction (not shown). PE and EW are energetically equivalent. **B** Volume-loaded Vo_2-PVA relation in a baseline contractile state (*thick line*) and Vo_2 components. The slope (*a*) is the oxygen (O_2) cost of PVA, the reciprocal of which (1/a) is contractile efficiency. Its y-intercept (*b*) is the PVA-independent Vo_2. The PVA-independent Vo_2 can be divided into two components: Ca^{2+} handling energy during excitation-contraction (E-C) coupling and basal metabolism. **C** Volume-loaded Vo_2-PVA relations in the baseline contractile state and in two altered contractile states (*thin solid lines*). **D** Upward or downward deviation of a Vo_2-PVA data point (*open circles*) from a baseline Vo_2-PVA relation (*solid circle*) with an increase of a decrease in Emax, respectively, at a constant LV volume during an inotropism run. We called this steeper Vo_2-PVA relation the composite Vo_2-PVA relation (*thick dashed line with arrowheads*). Vo_2 at the solid circle on the baseline Vo_2-PVA relation can be divided into two components: PVA-dependent Vo_2 above *b* and PVA-independent Vo_2 below *b*. Vo_2 at either open circle on another Vo_2-PVA relation can also be divided into the same two components, both of which have been changed according to the respective changes in PVA and Emax. **E** Relation between PVA-independent Vo_2 and Emax. The slope (*c*) of this relation is the O_2 cost of Emax, and the y-intercept (*d*) of this relation indicates the PVA-independent Vo_2 extrapolated to zero Emax. The *d* corresponds to basal metabolism

ever, one study [36] suggested this series resistance to be nonviscous and not to have an important role in ventricular energetics.

The total mechanical energy generated by contraction could eventually be quantified by the total number of CB cycles and the thermodynamic efficiency of each CB hydrolyzing ATP [37, 38]. Although the number of CB cycles per 1 ATP is generally considered to be 1—and hence the number of CB cycles is proportional to the number of ATP moles hydrolyzed [39]—there is evidence that the coupling ratio between CB cycling and ATP hydrolysis deviates from unity under certain loading conditions [40]. Moreover, the cycling rate of CB is calculated to be one to three cycles per beat [41], but direct determination of the total number of CB cycles in a twitch is not yet possible. Therefore until the day comes when CB kinetics and thermodynamics can be quantified more precisely, we can not predict the true total mechanical energy in a constitutive manner. At present, our method of determining total mechanical energy, though macroscopic and phenomenological, seems to be the best available in cardiac mechanoenergetics.

Vo_2–PVA Relation

Suga and co-workers have been studying whether and how PVA would correlate with Vo_2 of the left ventricle using the excised cross-circulated canine heart preparation [1, 7]. This preparation can be made without interrupting coronary flow and hence does not suffer from myocardial stunning and preconditioning. This point is an advantage over other types of excised heart preparation.

In our study the LV was installed with a thin water-filled balloon with a sufficient unstressed volume. LV volume was then measured and controlled with a custom-made servo pump system [18]. Emax and PVA of each contraction were determined on line. The LV PVA normalized for 100 g of LV was expressed as $mm Hg \cdot ml \cdot beat^{-1} \cdot 100 g^{-1}$.

The Vo_2 was determined as the product of coronary flow and arteriovenous oxygen content difference (AVo_2D). Coronary flow was measured with an electromagnetic flowmeter in the coronary venous return tube. Coronary AVo_2D was continuously measured with our custom-made flowing whole-blood spectrophotometric oximeter (PWA-200S; Shoe Technica, Chiba, Japan) [42]. The oximeter was calibrated against a blood O_2 content analyzer (IL-382 CO-Oximeter; Instrumentation Laboratory, Lexington, MA, USA) in each experiment. Both PVA and Vo_2 were determined in the steady state under varied loading, heart rate, and inotropic conditions.

In our studies, PVA refers only to the left ventricle, whereas the measured Vo_2 consists of left (LV) and right (RV) ventricular components. Because the RV was collapsed by continuous drainage of coronary venous return, we assumed the RV PVA-dependent Vo_2 to be practically zero and hence the RV Vo_2 to be only PVA-independent Vo_2 comprising its basal metabolism and myocardial activation. LV Vo_2 comprises both PVA-dependent Vo_2 and PVA-independent Vo_2. We assumed PVA-independent Vo_2 to be homogeneous in the right and left ventricles. RV PVA-independent Vo_2 was determined by multiplying unloaded RV and LV Vo_2 with the RV/ total ventricular weight ratio. This value was subtracted from the total Vo_2 to obtain the LV Vo_2. The LV Vo_2 per minute was divided by the heart rate and expressed as $ml O_2 \cdot beat^{-1}$. The LV Vo_2 normalized for 100 g left ventricle was expressed as $ml O_2 \cdot beat^{-1} \cdot 100 g^{-1}$.

End-diastolic LV volume (preload) was changed to obtain a volume-loaded Vo_2–PVA relation (Fig. 1B). Isovolumic and ejecting contractions in the steady state were produced at four or five LV volumes including V_0. Volume-loaded Vo_2–PVA relations were obtained before and after inotropic interventions such as Ca^{2+} or pentobarbital sodium, as described later [43] (Fig. 1C). During an inotropic intervention a different type of Vo_2–PVA relation at a constant LV volume was obtained as a composite Vo_2–PVA relation (Fig. 1D). The important general findings obtained from these studies in normal hearts are summarized as follows. We describe the individual findings in detail later.

1. The Vo_2 correlates closely and linearly with the PVA at different LV volumes in any stable contractile state, whether a control, enhanced by a positive inotropic agent such as Ca^{2+}, or depressed by a negative inotropic agent such as pentobarbital sodium in any given heart. The Vo_2 axis intercept value of the Vo_2-PVA relation is the same as the Vo_2 obtained during an unloaded contraction at V_0.

2. The slope of the Vo_2-PVA relation is the same irrespective of contraction mode whether isovolumic or ejecting in a given heart.

3. The slope of the Vo_2-PVA relation is relatively constant in different normal hearts in a stable contractile state.

4. During a graded inotropic intervention, the slope of the composite Vo_2-PVA relation is usually steeper than the slope of the volume-loaded Vo_2-PVA relation.

5. The volume-loaded Vo_2-PVA relation shifts upward or downward usually parallel with an enhanced or depressed contractile state.

6. The magnitudes of the upward or downward shift of the Vo_2-PVA relation are usually comparable to increases or decreases in contractility assessed by Emax.

These findings are essentially the same as previously reported [1, 7], but more recent studies showed a different type of mechanoenergetics in pathophysiological hearts, as mentioned later.

Load Independence of the Vo_2-PVA Relation

Isovolumic Versus Ejecting Contractions

In our previous studies the Vo_2-PVA relation was compared for the isovolumic and ejecting contractions in each canine ventricle [44]. For either mode of contraction, the relation was linear with a correlation coefficient of nearly unity ($r = 0.96$ on average). When the modes were pooled, the two relations were superimposable, and the resultant Vo_2-PVA relation was also linear with a similar correlation ($r = 0.96$ on average).

Hisano and Cooper [45] applied the concept of PVA, which was originally developed for a ventricular chamber, to a papillary muscle preparation. The linear muscle version of PVA was called the force–length area (FLA). They found that the correlation (r) between Vo_2 and FLA was 0.96 on average. Moreover, the Vo_2-FLA relation was common to the isometric and shortening contractions. These results indicate that the linear, load-independent Vo_2 versus total mechanical energy relation holds reasonably well in myocardium in the same manner as in the ventricle. That is, the load-independent linear Vo_2-PVA relation seems to be intrinsic to myocardium; so it is not necessary to consider in energetics the complex shape of the ventricular chamber and myocardial fiber orientation within the ventricular wall. This feature of the Vo_2-PVA (or FLA) relation seems to be closely related to the law of conservation of energy in that energy is a scalar variable and the total is a simple sum of all the parts.

Energy Equivalence of External Work and Potential Energy

After external mechanical work (EW) and end-systolic elastic potential energy (PE) values were obtained for ejecting and isovolumic contractions in each canine LV, they were multiplied by A and B, respectively, and their sum, $A \cdot EW + B \cdot PE$, was correlated with the Vo_2 to determine the best fit values for A and B in each canine heart with the ejecting and isovolumic data pooled [46]. The results showed that the values of A and B were virtually identical to each other in individual hearts [46]. Therefore the PVA (i.e., a simple sum of EW and PE) can reliably predict the Vo_2 of a given heart in a stable contractile state.

The load independence of the Vo_2–PVA relation was confirmed not only in the baseline contractile state without intervention but also in an enhanced contractile state so long as the contractile state was stable [21].

Hata et al. [47] found that, within a constant PVA, almost all the PE can be converted effectively to EW without affecting the Vo_2 by appropriately unloading the LV P-V load during the relaxation period. This result evidently indicates that the mechanical energy represented by PVA can be either PE or EW without affecting myocardial energetics; that is , PE and EW are energetically equivalent.

During an isovolumic contraction, PE stored in the ventricle at peak contraction is given by the PVA. If no external work is done, PE is released as heat, and hence the heat released during relaxation should be identical to the PVA. In the rabbit papillary muscle at 20°C, the energy (joules) contained by the FLA of the isometrically contracting muscle was compared with the heat (joules) liberated during relaxation. The resulting relation between FLA and heat liberated during relaxation was not significantly different from the identity line [48]. These results confirmed the energetic prediction of the time-varying elastance model developed for the whole left ventricle; PE (= PVA in an isovolumic contraction) is released as heat when unused.

Contractility Dependence of the Vo_2–PVA Relation

Calcium

Cytosolic Ca^{2-} is bound to troponin C, and this binding elicits CB cycling [39]. Increased concentration of extracellular Ca^{2-} increases sarcolemmal Ca^{2-} influx through voltage-dependent Ca^{2+} channels during membrane depolarization. The resultant increase in intracellular Ca^{2+} concentration augments total released Ca^{2-} from the SR and enhances contractility.

When intracoronary arterial administration of $CaCl_2$ (0.05–0.20 mmol/min) increased Emax by 50–100%, it also elevated the volume-loaded Vo_2–PVA relation parallel to the baseline volume-loaded Vo_2–PVA relation with a 50%–100% increase in the PVA-independent Vo_2 [21, 43]. This method is usually the standard basic protocol for examining the dependency of the Vo_2–PVA relation on Emax. Dobutamine can be used in place of Ca^{2+} [1, 7].

Nipradilol

Nipradilol [3,4-dihydro-8-(2-hydroxy-3-isopropylamino)propoxy-3-nitroxy-2H-1-benzopyran] is a newly synthesized chemical agent designed to possess β-adrenoceptor blocking and vasodilating actions [49]. Nipradilol decreased Emax by 40%. PVA and Vo_2 were each decreased by 30% [49]. These results indicate that nipradilol, like propranolol, depresses myocardial mechanoenergetics. Propranolol lowered the Vo_2–PVA relation parallel with a 30% decrease in PVA-independent Vo_2 [50]. This response is opposite to the already studied responses to positive inotropic interventions, such as with Ca^{2+}, dobutamine, denopamine, isoproterenol, and norepinephrine [1, 7].

Oxygen Cost of PVA and Contractile Efficiency

The slope of the Vo_2–PVA relation means the O_2 cost of PVA, or the O_2 cost of mechanical energy. When the slope is a, PVA -dependent Vo_2 is expressed by $aPVA$. Then Vo_2 is given as $Vo_2 = aPVA + PVA$-independent Vo_2 (Fig. 1B). From a large number of canine LVs (body weight 12–15 kg) in previous studies, we have obtained an average value of $1.8 \times 10^{-5}\,mlO_2 \cdot mm\,Hg^{-1} \cdot ml^{-1}$ for the O_2 cost of PVA [1, 7] whereas an average value of 1.4×10^{-5} to $1.6 \times 10^{-5}\,ml\,O_2 \cdot mm\,Hg^{-1} \cdot ml^{-1}$ was obtained in our more recent studies [43, 51, 52]. These findings mean that about 1.5×10^{-5} to $1.8 \times 10^{-5}\,ml\,O_2$ is needed to increase the PVA by $1\,mm\,Hg \cdot ml \cdot beat^{-1}$. One milliliter of O_2 is biochemically equivalent to approximately 20 J, or precisely 19.5–20.5 J depending on the metabolic substrate used [53]. PVA in the amount of $1\,mm\,Hg \cdot ml$ is physically equivalent to $1.33 \times 10^{-4}\,J$. Therefore the a value of 1.5×10^{-5} to $1.8 \times 10^{-5}\,ml\,O_2 \cdot mm\,Hg^{-1} \cdot ml^{-1}$ is convertible to about 2.3–2.7 (dimensionless) [1, 7]. Note that this value is independent of LV weight.

The reciprocal of the O_2 cost of PVA, $1/a$, means the efficiency of energy conversion from the PVA-dependent Vo_2 to PVA. This efficiency is called "contractile efficiency", to be differentiated from other efficiencies, such as mechanical work efficiency and CB efficiency [1, 7, 41]. The contractile efficiency is 40% on average, ranging between 30% and 50% in different hearts [1, 7, 41]. The contractile efficiency is the product of the chemomechanical efficiency of oxidative phosphorylation from Vo_2 to ATP production and the chemomechanical efficiency of CB cycling from ATP hydrolysis to mechanical energy. The efficiency of oxidative phosphorylation is related to the P/O ratio (the atomic ratio of produced ATP to consumed oxygen) in the mitochondria. The method for measuring the P/O ratio in mitochondria is described later.

From an oxidative phosphorylation efficiency of 64% and a contractile efficiency of 40%, we calculated that the chemomechanical efficiency of CB cycling is 63% (0.40/0.64 = 0.63) [7]. Thus introduction of the PVA concept and contractile efficiency has allowed us to elucidate the stoichiometry during the energy conversion step from oxygen consumption to total mechanical energy [1, 7, 41]; this efficiency is the maximum possible efficiency of mechanical work [47]. Therefore it seems vitally important to search for methods to improve contractile efficiency in failing hearts.

When the contractile efficiency changes, the efficiency of oxidative phosphorylation, the efficiency of CB cycling, or both may change. Unfortunately, in our present studies, we cannot determine which efficiency changes.

Oxygen Cost of Emax

The activation component of Vo_2 is considered to reflect the energy expenditure by both Na^+-K^+- and Ca^{2+}-ATPases. Because the total amount of released Ca^{2+} is considered to increase in an enhanced contractile state, it is easily conceivable that a larger amount of Ca^{2+} is removed mostly into the SR by the Ca^{2+}-ATPase consuming more ATP with a stoichiometry of $2Ca^{2+}:1ATP$ [54] and additionally to the outside by the Na^+-Ca^{2+} exchanger. More Ca^{2+} seems to flow into the myocardial cell through the voltage-dependent Ca^{2+} channel during membrane depolarization in an enhanced contractile state [55]. This amount of Ca^{2+} must be removed from the cell during repolarization [54]. The Na^+-Ca^{2+} exchange per se does not consume ATP in order to remove Ca^{2+} in exchange with influx Na^+ (stoichiometry = $3Na^+:1Ca^{2+}$) [55]. However, this influx Na^+ must be pumped out by the Na^+-K^+ pump ATPase with a stoichiometry of $3Na^+$:$2K^+$:$1ATP$. Therefore the net stoichiometry is $1Ca^{2+}$:$1ATP$, which is half that of the SR Ca^{2+}-ATPase. As a whole, enhancement of contractility is associated with increases in both the amount of Ca^{2+} handled during the excitation–contraction–relaxation cycle and its energy utilization.

Therefore our finding that PVA-independent Vo_2 is increased in proportion to the increase in Emax seems to be based on the stoichiometry between the amount of Ca^{2+} to be handled in the excitation–contraction–relaxation process and the amount of ATP consumed in the ion pumps [1, 7].

We have introduced the O_2 cost of Emax to quantify the requirement of PVA-independent Vo_2 per unit increase in Emax. This cost is expressed by the slope of the relation between PVA-independent Vo_2 and Emax obtained while Emax is changed by an inotropic intervention (Fig. 1E) [1, 7].

When Vo_2–PVA relations are obtained at different levels of Emax, they elevate differently although their slopes are virtually the same, as shown in Fig. 1C. The elevation increases in proportion with the increase in Emax. Burkhoff et al. [56] obtained these parallel Vo_2–PVA relations. This method, however, would bring about a large estimation error when only two sets of Vo_2–PVA data are taken for each Vo_2–PVA relation at each Emax. We prefer a different method. We fix the ventricular end-diastolic volume (EDV) and change the Emax gradually. This method does not require changes in the ventricular loading condition, but it does require the assumption that the Vo_2–PVA relations at different Emax levels virtually parallel each other [57], or we need to know how the Vo_2–PVA relation changes its slope [8]. We validated this parallelism in many studies using various inotropic agents [1, 7].

When Emax, and hence PVA and Vo_2, were increased gradually at constant EDV and end-systolic volume (ESV), and so at constant stroke volume, the Vo_2–PVA data points linearly moved right and upward (i.e., deviated upward from the baseline Vo_2–PVA relation line [57], as shown in Fig. 1D. We called the regression line of these Vo_2–PVA data points a composite Vo_2–PVA relation.

From this composite relation, we determined the PVA-independent Vo_2 for each Emax by drawing a line through the data point in parallel to the baseline Vo_2–PVA relation. PVA-independent Vo_2 values were plotted against the corresponding Emax values, and the relation was found to be linear, as shown in Fig. 1E. This relation could be formulated by an empirical equation: PVA-independent $Vo_2 = c$Emax$ + d$, where the slope coefficient c indicates the O_2 cost of Emax, and the constant d indicates the PVA-independent Vo_2 intercept of the relation. From our recent studies [43, 51, 52], the O_2 cost of Emax was approximately 0.0015–$0.0030\,ml\,O_2 \cdot mm\,Hg^{-1} \cdot beat^{-1} \cdot 100\,g^{-2}$. The reciprocal of c represents the economy of the E-C coupling.

PVA-Dependent and PVA-Independent Vo_2

Potassium Chloride (KCl)-arrested Vo_2 was not significantly affected by various inotropic agents when KCl was infused directly into the coronary circulation at a barely minimal level to cause cardiac arrest and prevent Ca^{2+} overload in myocardial cells [1, 7]. This result indicates that the fraction of Vo_2 that changed with Emax at V_0 (i.e., unloaded contraction with zero PVA) is related to myocardial activation, or E-C coupling, which primarily handles intracellular Ca^{2+} transport [3, 54]. Any contraction with a positive PVA requires an extra Vo_2 proportional to the PVA. Accordingly, the total Vo_2 is composed of the three major energy expenditures (i.e., mechanical contraction, activation, basal metabolism).

The horizontal division between the PVA-dependent and PVA-independent Vo_2 in Fig. 1B is based on the assumption that the energy expenditure of Ca^{2+} handling during activation is independent of PVA. In fact, we have found that unloaded Vo_2 is virtually independent of whether the unloaded contraction is either the isovolumic contraction at V_0 or completely systolic unloaded contractions from high EDVs [58].

The linear Vo_2–PVA relation indicates that Vo_2 for mechanical contraction is proportional to PVA. Therefore it is reasonable to call the Vo_2 above the unloaded Vo_2 "PVA-dependent Vo_2" and the Vo_2 below the unloaded Vo_2 "PVA-independent Vo_2" (Fig. 1B).

PVA-dependent Vo_2 is consumed for ATP production for myosin ATPase. PVA-independent Vo_2 is consumed during ATP production for Ca^{2+} pump ATPase at the SR [59], Na^+-K^+ pump ATPase at the sarcolemma, and basal metabolism. It remains unknown whether the PVA-independent Vo_2 is always constant regardless of PVA because this Vo_2 component cannot be separated from the PVA-dependent Vo_2 during contractions with positive PVA.

Energy for Electrical Activation

In the empirical equation

$$\text{PVA-independent } Vo_2 = c\text{Emax} + d$$

the constant d (i.e., the PVA-independent Vo_2 at zero Emax) represents the Vo_2 for both basal metabolism and electrical activation. The O_2 cost of electrical activation is due to energy utilization by the Na^+-K^+ pump ATPase, which during membrane repolarization pumps out Na^- that has entered during membrane depolarization. When complete electromechanical dissociation was effected by removing Ca^{2+} in a beating canine heart, the Vo_2 for electrical activation was about $0.0004\,\text{ml}\,O_2 \cdot 100$ $g^{-1} \cdot \text{stimulation}^{-1}$ [60]. It was less than 1% of the total O_2. Therefore this component of Vo_2 has usually been neglected in the analysis of the Vo_2–PVA relation. This small percentage may be an underestimation of the ATP hydrolysis by the Na^+-K^+ pump because the absence of Ca^{2+} would eliminate both Ca^{2+} influx (slow inward current) and the resultant Na^+-Ca^{2+} antitransport and consequently the Na^+-K^+ pump (net stoichiometry = $1Ca^{2+}$:1ATP) [61]. An upper limit of Vo_2 for Na^+-K^+ pump ATPase for Na^+ flux of $6.6\,\mu\text{mol} \cdot 100\,g^{-1} \cdot \text{stimulation}^{-1}$ [62] would be $0.01\,\text{ml}\,O_2 \cdot 100\,g^{-1}$ [63]. This value is 25 times more than the empirically determined values [60]. Consequently, Vo_2 for Na^+ flux at a heart rate of 100 beats per minute would be $1\,\text{ml}\,O_2 \cdot \text{min}^{-1} \cdot 100\,g^{-1}$ at most, comparable to basal metabolism under KCl arrest [60].

Basal Metabolism

The basal metabolism of myocardium is the energy utilization of myocardial activities other than electrical activation and mechanical contraction. Whole-heart preparations used in our study can be relaxed under high K^+ (10–20 mM) perfusion, and basal metabolic Vo_2 can be measured directly.

Nozawa et al. [64] found that the basal metabolic Vo_2 was 1.24 ± 0.59 ml O_2 at 5 min under KCl arrest, decreased to 1.01 ± 0.53 ml O_2 within the next 5 min, and did not significantly decrease thereafter until 30 min under KCl arrest. The KCl concentration in the coronary blood was about 13 mmol/L. The KCl-arrested basal metabolic Vo_2 did not significantly increase with increases in EDV from V_0 (about 7 ml) to 50 ml [64] or 50–100% increases in Emax by dobutamine.

The basal metabolic Vo_2 of myocardium seems to include ATP utilization for protein synthesis, such as healing over, maintenance of cell membrane polarization by the Na^+-K^+ pump ATPase, and phosphorylation of various proteins. The Na^+-K^+ pump ATPase contributes to only 5–20% of the basal metabolism [65]. Much remains to be elucidated as to the components of basal metabolic energy utilization.

E-C Coupling Ca^{2+} Handling Energy

In cardiac myocytes the transition from the resting relaxed state with a low intracellular concentration of Ca^{2+} to a contraction occurs because a small quantity of Ca^{2+} crosses the sarcolemma and induces much larger release of Ca^{2+} from the SR. The initial events that couple excitation to contraction are initiated by depolarization of the cell membrane, which causes opening of the voltage-gated Na^+ and Ca^{2+} channels. The initial upstroke of the action potential in ventricular cardiac myocytes is caused by Na^+ influx via the Na^+ channel, whereas the subsequent slow inward current maintaining the plateau of the action potential is caused primarily by Ca^{2+} influx via the L-type Ca^{2+} channel. Cumulative Na^+ influx via the Na^+ channel can influence intracellular Ca^{2+} concentration via Na^+–Ca^{2+} exchange (Ca^{2+} influx–Na^+ efflux). However, it is the Ca^{2+} influx via the Ca^{2+} channel that is considered to be of greatest importance for E-C coupling [66–69].

The Ca^{2+} that enters the cell activates the Ca^{2+} release channel of the SR, releasing Ca^{2+} from internal stores within the SR: calcium-induced calcium release (CICR) [70]. The probability of opening of the Ca^{2+} release channel in the SR is markedly increased by exposure to micromolar concentrations of Ca^{2+}. The SR Ca^{2+} channel has sites for phosphorylation, ATP binding, and calmodulin binding. The Ca^{2+} that is released from the SR binds to the contractile proteins and initiates contraction. In the resting state the interaction of actin and myosin is inhibited by the troponin–tropomyosin complex, which is bound to actin. When Ca^{2+} binds to troponin C, a conformational change of the troponin–tropomyosin complex is induced, relieving this inhibition and resulting in CB interaction and contractile element shortening [71]. Thus changes in the affinity of the contractile proteins to Ca^{2+} as well as the magnitude of the Ca^{2+} transient achieved during each beat can regulate force development by a myocyte [69].

The decay of the Ca^{2+} transient occurs primarily by reuptake of Ca^{2+} into the SR mediated by the SR Ca^{2+}-ATPase and, secondarily, extrusion of Ca^{2+} from the myocyte mostly by Na^+–Ca^{2+} exchange: Ca^{2+} efflux–Na^+ influx "forward" mode of operation. Contribution of the sarcolemmal Ca^{2+}-ATPase is practically negligible [69]. The Kca (a Km for Ca^{2+}) for Ca^{2+} transport of the SR Ca^{2+}-ATPase is 300–400 nM. Thus SR Ca^{2+}-ATPase is strongly activated in the range of physiological Ca^{2+} concentrations, which occur during the normal contraction-relaxation cycle. Regulation of SR Ca^{2+}-ATPase occurs primarily by phosphorylation of phospholamban [59].

Competition between Ca^{2+} extrusion by Na^+–Ca^{2+} exchange and Ca^{2+} uptake by the SR is physiologically important because the Ca^{2+} that is taken up by the SR is available to the Ca^{2+} transient during a subsequent beat and thus can contribute to force development. In the steady state, the amount of Ca^{2+} entering the cell equals that extruded from the cell, and the amount released by the SR equals that sequestered by the SR.

The Vo_2 for E-C coupling is used for removing sarcoplasmic Ca^{2+} from $1-10\,\mu M$ to $0.1\,\mu M$ by active transport, mainly by SR Ca^{2+}-ATPase, to relax contraction [72–74]. Changes in contractility are accompanied by proportional changes in the amount of Ca^{2+} involved in the E-C coupling unless Ca^{2+} sensitivity (or responsiveness) of the contractile proteins is altered [43, 52, 75–77]. Such Ca^{2+} changes would then change the energy required for Ca^{2+} sequestration by the following four Ca^{2+} transport systems: (1) SR Ca^{2+}-ATPase; (2) sarcolemmal Na^+–Ca^{2+} exchange (these two mechanisms are predominant); (3) sarcolemmal Ca^{2+}-ATPase; (4) mitochondrial Ca^{2+} uptake (the latter two mechanisms are about 50-fold slower than former two) [69, 78–80].

A tight coupling exists between 2 moles of Ca^{2+} transported and 1 mole of ATP hydrolyzed in myocardial SR unless the SR is leaky to Ca^{2+} [81, 82]. This tight Ca:ATP stoichiometry suggests that Vo_2 for Ca^{2+} handling by the SR is proportional to the amount of Ca^{2+} handled by the SR during E-C coupling regardless of the Ca^{2+} release and uptake speeds [19, 81]. Uncertainty about the amount of Ca^{2+} handling via Na^+–Ca^{2+} exchange makes it difficult to partition exactly the Ca^{2+} handling Vo_2 into the Vo_2 components of the SR Ca^{2+} pump and Na^+–Ca^{2+} exchange.

Low concentrations of ryanodine open the SR Ca^{2+} release channel and thus deplete the SR Ca^{2+} stores. In the presence of continued stimulation of myocardial cells, ryanodine does not completely deplete the SR. However, in rested cells exposed to ryanodine, the SR becomes completely depleted [69]. Therefore in the resting myocardium energy expenditure for sequestering leaked Ca^{2+} appears to be small [82].

The activation (or E-C coupling) energy of $0.4\,J/100\,g$ observed experimentally in a control contractile state corresponds to about $100\,nmol\ Ca^{2+}/g$ tissue to be released and sequestered per beat on the basis of a Ca^{2+} pump stoichiometry of 2 Ca^{2+}/ATP [83]. Then the Vo_2 for E-C coupling of about $0.3-0.4\,J{\cdot}beat^{-1}{\cdot}100\,g^{-1}$ in the excised cross-circulated canine heart [21] suggests the involvement of $60-100\,nmol\,Ca^{2+}/g$ tissue [4, 84, 85]. This amount of Ca^{2+} involved in E-C coupling varies among reports; for example, 20% and 70% maximum force developments require Ca^{2+} amounts of 17 and $26\,nmol/g$ wet muscle in ferret heart, respectively [86].

The parallel shifts of the Vo_2–PVA relation under varied Emax [19] are consistent with the contemporary concept that the primary cellular change accompanying changes in contractility is the amount of Ca^{2+} released to the myofilaments per beat. The close relation between unloaded Vo_2 and Emax seems consistent with the linearity of the relation between Ca^{2+} transients and contractility [86]. This close relation also seems consistent with a fixed, linear stoichiometry between Ca^{2+} uptake and ATP consumption by SR independent of the contractile state [74, 81, 85].

Residual CB Cycling O_2 Consumption

Even the unloaded ventricle contracting with zero PVA changes its shape. The shape change suggests the existence of myocardial shortening by residual CB cycling and some mechanical energy generation.

However, the V_{O_2} values of contractions that are mechanically unloaded throughout systole by quick release from large EDVs are close to the V_{O_2} of unloaded contractions at V_0 [58]. These V_{O_2} data may be called PVA-independent, because PVA is zero or almost zero during any of these contractions. Therefore the V_{O_2} attributable to the length (preload)-dependent activation seems negligible, at least in the canine LV [58]. Furthermore, V_{O_2} did not significantly decrease even when ventricular volume was decreased from V_0 to complete collapse with a negative pressure in the ventricle [87]. The former condition considerably increased ventricular shape and size changes, and the latter condition minimized ventricular shape changes. Both these observations indicate that ventricular shape changes that are produced by residual CB cycling at zero PVA require no significant V_{O_2}, as shown in Fig. 2A.

In contrast to this contention, a group of investigators [88–90] have claimed that mechanical unloading cannot unequivocally distinguish mechanical from nonmechanical V_{O_2} because the mechanically unloaded heart undergoes shape changes with each contraction and beat-to-beat pressure fluctuations in the negative range. They suspected that when the ventricle is unloaded there is an uncertain

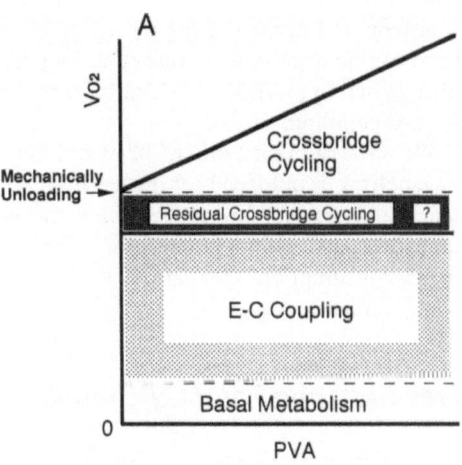

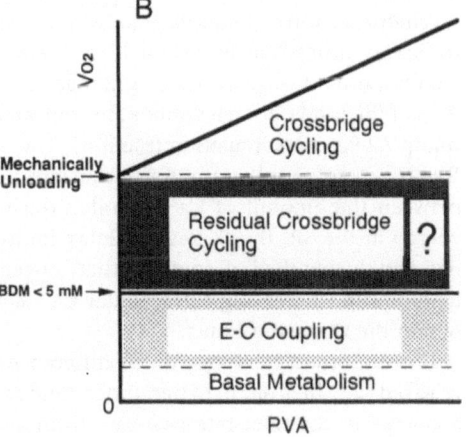

FIG. 2. V_{O_2} versus pressure–volume area (*PVA*) relation. **A** Our view of the mechanically unloading V_{O_2}, which is subdivided into a small amount of V_{O_2} for residual crossbridge cycling (negligible) and PVA-independent V_{O_2} for E-C coupling and basal metabolism. **B** LeWinter's view of mechanically unloading V_{O_2}, which is subdivided into a large amount of V_{O_2} for residual crossbridge cycling and that for nonmechanical activity (nonmechanical V_{O_2}). This nonmechanical V_{O_2}, estimated by the 2,3-butanedione monoxime (*BDM* < 5mM) method, consists of V_{O_2} for E-C coupling and basal metabolism. This diagram exaggerates the low range of LV V_{O_2} and PVA

amount of energy consumption for residual CB cycling, and that it has been incorrectly assigned to the nonmechanical Vo_2. Their contention is based on the method of Alpert et al. [88] in which heat output in rabbit papillary muscles is partitioned into tension-dependent (CB cycling) and tension-independent (E-C coupling) components using a negative inotropic drug, 2,3-butanedione monoxime (BDM). The principle of this approach is that at relatively low concentrations (<5 mM) in isolated rabbit muscles BDM inhibits CB cycling without affecting other energy-consuming processes [91, 92]. They considered that extrapolation of the Vo_2-force time integral (FTI) relation at BDM<5 mM to the Vo_2 axis provides an estimate of nonmechanical Vo_2, which includes Vo_2 for both E-C coupling and basal metabolism but not Vo_2 for residual CB cycling (Fig. 2B). Nonmechanical Vo_2 was estimated to be 0.00132–0.01370 ml O_2·beat^{-1}·100 g LV^{-1} [90]. In contrast, mechanically unloaded Vo_2 was estimated to be 0.0276 ml O_2·beat^{-1}·100 g LV^{-1} and about twice the value of the Vo_2-axis intercept of the Vo_2-FTI relation [90]. These results suggested that during mechanically unloaded conditions there is considerable energy utilization for "residual" CB cycling.

However, as suggested by Gwathmey et al. [93], in ferret papillary muscle BDM at concentrations even as low 1 mM reduced the Ca^{2+} current, reduced the peak Ca^{2+} transient, and decreased the sensitivity of the myofilaments. In excised cross-circulated canine hearts, de Tombe et al. [94] reported that a principal energetic mechanism of action of BDM (0.5–7.0 mM) is to reduce the energy related to Ca^{2+} handling for E-C coupling.

We observed that 5 mM of BDM did not affect Vo_2 for E-C coupling or the basal metabolism in unloaded rat myocardium in our newly developed experimental system [128]. This finding suggests that the Vo_2 for residual CB cycling in the totally unloaded myocardium in negligible. Therefore the partition of mechanically unloading O_2 consumption—the ratio of O_2 consumption to the residual CB cycling—is still controversial.

Free Ca^{2+} and Total Ca^{2+} Kinetics

The energy utilization for Ca^{2+} handling tends to be markedly underestimated on the basis of the popular observation that the peak Ca^{2+} transient required to activate mechanical contraction is 0.5–2.0 μM [75]. However, the amount of Ca^{2+} to be related to energy utilization is the total Ca^{2+} removed by both Ca^{2+} pump ATPase and a combination of the Na^+–Ca^{2+} exchange and the Na^+-K^+ pump ATPase. About 75%–95% of the total Ca^{2+} released to the contractile machinery is removed by the SR Ca^{2+} pump ATPase (recirculation fraction). This amount is 25–400 times greater than the free Ca^{2+} measured as the Ca^{2+} transient [75]. On the basis of the proportionality between the amount of Ca^{2+} handled during E-C coupling and the Ca^{2+} handling energy in the SR, the O_2 cost of Emax indirectly indicates the total amount of Ca^{2+} handled during the E-C coupling that is needed to cause a unit change in Emax. Ca^{2+} loading run (increasing extracellular Ca^{2+} concentration) is the standard protocol to obtain the O_2 cost of Emax.

It is important to recognize the difference between the Ca^{2+} transient and the total released Ca^{2+} in order to better understand cardiac energetics. The naive estimation of a change in the total released Ca^{2+} from an observed change in the Ca^{2+} transient easily leads to an incorrect conclusion.

Pathophysiology

Changes in Emax, O_2 cost of PVA, PVA-independent Vo_2, and O_2 cost of Emax have successfully characterized abnormal mechanoenergetics of various failing hearts [1]. Postischemic and postacidotic stunned hearts and hypercapnic acidotic hearts have shown one type of abnormality in mechanoenergetics [9-11]. Transient Ca^{2+} overload and pentobarbital sodium- and capsaicin-treated hearts have shown a different type of abnormal mechanoenergetics [43, 51, 52]. For a better understanding of mechanoenergetics of failing hearts, it is helpful to characterize the difference between these two types of mechanoenergetic abnormality.

Postischemic Stunned Myocardium

Myocardial stunning in the excised, cross-circulated canine heart was produced by 15 min of normothermic global ischemia followed by blood reperfusion for up to 2 h [9]. Coronary blood flow was markedly increased immediately after reperfusion, and Emax was considerably decreased compared to the control value. The depressed Emax and its rise to the control level with Ca^{2+} without myocardial necrosis qualify these postischemic hearts as stunned. This contractile reserve suggests that the depressed contractility was not due to the deficiency of energy supply. The Vo_2-PVA relation was only minimally shifted downward despite the decrease in Emax. The slope of the Vo_2-PVA relation was decreased after 20 min of reperfusion and returned toward the preischemic level at 60 min of reperfusion but was less than the control. After 1 or 2 h of reperfusion the Emax gradually recovered halfway (about 60% of control), but the PVA-independent Vo_2 recovered to almost the preischemic level (about 95% of the control). This result indicates that the PVA-independent Vo_2 increased in disproportion to the Emax.

In this stunned myocardium, the O_2 cost of Emax, determined with increased intracoronary Ca^{2+} infusion, was almost doubled compared to that of the preischemic control. For a given Emax, the PVA-independent Vo_2 in excess of basal metabolism was therefore about 2.2 times greater after stunning. This finding could be one reason for the hardly changed PVA-independent Vo_2 of the stunned hearts despite the decreased Emax. Therefore stunning is the first discovered intervention that significantly increased the O_2 cost of Emax [9].

The increased O_2 cost of Emax means that more Vo_2 is needed for Ca^{2+} handling to keep Emax constant. This condition occurs when the Ca^{2+} sensitivity of the contractile machinery is decreased, when the SR becomes leaky and futile Ca^{2+} cycling is increased, when the transsarcolemmal Na^+-Ca^{2+} exchange is increased, or with some or all of these conditions. In stunned myocardium a Ca^{2+} transient increased despite a decreased contractile force [95], which indicates decreased Ca^{2+} sensitivity of the contractile machinery. The SR is shown to be leaky during ischemia but to recover after reperfusion [96]. These findings suggest a key role of the decreased Ca^{2+} sensitivity of the contractile proteins in the increased O_2 cost of Emax in stunned myocardium. However, it is possible that either increased Ca^{2+} permeability of the SR membrane or increased Na^+-Ca^{2+} exchange may be a factor.

Hypercapnic Acidotic Myocardium

Acidosis is known to produce myocardial contractile dysfunction [97-100], and modification of the function of the SR [100, 101] has been proposed as the mechanism of the mechanical dysfunction during acidosis. The decreased Ca^{2+} sensitivity during acidosis suggests that an acidotic ventricle requires a higher intracellular Ca^{2+} concentration than a normal ventricle when the contractility is enhanced to the same level. Therefore a decrease in Ca^{2+} sensitivity may adversely increase the Vo_2 for Ca^{2+} handling during E-C coupling.

A stable acidosis of the excised cross-circulated canine LV was successfully induced and maintained without hypoxia by appropriately mixing CO_2 and air in a membrane oxygenator in the coronary arterial perfusion circuit [10]. The coronary venous blood from the right ventricle was exposed to room air so that CO_2 could freely leave the acidotic venous blood. This acidosis protocol had little effect on arterial blood gas and the general condition of the dog for 2–3 h.

Acidosis (pH 7.0, Pco_2 90 mm Hg in coronary arterial blood) decreased the Emax by about 45% and the PVA by about 50% at a fixed LV volume. There was a high, linear correlation between Vo_2 and PVA over a wide PVA range in each control volume run, acidosis volume run, and acidosis volume run during infusion of Ca^{2+}. The slope of the Vo_2–PVA relation was significantly decreased by acidosis without significantly decreasing PVA-independent Vo_2. It seems unlikely that the reciprocal of the slope of the linear Vo_2–PVA relation, contractile efficiency, was truly improved during acidosis. The decreased slope of the Vo_2–PVA relation during acidosis seems to be attributable to the insufficient autoregulatory increase in coronary blood flow in response to increasecd metabolic demands and to the nonlinear end-systolic P-V relation produced by acidotically depressed contractility [10]. When the preacidotic Emax level was restored by Ca^{2+} infusion during acidosis, unloaded Vo_2 exceeded the control value by about 20%, indicating that acidosis required a higher Vo_2 for nonmechanical activities at a matched Emax. Moreover, during acidosis the O_2 cost of Emax was 1.5 times higher than at preacidosis. Therefore acidosis produced LV contractile dysfunction accompanied by an increased O_2 cost of Emax. This increased energy cost of Emax can be due to decreased Ca^{2+} sensitivity of the contractile proteins during acidosis.

Stunned Myocardium After Rapid Correction of Acidosis

Left ventricular contractile dysfunction during acidosis has been reported to be almost reversible in crystalloid-perfused hearts after correction of acidosis [98, 102]. In contrast, in the excised cross-circulated canine heart during rapid correction of acidosis, a severe transient overshoot of Emax (400% of acidosis) occurred [11]. However, after the correction, Emax and PVA were lower than the preacidosis values by 46% and 44% at the same LV volume. When the preacidosis Emax level was restored by Ca^{2+} infusion, the Vo_2 intercept of the linear Vo_2–PVA relation exceeded the control value by 18% with an unchanged slope. Contractile efficiency was unchanged in the post-acidotic heart. In addition, the O_2 cost of Emax after correction of acidosis was 1.8 times higher than that of the control, indicating that postacidotic myocardium requires a higher Vo_2 for nonmechanical activities (basal metabolism and E-C coupling) for a unit increase in Emax. Because basal metabolic Vo_2 in the postacidotic myocardium was similar to the previously reported value in the normal heart, the increased Vo_2 for E-C coupling must be responsible for the increased PVA-independent Vo_2 in the postacidotic myocardium. It was hypothesized that these mechanoenergetic disorders after rapid correction of acidosis would result from transient Ca^{2+} overload that occurred within a few minutes via accelerated Na^+–Ca^{2+} exchange (reverse direction) due to the heavily operating Na^+–H^+ exchange to carry H^+ out of myocytes at the time of rapid pH recovery.

To examine this hypothesis, dimethylamiloride (DMA) $7\,\mu mol/L$ was administered for 3 min just before the correction of acidosis (CO_2 discontinuation). DMA is a potent, selective Na^+–H^+ exchange inhibitor. DMA completely prevented both the mechanical and energetic disorders after correction of acidosis. These results indicated that rapid recovery of pH paradoxically depressed myocardial contractility and increased the O_2 cost of Emax through activation of Na^+–H^+ exchange. That is, at the time of rapid pH recovery, intracellular Ca^{2+} increased transiently within a few minutes through accelerated Na^+–Ca^{2+} exchange due to an accumulation of Na^+ via the heavily operating Na^+–H^+ exchange to carry H^+ out of myocytes. The resultant transient Ca^{2+} overload caused severe contractile and energetic disorders.

The mechanoenergetic disorders demonstrated in the postacidotic myocardium are similar to those in the postischemic stunned myocardium; the O_2 cost of Emax in postacidotic stunned myocardium was 1.8 times higher than in the control. The underlying mechanism for the mechanoenergetic disorders of this pathological myocardium seems to be the transient Ca^{2+} overload resulting from accelerated Na^+–H^+ and Na^+–Ca^{2+} exchanges.

It is well known that Ca^{2+} sensitivity of the contractile protein is decreased by accumulated H^+ during acidosis. Under decreased Ca^{2+} sensitivity, more Ca^{2+} is needed to activate the contractile protein to the same force level, which means that the SR must hydrolyze more ATP by the Ca^{2+} pump ATPase to sequester more Ca^{2+}, which should lead to an increased PVA-independent Vo_2 at a given Emax during acidosis. This mechanism may account for the 1.5 times higher O_2 cost of contractility in acidotic myocardium [10].

In contrast, in postischemic stunned myocardium [9] the possibility of either a decreased molar coupling ratio of Ca^{2+}-ATP by SR Ca^{2+} pump ATPase or increased transsarcolemmal Na^+–Ca^{2+} exchange should be considered in addition to the decreased Ca^{2+} sensitivity of the contractile machinery as mentioned above. This additional mechanism would explain the somewhat higher O_2 cost of Emax in postischemic stunned myocardium than in acidotic myocardium (2.2 versus 1.5 times higher than normal) [9, 10]. Ryanodine also significantly decreased Emax by 42%, whereas PVA-independent Vo_2 remained disproportionately high (93% of control) [103]. This result suggests that ryanodine suppresses force generation of cardiac muscle for a given amount of total sequestered Ca^{2+} by SR similarly to that seen with myocardial ischemia and stunning [9, 11]. That is, ryanodine seems to make SR leaky for Ca^{2+}, thereby wasting energy for Ca^{2+} handling by SR [103].

Intermediately impaired O_2 cost of contractility in postacidotic stunned myocardium (1.8 times higher than normal) suggests that mechanisms of decreased Ca^{2+} sensitivity and SR dysfunction both exist. These results of O_2 cost of Emax are summarized in Fig. 3A.

Postacidotic stunned myocardium might be a pure expression of transient Ca^{2+} overload. Therefore we intended to produce the transient Ca^{2+}-overloaded myocardium alternatively by coronary perfusion with Ca^{2+}-free and high-Ca^{2+} Tyrode solution.

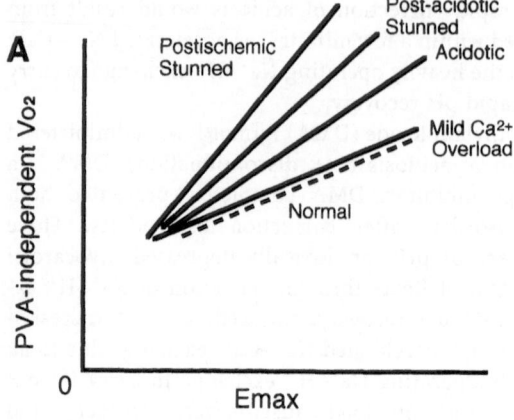

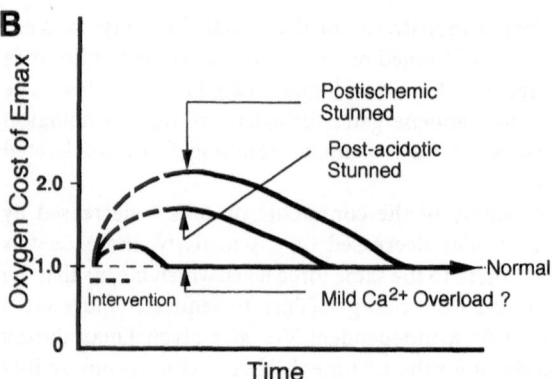

FIG. 3. **A** Oxygen costs of Emax enhanced with Ca^{2+} in normal hearts (*dashed line*), mild Ca^{2+} overloaded hearts, acidotic hearts, and postacidotic and postischemic stunned (*solid lines*) hearts, respectively. **B** Conceptual illustration of the time course and degrees of changes in oxygen costs of Emax (or the insult induced by Ca^{2+} overload) during and after each intervention in postischemic and postacidotic stunned hearts and mild Ca^{2+}-overloaded hearts

Ca^{2+}-Overloaded Myocardium

We tried to develop a new Ca^{2+}-overloading protocol to produce mild acute myocardial failure in the excised, cross-circulated canine heart preparation [52]. We initially could not produce cardiac dysfunction by either high Ca^{2+} (16 mmol/L) perfusion alone (to cause transient Ca^{2+} overload) or Ca^{2+}-free Tyrode perfusion alone for 10 min (to cause transient Ca^{2+} overload after Ca^{2+} depletion—(Ca^{2+} para-dox). We finally produced cardiac failure via a new, severer Ca^{2+}-overloading protocol that combined Ca^{2+} depletion with transient Ca^{2+} overload without ischemia. This new Ca^{2+}-overloading protocol consisted of coronary perfusion of Ca^{2+}-free Tyrode solution for 10 min followed by perfusion of high-Ca^{2+} Tyrode solution (16 mmol/L) for 5 min under a hydrostatic pressure of 80–90 cm H_2O intervening the blood cross-circulation. The last perfusion with normal-Ca^{2+} Tyrode solution (1.8 mmol/L) for 5 min before returning to the cross-circulation avoided any return of the high-Ca^{2+} solution into the support dog. We assessed cardiac mechanoenergetics and ultrastructural changes in these Ca^{2+}-overloaded failing hearts.

We succeeded in producing acute failing hearts (transiently Ca^{2+}-overloaded failing hearts) without myocardial ultrastructural changes using the Ca^{2+}-overloading proto-col. With this protocol LV contraction disappeared during the first Ca^{2+}-free Tyrode perfusion. The contraction was potentiated during the next high-Ca^{2+} Tyrode perfusion, but tonic contracture was not observed in any case. LV pressure during the high-Ca^{2+} period at the fixed LV volume reached about 160% of control. LV pressure fell markedly to about 30% by normal-Ca^{2+} Tyrode perfusion and recovered gradually over 50 min of blood recirculation to about 60% of control. Emax and PVA followed the same time course.

No significant changes in EDP were observed except for 10 min of blood recirculation when the EDP increased significantly to about 20% of control end-systolic pressure (ESP) and gradually returned toward control (2% of control ESP). Hence there were no significant differences between EDP in the control and Ca^{2+}-overload volume runs.

Coronary flow increased during the Ca^{2+}-free Tyrode perfusion, reaching maximum at about 400% of control. It then decreased during the high-Ca^{2+} Tyrode perfusion and increased during the normal-Ca^{2+} Tyrode perfusion. It then gradually decreased over 50 min of blood recirculation but remained above control in all the hearts.

The slopes of the Vo_2-PVA relation were 1.6×10^{-5} ml $O_2 \cdot$ mm Hg$^{-1} \cdot$ ml^{-1} for the control volume runs and 1.3×10^{-5} ml $O_2 \cdot$ mm Hg$^{-1} \cdot$ ml^{-1} for the Ca^{2+}-overload volume runs. There were no significant differences between these two slopes. PVA-independent Vo_2 values for the Ca^{2+}-overload volume runs were significantly smaller (70% of control) than those for the control volume runs. However, the O_2 cost of Emax, or the slope of the PVA-independent Vo_2-Emax relation, for the control Ca^{2+} run was close to that for the Ca^{2+}-overload run.

Therefore our Ca^{2+}-overloaded failing hearts had no increase in EDP at a given LV volume, a 40% decrease in Emax, and a proportional decrease in the PVA-independent Vo_2 for 1-4 h but no decrease in the O_2 cost of PVA defined as the slope of the Vo_2-PVA relation. $CaCl_2$ infusion normalized the depressed Emax and PVA-independent Vo_2. There was no difference in the O_2 cost of Emax for Ca^{2+} between the control and the present Ca^{2+}-overloaded hearts.

These results indicate that this protocol induced transient Ca^{2+} overload, probably due to sarcoplasmic Ca^{2+} repletion facilitated by an increased sarcolemmal Ca^{2+} permeability caused by Ca^{2+} depletion (Ca^{2+} paradox mechanism) [104, 105]. We concluded that even the transient Ca^{2+} overload without ischemia can produce mild acute heart failure.

The O_2 costs of PVA and Emax were not changed by the transient Ca^{2+} overload evoked by the present Ca^{2+} paradox (Ca^{2+} depletion)–Ca^{2+} overload protocol, as shown in Fig. 3A. The O_2 cost of PVA reflects the product of the PVA/ATP coupling ratio in the contractile machinery (CB cycling) and the ATP/Vo_2 coupling ratio in the mitochondria (mitochondrial oxidative phosphorylation) [7]. Therefore we believe that neither the PVA/ATP coupling ratio nor the ATP/Vo_2 coupling ratio was changed by the transient Ca^{2+} overload.

The O_2 cost of Emax reflects the product of the contractility/Ca^{2+} coupling ratio of the contractile machinery and the Ca^{2+}/ATP coupling ratio in the SR, and the ATP/Vo_2 coupling ratio. Therefore we believe that the transient Ca^{2+} overload neither produced decreased myofilament Ca^{2+} responsiveness (contractility/Ca^{2+} handling relation) nor increased the Ca^{2+} handling/ATP ratio. It seems likely that the amount of Ca^{2+} handled during E-C coupling is proportional to the myocardial contractility in the Ca^{2+}-overloaded failing heart. Therefore the decreased Emax seems to be due to a decreased amount of Ca^{2+} handled during E-C coupling.

We conclude that the present transient Ca^{2+} overload without ischemia induced LV contractile failure, primarily involving the suppression of Ca^{2+} handling energy for E-C coupling unlike the postischemic stunned, acidotic, and postacidotic stunned hearts.

In the mechanoenergetic study of the postischemic stunned heart by Ohgoshi et al. [9], PVA-independent Vo_2 did not decrease proportional to the Emax, and the O_2 cost of Emax was 2.2 times higher than that of the control. In acidotic myocardium, the O_2 cost of Emax was 1.5 times higher than in the control [10], and in postacidotic stunned myocardium it was 1.8 times higher than normal [11], as shown in Fig. 3A. The energetic changes in these pathological hearts were considered due to decreased responsiveness of the contractile machinery to Ca^{2+}, an increased Ca^{2+} handling/ATP ratio by futile Ca^{2+} cycling, or increased Na^+–Ca^{2+} exchange at the sarcolemma [9–11]. There are many studies suggesting the same mechanisms in the stunned, transient Ca^{2+}-overloaded myocardium [106–108].

However, transient Ca^{2+}-overloaded failing hearts produced by Ca^{2+} overloading after the Ca^{2+}-depleting protocol demonstrated mechanoenergetic aspects different from those of the postacidotic [11] and postischemic [9] stunned myocardium, although Emax was depressed to comparable degrees [9, 11]. The qualitatively different mechanoenergetics in these pathological hearts might derive from the different time courses and degrees of changes in O_2 cost of Emax or the degree of the insult induced by the Ca^{2+} overload, as shown in Fig. 3B.

Our transient Ca^{2+}-overloading protocol, like treatment with β-blockers such as propranolol [50] and nipradilol [49], lowered the Vo_2–PVA relation in a parallel manner. Therefore this failing heart could be characterized by a decrease in the total amount of Ca^{2+} handling during E-C coupling. Possible mechanisms responsible for this decreased Ca^{2+} handling include a depression in the transsarcolemmal Ca^{2+} flux (channel or pump mediated) and a reduction in the amount of Ca^{2+} stored in the SR.

Role of Na^+–H^+ and Na^+–Ca^{2+} Exchange Systems

The role of Na^+–Ca^{2+} and Na^+–H^+ exchanges in failing hearts are vitally important for their generation and recovery [9–11, 52, 79]. The Na^+–Ca^{2+} exchange is electrogenic and sensitive to membrane potential. The time course with which Ca^{2+} is extruded is influenced by the time course of the membrane potential. All the Ca^{2+} entering the cell during the initial depolarization seems to be extruded by the Na^+–Ca^{2+} exchange [69]. It appears that Ca^{2+} influx via Na^+–Ca^{2+} exchange (reverse mode) can also occur during the initial depolarization of cardiac cells. This process may be further stimulated by subsarcolemmal rises in Na^+ concentration caused by Na^+ influx via the cardiac Na^+ channel. However, whether it occurs during normal E-C coupling remains controversial [69].

As the intracellular Ca^{2+} concentration subsequently begins to rise as a result of Ca^{2+} release from the SR, the reverse potential for Na^+–Ca^{2+} exchange becomes greater than the plateau of the membrane potential. The Na^+–Ca^{2+} exchange then operates in a Ca^{2+} efflux–Na^+ influx "forward" mode. However, the weight of this Na^+–Ca^{2+} exchange during extrusion of cytosolic Ca^{2+}, especially in failing hearts, is still controversial [69, 79].

Mechanoenergetic disorders after rapid correction of acidosis [11] is considered to result from transient Ca^{2+} overload via accelerated Na^+–Ca^{2+} exchange (reverse mode) owing to the heavily operating Na^+–H^+ exchange to carry H^+ out of myocytes at the time of rapid pH recovery. The same mechanisms may be present in the postischemic stunned myocardium [9] and the transient Ca^{2+}-overloaded myocardium evoked by Ca^{2+}-free and high-Ca^{2+} Tyrode perfusion [52].

Pentobarbital Sodium-Treated Myocardium

Pentobarbital sodium (PS) is an anesthetic widely used in animal experiments. We have used it in our experiments as well. It is known as a cardiovascular depressant and a coronary dilator, but its effects on myocardial energetics with its negative or positive (due to Gregg's phenomenon) inotropism have not been reported. Therefore we wanted to clarify whether and how PS per se would affect cardiac mechanoenergetics compared with other negative inotropic agents.

We investigated the effects of graded doses of intracoronary infusions of PS on the mechanoenergetics in canine excised cross-circulated left ventricles [43]. PS increased Emax at low doses in 5 of 12 hearts. Marked coronary dilation was found in two of the five hearts. PS decreased Emax dose-dependently at high doses (>19 mg/ml blood) in all the hearts and lowered the Vo_2–PVA relation in a parallel manner with the same O_2 cost of PVA. The O_2 cost of Emax was comparable for PS and $CaCl_2$, which have opposite inotropism. These findings suggest that PS depresses myocardial mechanoenergetics, like β-blockers and Ca^{2+} antagonists, via suppression of total Ca^{2+} handling during E-C coupling.

We conclude that PS at low doses acts partly as a positive inotropic agent but at high doses acts as a negative inotropic agent on cardiac mechanoenergetics. At high doses PS produced an acute failing heart.

Capsaicin-Treated Myocardium

Capsaicin selectively acts on sensory nerve endings in cardiac muscles and coronary arterial smooth muscles. Capsaicin at high doses has cell-nonselective effects including both inhibition of cardiac muscle excitability and enhancement of vascular smooth muscle tone. We studied whether and how intracoronary infusion of capsaicin affects the mechanoenergetics of the excised blood-perfused canine heart and coronary vascular resistance. We found that capsaicin at low concentrations (0.4–2.8 μmol/L blood) increased the Vo_2 and Emax by 8–30% possibly due to a specific action on capsaicin-sensitive sensory nerves, such as releasing a neuropeptide, calcitonin gene-related polypeptide (CGRP) in LV muscles, though in only 3 of 10 hearts [51]. This result coincides with the reported histochemical observations that the distribution of capsaicin-sensitive sensory nerves in the canine left ventricle is not dense. Capsaicin at high doses dose-dependently halved Emax and proportionally decreased coronary flow. The maximum intracoronary infusion rate of capsaicin was 77 ± 40 μg/min, which corresponded to 7.4 ± 5.3 μmol/L blood at a coronary blood flow of 58 ± 37 ml/min.

It also lowered the linear Vo_2–PVA relation with the same O_2 cost of PVA, decreasing unloaded Vo_2. These effects of capsaicin at high doses seem to be a direct negative inotropic action on cardiac muscles associated with enhancement of coronary arterial smooth muscle tone, as these effects were not desensitized. No morphological changes in myocardial cells or mitochondria were detected. Therefore the negative inotropic action is not due to the toxic effect of capsaicin.

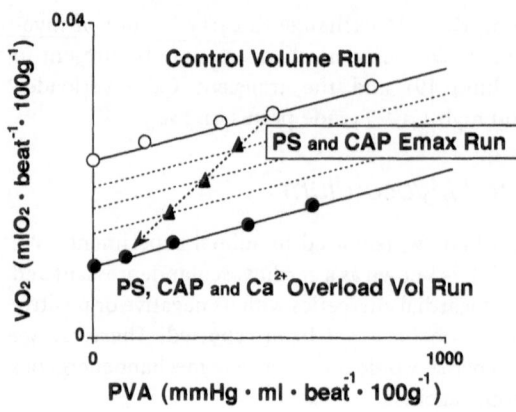

FIG. 4. Vo_2–PVA relations during a control volume loading run (*open circles*), during a pentobarbital (*PS*) and capsaicin (*CAP*) inotropism run (*Emax run*) (*solid triangles*), and during a PS, CAP, and Ca^{2+} overload volume loading run (*solid circles*)

Capsaicin also produced an acute failing heart, the mechanoenergetics of which are qualitatively similar to PS-treated acute failing hearts. These results are shown in Fig. 4.

Assessment of Mitochondrial Respiratory Function

The O_2 cost of PVA and the contractile efficiency can be considered to represent the overall efficiency of the energy conversion from O_2 to PVA via oxidative phosphorylation and CB cycling [7]. A greater coefficient a of the PVA-dependent Vo_2 (i.e., aPVA) means a greater O_2 cost of PVA and less contractile efficiency, suggesting increased inefficiency of oxidative phosphorylation or CB cycling, or both [7]. The efficiency of oxidative phosphorylation is related to the P/O ratio (the atomic ratio of ATP produced to O_2 consumed in the mitochondria). Therefore we considered that measuring the P/O ratio in the mitochordria (Mt) would help us to better understand the underlying mechanisms of altered contractile efficiency.

Left ventricular myocardial Mt were prepared from excised canine hearts. Differential centrifugation was used according to the method of Hatefi et al. [109]. Immediately after Mt preparation, the Mt Vo_2 was measured polarographically with an O_2 electrode installed in a closed cell (UC-12; Central Kagaku, Tokyo, Japan) at 25°C. The incubation medium contained 0.3 M mannitol, KH_2PO_4, 10 mmol/L, $MgCl_2$ 2.5 mmol/L, and ethylenediaminetetra-acetate (EDTA) 0.25 mmol/L at pH 7.4 in a total solution of 0.7 ml. Respiration was initiated by adding 0.03 ml of Mt suspension (15.6 ± 3.7 mg protein/ml); 0.2 M succinic acid (0.03 ml) as substrate and 10 mmol/L adenosine diphosphate (ADP) (0.03 ml = 300 ng atom) were added. The rate of Vo_2 in state III (state III O_2), the P/O ratio (i.e., ADP/O ratio), and the respiratory control index (RCI) were determined. State III O_2 was calculated from Mt Vo_2 in nanogram atoms (1 mol O_2 = 2 g atoms O) of O_2 consumed per minute per milligram of Mt protein during state III respiration. The ADP/O ratio was calculated as 300 ng atom/VO_2 in nanogram atoms of O_2 in state III. RCI (dimensionless) was taken as the ratio between the rates of Vo_2 before and after the addition of ADP. Succinate was used as a metabolic substrate.

State III Oxygen

Mitochondria oxidize the substrate in the electron transmission system and perform oxidative phosphorylation using the oxidation-reduction energy released during this process. Physiologically, electron transport and ATP synthesis are coupled. When the ADP supply for Mt is insufficient, the electron transport reaction is strongly depressed. Chance's state III is obtained by adding the substrate and ADP. In this state oxidative phosphorylation proceeds most effectively and results in the most active Mt respiration. State III O_2 reflects the activity of the entire electron transport system. State III O_2, at least in canine normal Mt, ranges between about 300 and 400 ng atom·min^{-1}·mg protein^{-1}.

Respiratory Control Index

A high RCI indicates good coupling of Mt oxidative phosphorylation and a high rate of oxidative phosphorylation. RCI also indicates the intactness of the Mt. When succinate is used as a substrate, which enters the citric acid (or tricarboxylic acid, TCA) cycle on its way, the RCI ranges between 4 and 5 (dimensionless).

P/O Ratio

The P/O ratio can be used as an index of the efficiency of oxidative phosphorylation. This value depends on the substrate used. Theoretically, succinate yields a value of 2, ascorbic acid 1, and pyruvic acid 3. P/O is obtained as the ADP/O ratio in normal Mt. However, in pathophysiological Mt, phosphorylation is depressed. In such a state, obtaining P/O ratio by this method is meaningless. Therefore we used state III O_2 and the RCI for estimating Mt respiratory function in pathophysiological mitochondria.

Mitochondria from Transient Ca^{2+}-Overloaded Myocardium

We prepared Mt from canine normal hearts and the transient Ca^{2+}-overloaded acute failing canine hearts produced by intracoronary perfusion of Ca^{2+}-free and high-Ca^{2+} Tyrode solution mentioned above. The RCI and state III O_2 of these two Mt preparations were compared. In the transient Ca^{2+}-overloaded myocardial Mt the RCI was about 76% of normal, and state III O_2 was about 54% of normal—significantly different results. These results, shown in Fig. 5 [129], indicate that the rate of oxidative phosphorylation in the Mt from transient Ca^{2+}-overloaded hearts was depressed, but they did not provide any information about the changes in the P/O ratio.

Remaining Problems and Perspectives

Analysis of Cardiac Function in Small Animals

An eight-electrode conductance catheter (7F, 10 cm) developed by Baan et al. [110] has been applied to large animals such as dogs and to humans to measure instantaneously the absolute LV volume quantitatively. For calibration Baan et al. developed the formula

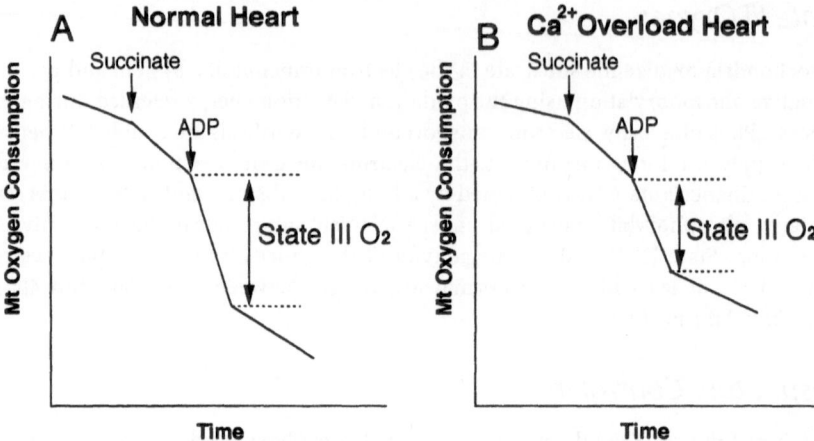

FIG. 5. Mitochondrial (*Mt*) oxygen consumption curves in normal heart and transient Ca^{2+}-overloaded heart. Succinate is added as a substrate. After addition of adenosine diphosphate (*ADP*), Mt respiration is enhanced. Oxygen consumption during this period (*state III O₂*) is measured as an index of Mt respiratory function. The ratio of the slope of the oxygen consumption curve after addition of ADP versus the control slope is also calculated as the respiratory control index (RCI). State III O_2 and RCI in the Ca^{2+}-overloaded heart (**B**) were smaller than those in normal heart (**A**)

$$V(t) = (1/\alpha)(L^2/\sigma_b)G(t) - V_c$$

where $V(t)$ is the time-varying LV volume, α is a dimensionless constant, L is the electrode separation, σ_b is the conductivity of blood obtained by a sampling cuvet, and $G(t)$ is the measured conductance within the LV cavity. V_c is a correction term needed because of the parallel conductance of structures surrounding the cavity; it is measured by transiently changing σ_b by injecting a small bolus of hypertonic saline into the left ventricle. Only when appropriately installed does this conductance catheter provide a reliable, simple method for measuring instantaneously the LV volume [110–112]. When the pressure was recorded simultaneously, we were able to assess LV pump performance by displaying P-V loops. For rabbits, a miniaturized conductance catheter (3.5F, 3 cm) was devised by Solda et al. [113]. It was equipped with six equidistant cylindrical electrodes that were 5 mm from each other. Using this conductance catheter, it is easy to monitor beat-to-beat LV volume changes in smaller, less expensive experimental animals than dogs.

We have instituted use of a miniaturized conductance catheter (3F, 1.2 cm) for rats. It is equipped with six equidistant (3 mm) ring electrodes. The current is delivered by a signal conditioner-processor (our custom-made apparatus for rats; S·I Medicotech Co., Osaka, Japan). With this conductance catheter system and a micromanometer-tipped transducer, we obtained dynamic P-V loops by changing the afterload with a temporary aortic occlusion, as shown in Fig. 6 [130]. This procedure enables us to obtain Emax so as to assess contractile states in situ in small experimental animals such as rats. Furthermore, this conductance catheter system is expected to be developed for mice and hamsters smaller than rats. When the conductance catheter system for these small animals is instituted, it will be easy to obtain dynamic P-V loops and

FIG. 6. Example of rat LV pressure–volume loops obtained with our newly developed conductance catheter while changing the afterload using a temporary aortic occlusion

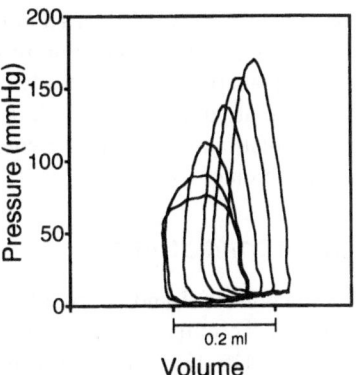

Volume

estimate cardiac pump function more appropriately. For example, various types of transgenic mice (e.g., those with Na^+/H^+ antiporter over-expression and endothelin-1 deficiency) can be used for analyzing the function of a specific gene at the whole-body level. Pathological model animals, such as cardiomyopathic hamsters (Bio 14.6 & Bio 53.58), can also be used for analyzing pathological features at the whole-body level.

Simulation Studies

Our recent simulation study yielded quantitative relations between the energy consumption specifically for intramyocardial Ca^{2+} handling during E-C coupling and the contractile force at different Ca^{2+} sensitivities of contractile machinery [114]. Although intracellular Ca^{2+} is measurable, neither the total amount of Ca^{2+} released and then removed nor the Ca^{2+} bound with troponin C is easily measurable in beating myocardium. Therefore this simulation study was conducted to visualize quantitatively how the total Ca^{2+} handling would change with Ca^{2+} sensitivity. The model consisted simply of the SR, sarcoplasm, troponin C (Tn), and CB. The relations among the released Ca^{2+} from the SR, peak concentrations of sarcoplasmic Ca^{2+} and Ca^{2+}-bound troponin ([TnCa]), and peak contractile force were computed based on the assumptions that the released Ca^{2+} diffuses as free Ca^{2+} in the sarcoplasm, binds kinetically with Tn with an association rate constant of k1, dissociates from TnCa with a dissociation rate constant of k2, and is sequestered into the SR with ATP consumption. TnCa was associated with CB cycling to develop force with a set of given on-and-off rate constants. When the association constant ka (= k1/k2) of Tn as an index of Ca^{2+} sensitivity of Tn was varied 32 fold from 0.25 to 8.00/μM around a normal value of 2.00/μM, the Ca^{2+} handling energy at any given peak force level decreased more steeply in the subnormal range of Ka than in the normal range of Ka. This nonlinearity indicates that the Ca^{2+} handling energy saving for a given increase in Ka is considerably greater in a subnormal Ka range.

This simulation suggests the possibility that the O_2 cost of Emax is variably improved by a Ca^{2+} sensitizer; the improvement is more effective below a normal Ka level. This nonlinearity may partly account for the consistent failure to observe a decreased O_2 cost of Emax for new cardiotonic agents with Ca^{2+}-sensitizing effects, such as pimobendan and EMD-53998 [115–118]. However, the Ca^{2+} sensitivity of the contractile elements decreased in failing hearts, such as stunned [9, 11] and acidotic hearts [10, 95]. The simulation results suggest that Ca^{2+} sensitization may save Ca^{2+} handling energy more effectively in these failing hearts than in normal hearts. If the cooperativity during Ca^{2+} binding to Tn and CB attachment were incorporated into the simulation, Ca^{2+} handling energy would be more effectively reduced with Ca^{2+} sensitization of troponin C.

Arrhythmia Studies

Both exponential and alternans decays of postextrasystolic potentiation have been shown to accompany corresponding changes in Ca^{2+} transients during individual beats [86, 119–122]. The exponential decay of Ca^{2+} transients has been explained by the delay of Ca^{2+} transfer from Ca^{2+} uptake to its release in the SR [86, 119, 123, 124]. The recirculation fraction of intracellular Ca^{2+} within the myocardium is also considered to be involved in exponential decay [119]. Dependence of the action potential duration, and hence Ca^{2+} influx, on contractility during each individual beat and its influence on the next beat might also be involved in exponential decay [125, 126].

The Ca^{2+} transfer delay within the SR can also account for both sustained and transient alternans [120, 126]. When the SR was made permeable to Ca^{2+} by caffeine or ryanodine, both sustained and transient alternans, were abolished [120]. The Ca^{2+} handling function of the SR is therefore considered to be indispensable to the generation and maintenance of the alternans [120]. Therefore assessment of both exponential and alternans decays of postextrasystolic potentiation would be helpful for better understanding of the intracellular Ca^{2+} dynamics within the myocardium.

We found that postextrasystolic potentiated contractility after a spontaneous extrasystole most frequently decayed as a transient alternans over several beats in excised, cross-circulated, atrially paced canine hearts [127]. This type of heart preparation, which we have been using consistently in mechanoenergetic studies [1, 7, 43, 51, 52], had normal coronary blood perfusion pressure and mechanoenergetic performance. Spontaneous atrial and ventricular extrasystoles occurred occasionally in every heart. Postextrasystoles usually decayed as transient alternans, whereas they rarely decayed exponentially against the general finding mentioned above. The compensatory pause after either an atrial or ventricular extrasystole was essential for the postextrasystolic transient alternans. Artificially produced atrial or ventricular extrasystoles showed the same pattern as the postextrasystolic transient alternans.

We concluded that the alternans decays of atrial and ventricular extrasystoles occurred even in the normal heart. Additional studies of the postextrasystolic transient alternans would provide us with new insights into not only intracellular Ca^{2+} dynamics within the normal and failing myocardium but also energetics related to Ca^{2+} handling via the Ca^{2+} pumps and the Na^{+}–Ca^{2+} exchange during E-C coupling.

Acknowledgments. We greatly thank Dr. T. Akashi, a postgraduate student, and Drs. T. Namba and K. Ishioka, anesthesiologists, for surgical assistance. This study was partly supported by Grants-in-Aid for Scientific Research (04237219, 04454267, 04557041, 05305007, 06213226, 06770494, 07508003, 07770508) from the Ministry of

Education, Science, and Culture; Research Grants for Cardiovascular Diseases (3A-2, 4C-4, 7C-2) and on Aging and Health from the Ministry of Health and Welfare; 1994 and 1995 Joint Research Grant Utilizing Scientific and Technological Potential in Regions from the Science and Technology Agency; and a Research Grant from the Foundation of Sanyo Broadcasting, all of Japan.

References

1. Suga H, Goto Y (1991) Cardiac oxygen costs of contractility (Emax) and mechanical energy (PVA): new key concepts in cardiac energetics. In: Sasayama S, Suga H (eds) Recent progress in failing heart syndrome. Springer, Berlin Heidelberg New York Tokyo, pp 61–115
2. Drake-Holland AJ, Noble MIM (1983) Cardiac metabolism, Wiley, New York
3. Gibbs CL (1978) Cardiac energetics. Physiol Rev 58:174–254
4. Gibbs CL, Chapman JB (1979) Cardiac energetics. In: Bern RM, Sperelakis N, Geiger SR (eds) Handbook of physiology: the cardiovascular system 1. American Physiological Society, Bethesda, pp 775–804
5. Gibbs CL (1982) Modification of the physiological determinants of cardiac energy expenditure by pharmacological agents. Pharmacol Ther 18:133–157
6. Chapman JB (1983) Heat production. In: Drake-Holland AJ, Noble MIM (eds) Cardiac metabolism. Wiley, New York, pp 239–256
7. Suga H (1990) Ventricular energetics. Physiol Rev 70:247–277
8. Takaki M, Namba T, Araki J, Ishioka K, Ito H, Akashi T, Zhao L-Y, Zhao D-D, Liu M, Fujii W, Suga H (1993) How to measure cardiac energy expenditure. In: Preusse CJ, Piper HM (eds) Ischemia-reperfusion in cardiac surgery. Kluwer Academic, Dordrecht, pp 403–419
9. Ohgoshi Y, Goto Y, Futaki S, Yaku H, Kawaguchi O, Suga H (1991) Increased oxygen cost of contractility in stunned myocardium of dog. Circ Res 69:975–988
10. Hata K, Goto Y, Kawaguchi O, Takasago T, Saeki A, Nishioka T, Suga H (1994) Hypercapnic acidosis increases oxygen cost of contractility in the dog left ventricle. Am J Physiol 266:H730–H740
11. Hata K, Takasago T, Saeki A, Nishioka T, Goto Y (1994) Stunned myocardium after rapid correction of acidosis. Circ Res 74:794–805
12. Coleman HN, Sonnenblick EH, Braunwald E (1969) Myocardial oxygen consumption associated with external work: the Fenn effect. Am J Physiol 217:291–296
13. Suga H (1979) Total mechanical energy of a ventricular model and cardiac oxygen consumption. Am J Physiol 236:H498–H505
14. Suga H (1990) Cardiac mechanics and energetics—from Emax to PVA. Front Med Biol Eng 2:3–22
15. Suga H (1969) Time course of left ventricular pressure-volume relationship under various end-diastolic volumes. Jpn Heart J 10:509–515
16. Suga H (1971) Theoretical analysis of a left ventricular pumping model based on the systolic time-varying pressure/volume ratio. IEEE Trans Biomed Eng 18:47–55
17. Sunagawa K, Sagawa K (1982) Models of ventricular contraction based on time-varying elastance. CRC Crit Rev Biomed Eng 7:193–228
18. Sagawa K, Maughan L, Suga H, Sunagawa K (1988) Cardiac contraction and the pressure-volume relationship. Oxford University Press, New York
19. Suga H, Sagawa K, Shoukas AA (1973) Load independence of the instantaneous pressure-volume ratio of the canine left ventricle and effects of epinephrine and heart rate on the ratio. Circ Res 32:314–322
20. Suga H, Sagawa K (1974) Instantaneous pressure-volume relationships and their ratio in the excised, supported canine left ventricle. Circ Res 35:117–126
21. Suga H, Hisano R, Goto Y, Yamada O, Igarashi Y (1983) Effect of positive inotropic agents on the relation between oxygen consumption and systolic pressure-volume in canine left ventricle. Circ Res 53:306–318

22. Sagawa K (1978) The ventricular pressure-volume diagram revised. Circ Res 43:677–687
23. Sagawa K (1981) The end-systolic pressure-volume relation of the ventricle: definition, modification and clinical use. Circulation 63:1223–1227
24. Sagawa K, Sunagawa K, Maughan WL (1985) Ventricular end-systolic pressure-volume relations. In: Levin HJ, Gaasch WH (eds) The ventricle: basic and clinical aspects. Nijhoff, Boston, pp 79–103
25. Suga H, Sagawa K (1972) Mathematical interrelationship between instantaneous ventricular pressure-volume ratio and myocardial force-velocity relation. Ann Biomed Eng 1:160–181
26. Shroff SG, Janicki JS, Weber KT (1983) Left ventricular systolic dynamics in terms of its chamber mechanical properties. Am J Physiol 245:H110–H124
27. Suga H, Yamada O, Goto Y (1984) Comments on "pressure-volume relationship in isolated cat trabecular which appeared in Circ Res 49:388–394, 1981." Circ Res 54:208–209
28. Suga H (1979) External mechanical work from relaxing ventricle. Am J Physiol 236:H494–H497
29. Suga H (1980) Relaxing ventricle performs more external work than quickly released elastic energy. Eur Heart J 1(suppl A):131–137
30. Suga H (1979) Total internal mechanical work of ventricle assessed from quick release pressure-volume curve. Jpn J Physiol 29:227–237
31. Suga H, Sagawa K, Demer L (1980) Determinants of instantaneous pressure in canine left ventricle: time and volume specification. Circ Res 46:256–263
32. Yasumura Y, Nozawa T, Futaki S, Tanaka N, Suga H (1989) Time-invariant oxygen cost of mechanical energy in dog left ventricle: consistency and inconsistency of time-varying elastance model with myocardial energetics. Circ Res 64:763–778
33. Hunter WC, Janicki JS, Weber KT, Noodergraaf A (1983) Systolic mechanical properties of the left ventricle: effects of volume and contractile state. Circ Res 52:319–327
34. Little WC, Freeman GL (1987) Description of LV pressure-volume relations by time-varying elastance and source resistance. Am J Physiol 253:H83–H90
35. Vaartjes SR, Boom HBK, Boom BK (1987) Left ventricular internal resistance and unloaded ejection flow assessed from pressure-flow relations: a flow-clamp study on isolated rabbit hearts. Circ Res 60:727–737
36. Kawaguchi O, Goto Y, Futaki S, Ohgoshi Y, Yaku H, Hata K, Takasago T, Saeki A, Suga H (1993) Ejecting deactivation does not affect O_2 consumption-pressure-volume area relation in dog hearts. Am J Physiol 265:H934–H942
37. Yasumura Y, Suga H (1988) Cross-bridge model compatible with the linear relation between left ventricular oxygen consumption and pressure-volume area. Jpn Heart J 29:335–347
38. Taylor TW, Goto Y, Suga H (1993) Variable cross-bridge cycling-ATP coupling accounts for cardiac mechanoenergetics. Am J Physiol 264:H994–H1004
39. Woledge RC, Curtin NA, Homsher E (1985) Energetic aspects of muscle contraction. Academic, London
40. Yanagida T, Arata T, Oosawa F (1985) Sliding distance of actin filament induced by a myosin cross-bridge during one ATP hydrolysis cycle. Nature 316:366–369
41. Suga H, Goto Y, Kawaguchi O, Hata K, Takasago T, Saeki A, Taylor TW (1993) Ventricular perspective on efficiency. Basic Res Cardiol 88(suppl 2):43–65
42. Suga H, Futaki S, Ohgoshi Y, Yaku H, Goto Y (1989) Arteriovenous oximeter for O_2 content difference, O_2 saturations, and hemoglobin content. Am J Physiol 257:H1712–H1716
43. Namba T, Takaki M, Araki J, Ishioka K, Suga H (1994) Energetics of the negative and positive inotropism of pentobarbitone sodium in the canine left ventricle. Cardiovasc Res 28:557–564
44. Suga H, Hayashi T, Shirahata M (1981) Ventricular systolic pressure-volume area as predictor of cardiac oxygen consumption. Am J Physiol 240:H39–H44
45. Hisano R, Cooper G IV (1987) Correlation of force-length area with oxygen consumption in ferret papillary muscle. Circ Res 61:318–328

46. Suga H, Hayashi T, Shirahata M, Suehiro S, Hisano R (1981) Regression of cardiac oxygen consumption on ventricular pressure-volume area in dog. Am J Physiol 240:H320–H325

47. Hata K, Goto Y, Suga H (1991) External mechanical work during relaxation period does not affect myocardial oxygen consumption. Am J Physiol 261:H1778–H1784

48. Mast F, Elzing G (1990) Heat released during relaxation equals force-length area in isometric contractions of rabbit papillary muscle. Circ Res 67:893–901

49. Zhao DD, Namba T, Araki J, Ishioka K, Takaki M, Suga H (1993) Nipradilol depresses cardiac contractility and O_2 consumption without decreasing coronary resistance in dogs. Acta Med Okayama 47:29–33

50. Suga H, Goto Y, Yasumura Y, Nozawa T, Futaki S, Tanaka N, Uenishi M (1988) O_2 consumption of dog heart under decreased coronary perfusion and propranolol. Am J Physiol 254:H292–H303

51. Takaki M, Akashi T, Ishioka K, Kikuta A, Matsubara H, Yasuhara S, Fujii W, Suga H (1994) Effects of capsaicin on mechanoenergetics of excised cross-circulated canine left ventricle and coronary artery. J Mol Cell Cardiol 26:1227–1239

52. Araki J, Takaki M, Namba T, Mori M, Suga H (1995) Short-term Ca^{2+} free-high Ca^{2+} coronary perfusion suppresses contractility and excitation-contraction coupling energy in canine hearts. Am J Physiol 268:H1061–H1070

53. Elzinga G (1983) Cardiac oxygen consumption and the production of heat and work. In: Drake-Holland AJ, Noble MIM (eds) Cardiac metabolism. Wiley, New York, pp 173–194

54. Suga H, Goto Y, Futaki S, Kawaguchi O, Yaku H, Hata K, Takasago T (1991) Calcium kinetics and energetics in myocardium: simulation study. Jpn Heart J 32:57–67

55. Ruegg JC (1988) Calcium in muscle activation. Springer, Berlin

56. Burkhoff D, Yue D, Oikawa RY, Franz MR, Schaefer J, Sagawa K (1987) Influence of ventricular contractility on non-work-related myocardial oxygen consumption. Heart Vessels 3:66–72

57. Ohgoshi Y, Goto Y, Futaki S, Yaku H, Kawaguchi O, Suga H (1990) New method to determine oxygen cost for contractility. Jpn J Physiol 40:127–138

58. Yasumura Y, Nozawa T, Futaki S, Tanaka N, Suga H (1989) Minor preload dependence of O_2 consumption of unload contraction in dog heart. Am J Physiol 256:H1289–H1294

59. Tada M, Shigekawa M, Kadoma M, Nimura Y (1989) Uptake of calcium by sarcoplasmic reticulum and its regulation and functional consequences. In: Sperelakis N (ed) Physiology and pathophysiology of the heart, 3rd edn. Kluwer Academic, Boston, pp 267–290

60. Klocke FJ, Braunwald E, Ross J (1966) Oxygen cost of electrical activation of the heart. Circ Res 18:357–365

61. Langer G (1974) Ionic movements and the control of contraction. In: Langer GA, Brady AJ (eds) The mammalian myocardium. Wiley, New York, pp 193–217

62. Langer GA (1968) Ion fluxes in cardiac excitation and contraction and their relation to myocardial contractility. Physiol Rev 48:708–757

63. Chapman JB (1983) Heat production. In: Drake AJ, Noble MIM (eds) Cardiac metabolism. Wiley, Chichester, pp 239–256

64. Nozawa T, Yasumura Y, Futaki S, Tanaka N, Suga H (1988) No significant increase in O_2 consumption of KCl-arrested dog heart with filling and dobutamine. Am J Physiol 255:H807–H812

65. Gibbs CL (1982) Modification of physiological determinants of cardiac energy expenditure by pharmacological agents. Pharmacol Ther 18:133–157

66. DuBell WH, Houser SR (1989) Voltage and beat dependence of the Ca^{2+} transient in feline ventricular myocytes. Am J Physiol 257:H746–H759

67. Beukelmann DJ, Wier WG (1988) Mechanism of release of Ca^{2+} from sarcoplasmic reticulum of guinea-pig cardiac cells. J Physiol (Lond) 405:233–255

68. Niggli E, Lederer WJ (1990) Voltage-independent calcium release in heart muscle. Science 250:565–568

69. Barry WH, Bridge JHB (1993) Intracellular calcium homeostasis in cardiac myocytes. Circulation 87:1806–1815

162   M. Takaki et al.

70. Fabiato A (1983) Calcium induced release of calcium from the cardiac sarcoplasmic reticulum. Am J Physiol 245:C1–C14
71. Moss RL (1992) Ca²⁺ regulation of mechanical properties of striated muscle. Circ Res 70:865–884
72. Fabiato A (1985) Time and calcium dependence of activation and inactivation of calcium-induced release of calcium from sarcoplasmic reticulum of a skinned canine cardiac Purkinje cell. J Gen Physiol 85:247–289
73. Tada M, Katz AM (1982) Phosphorylation of the sarcoplasmic reticulum and sarcolemma. Annu Rev Physiol 44:401–423
74. Tada M, Yamamoto T, Tonomura Y (1978) Molecular mechanism of active calcium transport by sarcoplasmic reticulum. Physiol Rev 58:1–79
75. Allen DG, Kurihara S (1980) Calcium transients in mammalian ventricular muscle. Eur Heart J 1(suppl A):5–15
76. Endoh M, Blinks JR (1988) Actions of sympathomimetic amines on the Ca²⁺ transients and contractions of rabbit myocardium: reciprocal changes in myofibrillar responsiveness to Ca²⁺ mediated through α- and β-adrenoceptors. Circ Res 62:247–265
77. Yue DT, Burkhoff D, Franz MR, Hunter WC, Sagawa K (1985) Postextrasystolic potentiation of the isolated canine left ventricle: relationship to mechanical restitution. Circ Res 56:340–350
78. Katz AM, Repke DI (1985) Calcium-membrane interactions in the myocardium: effects of ouabain, epinephrine, and 3′,5′-cyclic adenosine monophosphate. Am J Cardiol 31:193–201
79. Bassani RA, Bassani JW, Bers DM (1992) Mitochondrial and sarcolemmal Ca²⁺ transports reduce [Ca]ᵢ during caffeine contractures in rabbit cardiac myocytes. J Physiol (Lond) 453:591–608
80. Bers DM, Lederer WJ, Berlin JR (1990) Intracellular Ca transients in rat cardiac myocytes: role of Na-Ca exchange in excitation-contraction coupling. Am J Physiol 258:C944–C954
81. Gibbs CL, Chapman JB (1985) Cardiac mechanics and energetics: chemomechanical transduction in cardiac muslce. Am J Physiol 249:H199–H206
82. Hasselbach W, Oetliker H (1983) Energetics and electrogenicity of the sarcoplasmic reticulum calcium pump. Annu Rev Physiol 45:325–339
83. Gibbs CL (1987) Cardiac energetics. In: Ter Keurs HEDJ, Tyberg JV (eds) Mechanics of the circulation. Nijhoff, Dordrecht, pp. 69–86
84. Pierce GN, Philipson KD, Langer GA (1985) Passive calcium-buffering capacity of a rabbit ventricular homogenate preparation. Am J Physiol 249:C248–C255
85. Solaro RJ, Briggs FN (1974) Estimating the functional capabilities of sarcoplasmic reticulum in cardiac muscle: calcium binding. Circ Res 34:531–540
86. Wier WG, Yue DT (1986) Intracellular calcium transients underlying the short-term force-interval relationship in ferret ventricular myocardium. J Physiol (Lond) 376:507–530
87. Suga H, Yasumura Y, Nozawa T, Futaki S, Tanaka N, Uenishi M (1988) Pressure-volume relationship around zero transmural pressure in excised cross-circulated dog left ventricle. Circ Res 63:361–372
88. Alpert NR, Blanchard EM, Mulieri LA (1989) Tension-independent heat in rabbit papillary muscle. J Physiol (Lond) 414:433–453
89. Yaku H, Slinker BK, Mochizuki T, Lorell BH, Lewinter MM (1993) Use of 2,3-butanedione monoxime to estimate nonmechanical Vo₂ in rabbit hearts. Am J Physiol 265:H834–H842
90. Higashiyama A, Watkins MW, Chen Z, LeWinter MM (1994) Preload does not influence nonmechanical O₂ consumption in isolated rabbit heart. Am J Physiol 266:H1047–H1054
91. Blanchard EM, Smith GL, Allen DG, Alpert NR (1990) The effects of, 2,3-butanedione monoxime on initial heat, tension, and aequorin light output of ferret papillary muscles. Pflugers Arch 416:219–221
92. Perreault CL, Mulieri LA, Alpert NR, Ransil BJ, Allen PD, Morgan JP (1992) Cellular basis of 2,3-butanedione monoxime in human myocardium. Am J Physiol 263:H503–H510
93. Gwathmey JK, Hajjar RJ, Solaro RJ (1991) Contractile deactivation and uncoupling of crossbridges: effects of 2,3-butanedione monoxime on mammalian myocardium. Circ Res 69:1280–1292

94. De Tombe PP, Burkhoff D, Hunter WC (1992) Comparison between the effects of 2–3 butandione monoxime (BDM) and calcium chloride on myocardial oxygen consumption. J Mol Cell Cardiol 24:783–797
95. Kusuoka H, Porterfield JK, Weisman HF, Weisfeldt ML, Marban E (1987) Pathophysiology and pathogenesis of stunned myocardium: depressed Ca^{2+} activation of contraction as a consequence of reperfusion-induced cellular calcium overload in ferret hearts. J Clin Invest 79:950–961
96. Krause SM, Jacobus WE, Becker LC (1989) Alterations in cardiac sarcoplasmic reticulum calcium transport in the postischemic "stunned" myocardium. Circ Res 65:526–530
97. Blanchard EM, Solaro RJ (1984) Inhibition of the activation and troponin calcium binding of dog cardiac myofibrils by acidic pH. Circ Res 55:382–391
98. Cingolani HE, Koretsune Y, Marban E (1990) Recovery of contractility and pHi during respiratory acidosis in ferret hearts: role of Na^+-H^+ exchange. Am J Physiol 259:H843–H848
99. Marban E, Kusuoka H (1987) Maximal Ca^{2+}-activated force and myofilament Ca^{2+} sensitivity in intact mammalian hearts: differential effects of inorganic phosphate and hydrogen ions. J Gen Physiol 90:609–623
100. Orchard CH (1987) The role of the sarcoplasmic reticulum in the response of ferret and rat heart muscle to acidosis. J Physiol (Lond) 436:559–578
101. McCall E, Orchard CH (1991) The effect of acidosis on the interval-force relation and mechanical restitution in ferret papillary muscle. J Physiol (Lond) 432:45–63
102. Shimizu M, Kimura S, Myerburg RJ, Bassett AL (1990) Effects of hypoxia, acidosis, and simulated ischemia on repriming of caffeine contracture in rat myocardium. J Mol Cell Cardiol 22:687–705
103. Takasago T, Goto Y, Kawaguchi O, Hata K, Saeki A, Nishioka T, Suga H (1993) Ryanodine wastes oxygen consumption for Ca^{2+} handling in the dog heart: a new pathological heart model. J Clin Invest 92:823–830
104. Frank JS, Rich TL, Beydler S, Kreman M (1982) Calcium depletion in rabbit myocardium. Circ Res 51:117–130
105. Rich TL, Langer GA (1982) Calcium depletion in rabbit myocardium. Circ Res 51:131–141
106. Hoffman PA, Miller WP, Moss RL (1993) Altered calcium sensitivity of isometric tension in myocyte-sized preparations of porcine postischemic stunned myocardium. Circ Res 72:50–56
107. Kitakaze M, Weisman HF, Marban E (1988) Contractile dysfunction and ATP depletion after transient calcium overload in perfused ferret hearts. Circulation 77:685–695
108. Kusuoka H, Marban E (1992) Cellular mechanism of myocardial stunning. Annu Rev Physiol 54:243–256
109. Hatefi Y, Jurtshuk P, Haavik AJ (1961) Studies on the electron transport system. Arch Biochem Biophys 94:148–155
110. Baan J, van der Velde ET, de Bruin HG, Smeenk GJ, Koops J, van Dijk AD, Temmerman D, Senden J, Buis B (1984) Continuous measurement of left ventricular volume in animals and humans by conductance catheter. Circulation 70:812–823
111. Burkhoff D, van der Velde E, Kass D, Baan J, Maughan WL, Sagawa K (1985) Accuracy of volume measurement by conductance catheter in isolated, ejecting canine hearts. Circulation 72:440–447
112. Nozawa T, Yasumura Y, Futaki S, Tanaka N, Uenishi M, Suga H (1988) Efficiency of energy transfer from pressure-volume area to external mechanical work increases with contractile state and decreases with afterload in the left ventricle of the anesthetized closed-chest dog. Circulation 77:1116–1124
113. Solda PL, Perlini S, Piepoli M, Crandi A, Paroni G, Barzizza F, Finardi G, Bernardi L (1990) Measuring left ventricular dimensions by conductance catheter in the rabbit. Eur Heart J 11:925–935
114. Namba T, Takaki M, Araki J, Ishioka K, Akashi T, Zhao LY, Matsushita T, Ito H, Fujii W, Matsubara H, Suga H (1993) Ca^{2+} sensitivity of contractile machinery and Ca^{2+} handling energy: simulation. Jpn Heart J 34:601–616

115. Futaki S, Nozawa T, Yasumura Y, Tanaka N, Suga H (1988) A new cardiotonic agent, OPC-8212, elevates the myocardial oxygen consumption versus pressure-volume area (PVA) relation in a similar manner to catecholamine and Ca^{2+} in canine hearts. Heart Vessels 4:153–161

116. Futaki S, Goto Y, Ohgoshi Y, Yaku H, Suga H (1992) Similar oxygen cost of myocardial contractility between DPI 201–106 and epinephrine despite different subcellular mechanisms of action in dog hearts. Heart Vessels 7:8–17

117. Hata K, Goto Y, Futaki S, Ohgoshi Y, Yaku H, Kawaguchi O, Takasago T, Saeki A, Taylor TW, Nishioka T, Suga H (1992) Mechanoenergetic effects of pimobendan in canine left ventricles: comparison with dobutamine. Circulation 86:1291–1301

118. De Tombe, Burkhoff D, Hunter WC (1992) Effects of calcium and EMD-53998 on oxygen consumption in isolated canine hearts. Circulation 86:1945–1954

119. Ter Keurs HEDJ, Gau WD, Bosker H, Drake-Holland AJ, Noble MIM (1990) Characterisation of decay of frequency induced potentiation and postextrasytolic potentiation. Cardiovasc Res 24:903–910

120. Lab MJ, Lee JA (1990) Changes in intracellular calcium during mechanical alternans in isolated ferret ventricular muscle. Circ Res 66:585–595

121. Hess OM, Surber EP, Ritter M, Krayenbuehl HP (1984) Pulsus alternans: its influence on systolic and diastolic function in aortic valve disease. J Am Coll Cardiol 4:1–7

122. Kihara Y, Grossman W, Morgan JP (1989) Direct measurement of changes in intracellular calcium transients during hypoxia, ischemia, and reperfusion of the intact mammalian heart. Circ Res 65:1029–1044

123. Yue DT, Burkhoff D, Franz MR, Hunter WC, Sagawa K (1985) Postextrasystolic potentiation of the isolated canine left ventricle: relationship to mechanical restitution. Circ Res 56:340–350

124. Burkhoff D, Sagawa K (1986) Influence of pacing site on canine left ventricular force-interval relationship. Am J Physiol 250:H414–H418

125. Wohlfart B (1979) Relationships between peak force, action potential duration and stimulus interval in rabbit myocardium. Am J Physiol 244:395–409

126. Elzinga G, Lab MJ, Noble MIM, Papadoyannis DE, Pidgeon J, Seed A, Wohlfart B (1981) The action potential duration and contractile response of the intact heart related to the preceding interval and the preceding beat in the dog and cat. J Physiol (Lond) 314:481–500

127. Araki J, Takaki M, Matsushita T, Matsubara H, Suga H (1994) Postextrasystole transient contractile alternans in canine hearts. Heart Vessels 9:241–248

128. Yasuhara S, Takaki M, Kikuta A, Ito H, Suga H (1995) Myocardial oxygen consumption of mechanically unloaded contraction of rat ventricular slices by a new approach. Am J Physiol (in press)

129. Takaki M, Zhao DD, Zhao LY, Araki J, Mori M, Suga H (1995) Suppression of myocardial mitochondrial respiratory function in acute failing hearts made by a short-term Ca^{2+} free-high Ca^{2+} coronary perfusion. J Mol Cell Cardiol 27:2009–2013

130. Ito H, Takaki M, Yamaguchi H, Tachibana H, Suga H (1995) Left ventricular volumetric conductance catheter for rats. Am J Physiol (in press)

Left Ventricular Contractile and Energetic Dysfunction After Recovery from Acidosis

Yoichi Goto[1] and Katsuya Hata[2]

Abstract. It has been generally recognized that left ventricular (LV) contractile dysfunction during acidosis is almost reversible after correction of acidosis in crystalloid-perfused hearts. In contrast, we have found that LV contractile function is paradoxically depressed after rapid correction of acidosis in blood-perfused hearts. To determine the mechanism of this phenomenon, we measured LV contractility (Emax), total mechanical energy (PVA), and myocardial oxygen consumption (Vo_2) before and after correction of hypercapnic acidosis in isolated cross-circulated dog hearts. During acidosis with CO_2 loading, Emax decreased significantly. During rapid correction of acidosis by CO_2 unloading, a transient overshoot of Emax and concomitant ventricular arrhythmias were followed by a paradoxical decrease in Emax and a significant increase in the oxygen cost of contractility. This result indicates that the postacidotic failing heart requires higher Vo_2 for a unit increase in Emax than the normal heart, which energetically resembles postischemic stunned myocardium. When dimethylamiloride, a selective Na^+-H^+ exchange inhibitor, was administered just before the correction of acidosis, the development of contractile and energetic abnormalities after correction of acidosis was almost completely prevented. Thus rapid correction of acidosis paradoxically depresses myocardial contractility and increases the oxygen cost of contractility through activation of the Na^+-H^+ exchange system. In addition, the blood-perfused heart behaves differently from the crystalloid-perfused heart during the process of recovery from acidosis.

Key words. Acidosis—Stunned myocardium—Pressure-volume area—Myocardial oxygen consumption—Na^+-H^+ exchange system

Introduction

It has been recognized for more than 100 years that acidosis decreases the contractility of the heart [1]. This contractile dysfunction during acidosis has been attributed mainly to a decrease in Ca^{2+} responsiveness of contractile protein [2, 3]. However,

---

[1] Division of Cardiology, Department of Medicine, National Cardiovascular Center, 5-7-1 Fujishiro-dai, Suita, Osaka 565, Japan
[2] First Department of Internal Medicine, Kobe University School of Medicine, 7-5-2 Kusunoki-cho, Chuo-ku, Kobe 650, Japan

165

myocardial contractile function after recovery from acidosis has not been well understood. Studies in crystalloid-perfused hearts have indicated that the influence of
acidosis on myocardium is reversible [4, 5], whereas studies using in situ hearts
have suggested that rapid correction of acidosis results in myocardial damage [6].
Furthermore, the mechanism of the myocardial damage after correction of acidosis is
not known.

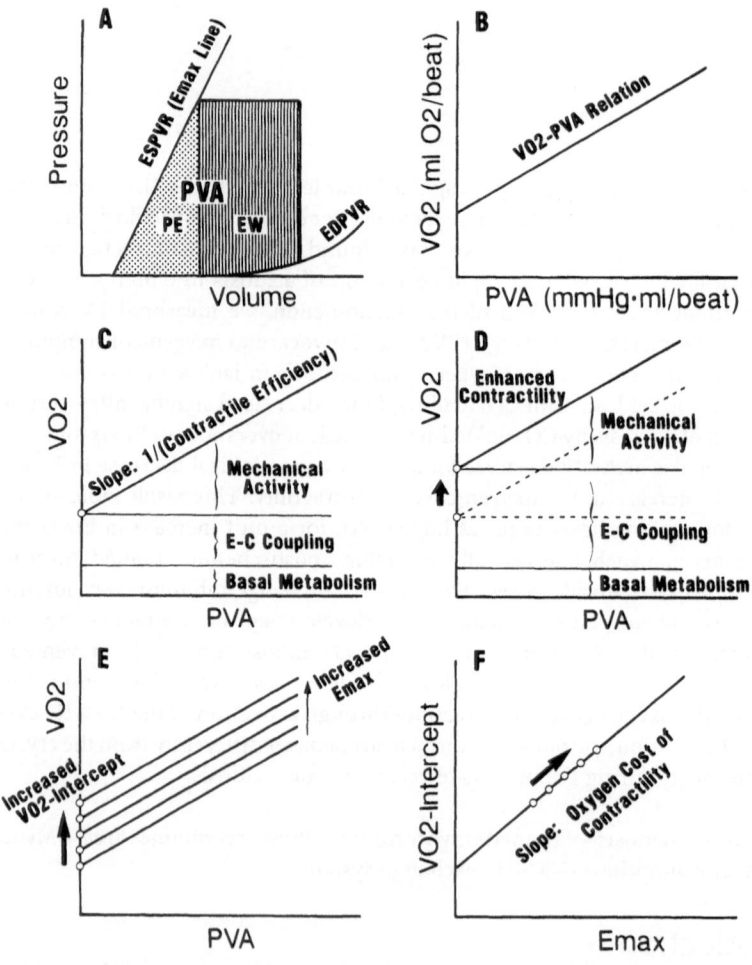

Fig. 1. Left ventricular (LV) pressure-volume (P-V) area (*PVA*) and the related
mechanoenergetic indexes. PVA is the area surrounded by the end-systolic (*ESPVR*) and end-
diastolic P-V relations (*EDPVR*) and the systolic P-V trajectory. It consists of potential energy
(*PE*) and external work (*EW*) in an ejecting contraction (**A**). The Vo_2-PVA relation is linear (**B**),
and the reciprocal of the slope indicates contractile efficiency, whereas the Vo_2 intercept (or
PVA-independent Vo_2) reflects Vo_2 for excitation-contraction (*EC*) coupling and basal metabolism (**C**). When ventricular contractility (*Emax*) is enhanced by catecholamines or calcium, the
Vo_2-PVA relation shifts upward in a parallel manner with an increased Vo_2 for E-C coupling
(**D**). As Emax is progressively enhanced in multiple steps, the Vo_2 intercept also increases
progressively (**E**), constructing a linear relation between the Vo_2 intercept and Emax (**F**). The
slope is called the oxygen cost of contractility. (From [12], with permission)

In recent decades, Emax, the slope of the left ventricular (LV) end-systolic pressure–volume relation, has been used as a measure of LV contractility for the most part independent of loading conditions [7]. In addition, LV pressure–volume area (PVA)—a specific area in the pressure–volume diagram circumscribed by the end-systolic and end-diastolic pressure–volume relations and the systolic segment of the pressure–volume trajectory (Fig. 1A)—has been shown to correlate linearly with myocardial oxygen consumption (Vo_2) of the left ventricle [8] (Fig. 1B). Using the framework of the Emax–PVA–Vo_2 relation, one can assess the relation between LV contractile function and its energy cost during various inotropic interventions [9-14].

In this chapter we present our data for the Emax–PVA–Vo_2 relation during the recovery process from acidosis in the isolated cross-circulated dog heart and discuss the mechanism of contractile and energetic dysfunction of the left ventricle after rapid correction of acidosis [15].

Background

Previous studies have shown that PVA linearly correlates with Vo_2 per beat in a load-independent manner [8, 9] (Fig. 1B). The reciprocal of the slope of the linear Vo_2–PVA relation is called "contractile efficiency" [8, 11] and has been considered to indicate chemomechanical energy transduction efficiency of contractile machinery from oxygen to total mechanical energy generated by an LV contraction (Fig. 1C). On the other hand, the Vo_2 intercept of the Vo_2–PVA relation (PVA-independent Vo_2) consists of Vo_2 for nonmechanical activities such as excitation–contraction (E-C) coupling and basal metabolism [8].

Enhanced ventricular contractility (Emax) with calcium or epinephrine increases Vo_2 for E-C coupling without affecting contractile efficiency, resulting in a parallel upward shift of the Vo_2–PVA relation [9] (Fig. 1D). However, enhanced contractility with calcium or epinephrine does not affect Vo_2 for basal metabolism. When LV contractility is enhanced in several steps, as in Fig. 1E, the increases in PVA-independent Vo_2 linearly correlate with the increases in Emax (Fig. 1F). The slope of the linear relation between PVA-independent Vo_2 and Emax is called the oxygen cost of contractility, which indicates an oxygen requirement during E-C coupling for a unit increase in Emax [8, 11, 13].

We have demonstrated that the oxygen cost of contractility is 2.2 times higher in the postischemic stunned myocardium than in the normal heart [13]. In another study we developed a stable acidotic heart model in the blood-perfused dog heart and found that the oxygen cost of contractility is 1.5 times higher in the acidotic heart than in the normal heart [14]. During the course of the latter study, we found that rapid normalization of arterial blood pH from approximately 7.0 to 7.4 produced a marked, transient overshoot of LV contractility, followed by severe LV contractile dysfunction that can be referred to as postacidotic stunned myocardium [15].

Hypothesis

We hypothesized that contractile dysfunction after rapid correction of acidosis may be attributed to intracellular Ca^{2+} overload resulting from the accelerated Na^+–Ca^{2+} exchange due to accumulation of intracellular Na^+ via the heavily operating Na^+–H^+ exchange system to carry H^+ out of the myocyte. This mechanism may be similar to that proposed for reperfusion injury in postischemic myocardium [16, 17]. If the mechanism of postacidotic contractile dysfunction is the same as that of postischemic stunned myocardium, the oxygen cost of contractility would also be higher than that in normal myocardium. In addition, if this hypothesis is correct, the administration of an inhibitor of the Na^+-H^+ exchange system during the correction of acidosis would prevent postacidotic contractile dysfunction because studies have indicated that inhibition of the Na^+-H^+ exchange system attenuates ischemia–reperfusion injury [16–18].

Heart Preparation

Experiments were performed on isolated, blood-perfused dog hearts supported by cross-circulation with an intact animal. The surgical procedure of the cross-circulated heart preparation has been described previously [9, 13]. After cross-circulation was started, a thin balloon was inserted into the left ventricle of the isolated heart and connected to our custom-made volume servo pump to control and measure the LV volume. Coronary blood flow (CBF) and coronary arteriovenous oxygen content difference were measured to calculate the Vo_2 per beat. The temperature of the excised heart was maintained at 35–37°C throughout the experiment. The systemic arterial pressure of the support dog, which served as the coronary perfusion pressure of the excised heart, was kept above 80 mm Hg throughout the experiment. Arterial pH, Po_2, and Pco_2 of the support dog were maintained within their physiological ranges using supplemental oxygen and intravenous sodium bicarbonate as needed.

Experimental Protocol

First, the LV pressure, volume, CBF, and arteriovenous oxygen content difference were measured during steady-state isovolumic contractions at various LV volumes to calculate LV Emax, PVA, and Vo_2 at a stable baseline contractility (control volume run). After the control volume run, LV contractility was enhanced in steps by infusing 1% $CaCl_2$ into the coronary arterial perfusion tube until Emax was nearly doubled while the LV volume was kept constant. Data for Emax, PVA, and Vo_2 were collected during steady-state contractions at several levels of contractility (control Ca^{2+} run).

When contractility returned to the baseline level after discontinuation of $CaCl_2$, acidosis was induced by aerating a membrane oxygenator placed in the arterial perfusion circuit with CO_2. Stable acidosis was maintained for at least 15 min, after which the CO_2 was discontinued; the recovery process from acidosis was continuously monitored. When all variables were stabilized, approximately 30 min after CO_2 discontinuation, a second volume run (postacidosis volume run) and Ca^{2+} run (postacidosis Ca^{2+} run) were performed in a manner similar to the control runs.

To determine if the Na^+-H^+ exchange system plays an essential role in the development of postacidotic contractile dysfunction, 5-(N,N-dimethyl)-amiloride (DMA), a selective Na^+-H^+ exchange inhibitor [19], at a concentration of 7 µmol/L in 0.04% dimethylsulfoxide (DMSO) was infused into the coronary arterial perfusion tube for 3 min starting just before CO_2 discontinuation in seven hearts [DMA(+) group] but not in an other six hearts [DMA(−) group]. DMA at this concentration has been reported to inhibit Na^+-H^+ exchange by approximately 50% [20].

In each volume run, contractile efficiency was determined from the reciprocal of the slope of the Vo_2–PVA relation. The oxygen cost of contractility was determined from the slope of the relation between PVA-independent Vo_2 and Emax for each Ca^{2+} run before and after producing postacidotic contractile dysfunction.

Results

Figure 2 shows typical tracings of LV pressure, volume, electrocardiogram (ECG), coronary blood flow, and arteriovenous oxygen content difference (top panels), as well as LV pressure–volume diagrams (bottom panels) during control (Fig. 2A), acidosis (Fig. 2B), and postacidosis (Fig. 2C) periods in one heart of the DMA(−) group. During acidosis, peak LV pressure at a constant LV volume decreased, and hence Emax (the diagonal line in the bottom panel of Fig. 2) decreased. Shortly after discontinuing CO_2, the peak LV pressure increased rapidly and markedly, accompanying ventricular arrhythmias, and peaked at a level far beyond the control level within a few minutes. It then decreased gradually over 30 min and reached a new postacidotic level that was lower than the control level. Based on the average of six hearts in the DMA (−) group, postacidosis Emax was significantly lower than the control value ($P < 0.05$) (Table 1) after the severe transient overshoot during the early recovery phase (304 ± 89% of acidosis Emax).

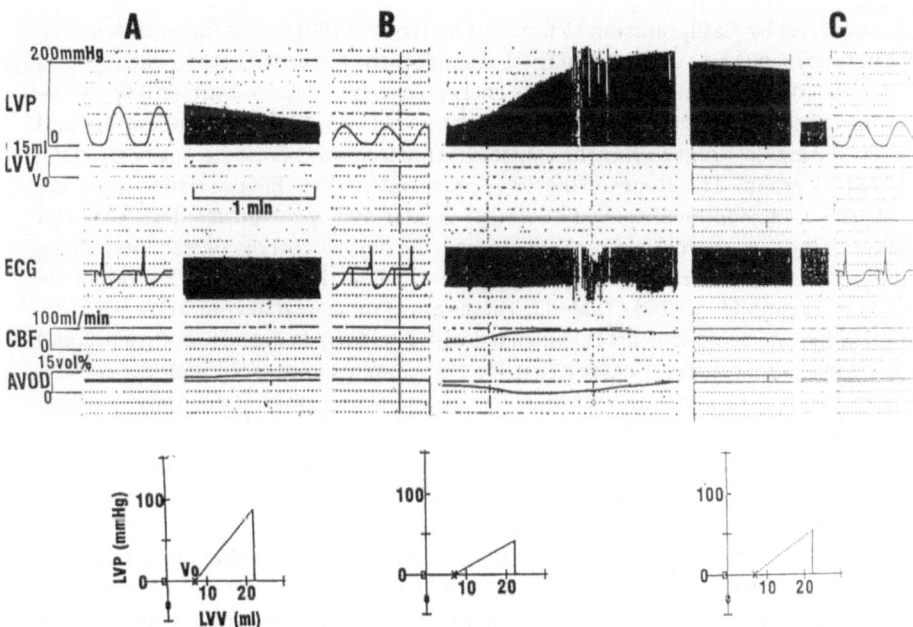

FIG. 2. *Top.* Simultaneous tracings of LV isovolumic pressure (*LVP*), volume (*LVV*), electrocardiogram (*ECG*), coronary blood flow (*CBF*), and arteriovenous oxygen content difference (*AVOD*) during the control (**A**), acidosis (**B**), and postacidosis (**C**) periods in a representative heart of the DMA(−) group. *Bottom.* LV pressure-volume diagrams for the corresponding periods of **A**, **B**, and **C**. Note that Emax during the postacidosis period was lower than that during the control period. (From [15], with permission)

TABLE 1. Experimental results

Parameter	Control	Acidosis	Peak recovery	Postacidosis
DMA (−) group				
E_{max} (mm Hg·ml^{-1}·100 g)	5.5 ± 1.8	2.8 ± 0.6*	11.2 ± 4.0*	2.9 ± 0.6*
VO_2–PVA relation				
Slope (10^{-5} ml O_2·mm Hg^{-1}·ml^{-1})	1.84 ± 0.26	–	–	1.61 ± 0.15
PVA-independent Vo_2 (ml O_2·beat^{-1}·100 g^{-1})	0.029 ± 0.004	–	–	0.026 ± 0.005*
Oxygen cost of contractility (ml O_2·mm Hg^{-1}·ml·beat^{-1}·100 g^{-2})	0.0015 ± 0.0006	–	–	0.0028 ± 0.0014*
DMA (+) group				
E_{max} (mm Hg·ml^{-1}·100 g)	5.3 ± 1.6	3.3 ± 1.0*	9.6 ± 2.4*	4.5 ± 1.5
VO_2–PVA relation				
Slope (10^{-5} ml O_2·mm Hg^{-1}·ml^{-1})	1.74 ± 0.26	–	–	1.70 ± 0.34
PVA-independent Vo_2 (ml O_2·beat^{-1}·100 g^{-1})	0.027 ± 0.005	–	–	0.025 ± 0.004
Oxygen cost of contractility (ml O_2·mm Hg^{-1}·ml·beat^{-1}·100 g^{-2})	0.0020 ± 0.0005	–	–	0.0019 ± 0.0006

DMA(−) group, group not treated with 5-(N,N-dimethyl)amiloride (DMA); *Emax*, left ventricular contractility index; Vo_2, myocardial oxygen consumption; *PVA*, pressure-volume area; *DMA(+) group*, group treated with DMA.
*$P < 0.05$ compared with the respective control value.

Despite the significant decrease in Emax during the postacidosis period, the slope of the Vo_2–PVA relation was unchanged and PVA-independent Vo_2 decreased only slightly (Table 1). When postacidosis Emax was enhanced and matched with the control level by $CaCl_2$ infusion (5.6 ± 1.9 mm Hg·ml^{-1}·100 g), PVA-independent Vo_2 (0.034 ± 0.004 ml O_2·beat^{-1}·100 g^{-1}) significantly exceeded the control level ($P < 0.05$), suggesting an increased energy cost for a given contractility in the postacidotic heart. Figure 3A depicts the relation between PVA-independent Vo_2 and Emax during Ca^{2+} runs during the control and postacidosis periods in one heart of the DMA(−) group. The slope of the PVA-independent Vo_2–Emax relation (i.e., the oxygen cost of contractility) was obviously greater during the postacidosis Ca^{2+} run than during the control Ca^{2+} run. On average, the oxygen cost of contractility during the postacidosis Ca^{2+} run was 83 ± 23% greater than that in the control Ca^{2+} run in the DMA(−) group ($P < 0.01$) (Table 1). These results indicate that contractile dysfunction in the postacidotic heart is associated with unchanged contractile efficiency and increased nonmechanical energy cost for E-C coupling compared with the normal heart. Thus postacidotic myocardium resembles postischemic stunned myocardium in terms of both mechanics and energetics.

When DMA was administered just before CO_2 discontinuation in the DMA(+) group, the increase in peak LV pressure was milder and more gradual and was accompanied by fewer arrhythmias. The relative magnitude of the overshoot of Emax (199 ± 69% of the acidosis Emax) was significantly smaller than that in the DMA(−) group (304 ± 89%) ($P < 0.05$). After this milder contractile overshoot, the steady-state postacidosis Emax level was not significantly different from the control Emax (Table 1). Thus no contractile dysfunction occurred during the postacidosis period in the DMA(+) group.

Figure 3B depicts the relation between PVA-independent Vo_2 and Emax during Ca^{2+} runs for the control and postacidosis periods in one heart of the DMA(+) group. The two lines were almost superimposable, indicating that the oxygen cost of contractility was similar in the two runs. On average, the oxygen cost of contractility

FIG. 3. **A** Relations between PVA-independent oxygen consumption (Vo₂) and Emax in the control Ca²⁺ run (*open circles*) and postacidosis Ca²⁺ run (*closed circles*) in a representative heart of the DMA(−) group. **B** Same relations in a representative heart of the DMA(+) group. Note that the oxygen cost of contractility, indicated by the slope of the regression line, is greater during the postacidosis period than during the control period in the DMA(−) group but not in the DMA(+) group. (From [15], with permission)

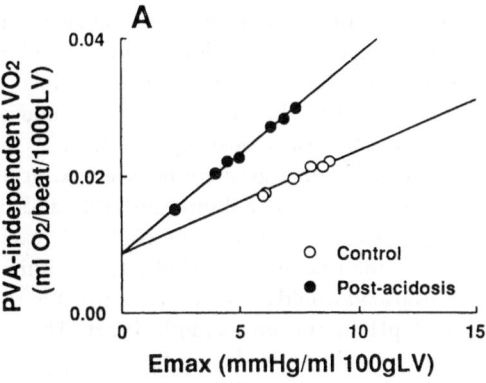

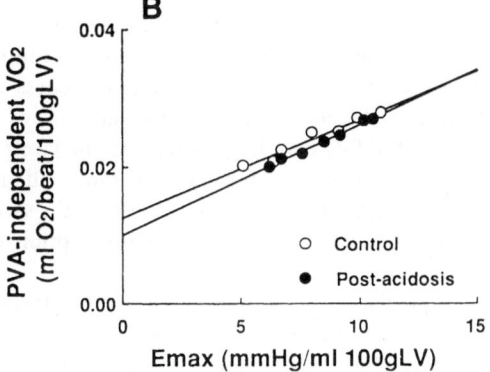

during the postacidosis Ca²⁺ run was close to that during the control Ca²⁺ run in the DMA(+) group (Table 1). Thus DMA successfully prevented both contractile and energetic dysfunction that would occur after rapid correction of acidosis.

Discussion

The major findings of the present study were as follows: (1) Rapid correction of acidosis resulted in severe contractile dysfunction (postacidotic stunned myocardium) in the blood-perfused heart. (2) In the postacidotic myocardium, the oxygen cost of contractility (reflecting the energy cost of E-C coupling) was significantly elevated, while contractile efficiency (reflecting the efficiency of crossbridge cycling) was unchanged. (3) Inhibition of the Na⁺-H⁺ exchange system with DMA almost completely prevented contractile and energetic dysfunction in the postacidotic heart. These findings indicate that rapid recovery of pH from acidosis results in both mechanical and energetic dysfunction through activation of the Na⁺-H⁺ exchange system.

Dimethylamiloride is a potent, selective Na⁺-H⁺ exchange inhibitor [19]. In addition, DMA at this concentration would not directly affect the intracellular Ca²⁺ concentration or E-C coupling in our preparation because we confirmed in preliminary experiments that it did not affect LV contractility or Vo₂ in the normal heart.

Therefore the mechanism of the beneficial effect of only a 3-min infusion of DMA could be explained as follows: During acidosis the accumulated intracellular H^+ would not be eliminated because extracellular H^+ is also elevated, so there would be no gradient of H^+ between intracellular and extracellular spaces. However, during rapid correction of acidosis, extracellular H^+ would be normalized first, resulting in an acute substantial gradient between extracellular and intracellular H^+ concentration. This H^+ gradient should instantly and maximally accelerate the Na^+–H^+ exchange system, and hence the Na^+–Ca^{2+} exchange system, leading to a transient excessive increase in intracellular Ca^{2+} within a few minutes. This acute, excessive Ca^{2+} overload would cause severe contractile and energetic disorders after normalization of pH in the postacidotic heart. Thus by inhibiting the Na^+–H^+ exchange system for only 3 min during the early phase of recovery from acidosis, the rapid, excessive rise of intracellular Ca^{2+} and subsequent mechanoenergetic dysfunction can be prevented.

It has been shown that oxygen cost of contractility is also elevated in acidotic myocardium [14] and postischemic stunned myocardium [13]. In acidotic myocardium, decreased Ca^{2+} responsiveness of the contractile protein [2, 3] may be responsible for the increased oxygen cost of contractility because more free Ca^{2+} is needed for E-C coupling to activate the contractile protein to the same force level [14]. This situation means that more adenosine triphosphate (ATP) must be hydrolyzed by the Ca^{2+} pump ATPase in the sarcoplasmic reticulum (SR) to sequester more Ca^{2+}, leading to greater consumption of PVA-independent Vo_2 for a unit increase in Emax [14].

In postischemic stunned myocardium the mechanism responsible for increased oxygen cost of contractility is considered to be not only decreased Ca^{2+} responsiveness [21] but also a decreased molar coupling ratio of net sequestered Ca^{2+}/ATP consumed by the Ca^{2+} pump ATPase due to increased Ca^{2+} permeability of the SR membrane [22]. [13]. The latter mechanism means that more ATP would be consumed by the Ca^{2+} pump ATPase to lower intracellular Ca^{2+} and to relax the stunned myocardium to the same extent as the normal myocardium during each cardiac cycle. Because accelerated Na^+–H^+ exchange and subsequent Ca^{2+} overload have been considered the important mechanisms of postischemic stunned myocardium [16–19], the mechanisms of the contractile and energetic disorders in the postacidotic and postischemic stunned myocardium are likely to be similar.

In the postacidotic heart, contractile efficiency was unchanged from the control value. Because contractile efficiency is the product of the mitochondrial oxidative phosphorylation efficiency (Vo_2 to ATP) and the crossbridge cycling efficiency (ATP to PVA) [8, 11, 13], this result may indicate either that both efficiencies remained constant or that a decrease in either efficiency might have been offset by a balanced increase in the other efficiency. We believe that the latter possibility is remote because the contractile efficiency was unchanged in both DMA($-$) and DMA($+$) groups regardless of the changes in Emax and the oxygen cost of contractility.

One important message from the present study is that the functional response to rapid correction of acidosis differs between blood-perfused and crystalloid-perfused hearts (i.e., a severe transient overshoot of contractility and subsequent contractile dysfunction in he blood-perfused heart versus only slight contractile overshoot and almost complete reversibility in the crystalloid-perfused heart). Differences in the oxygen-carrying capacity, buffering mechanism, and ionic and hormonal environments may be responsible for the different responses [23]. Although the precise mechanism of the responses of the two perfusion modalities is still to be determined, the postacidotic stunned myocardium observed in the blood-perfused heart is compatible with the findings reported for the in situ heart—that rapid correction of acidosis with sodium bicarbonate produces myocardial damage [6].

In summary, the effects of rapid correction of acidosis on LV mechanics and energetics were assessed in excised cross-circulated dog hearts utilizing the framework of the Emax–PVA–Vo$_2$ relation. The results indicate that rapid correction of acidosis causes a transient overshoot of contractility followed by severe contractile dysfunction (postacidotic stunned myocardium) and an increased oxygen cost of contractility, reflecting an increased energy cost of E-C coupling. Inhibition of the Na$^+$–H$^+$ exchange system with DMA can prevent not only the contractile but also the energetic disorders in the postacidotic heart. Therefore rapid recovery of pH from acidosis likely results in both mechanical and energetic dysfunction through activation of the Na$^+$–H$^+$ exchange system.

Acknowledgments. This study was supported in part by Research Grants for Cardiovascular Diseases (4A-1 and 4C-4) from the Ministry of Health and Welfare of Japan.

References

1. Gaskell WH (1880) On the tonicity of the heart and blood vessels. J Physiol (Lond) 3:48–75
2. Solaro RJ, Lee JA, Kentish JC, Allen DG (1988) Effects of acidosis on ventricular muscle from adult and neonatal rats. Circ Res 63:779–787
3. Orchard CH, Kentish JC (1990) Effects of changes of pH on the contractile function of cardiac muscle. Am J Physiol 258:C967–C981
4. Shimizu M, Kimura S, Myerburg RJ, Bassett A (1990) Effects of hypoxia, acidosis, and simulated ischemia on repriming of caffeine contracture in rat myocardium. J Mol Cell Cardiol 22:697–705
5. Cingolani HE, Koretsune Y, Marban E (1990) Recovery of contractility and pH$_i$ during respiratory acidosis in ferret hearts: role of Na$^+$–H$^+$ exchange. Am J Physiol 259:H843–H848
6. Shapiro JI (1990) Functional and metabolic responses of isolated hearts to acidosis: effects of sodium bicarbonate and Caribarb. Am J Physiol 258:H1835–H1839
7. Suga H, Sagawa K (1974) Instantaneous pressure-volume relationships and their ratio in the excised supported canine left ventricle. Circ Res 35:117–126
8. Suga H (1990) Ventricular energetics. Physiol Rev 70:247–277
9. Suga H, Hisano R, Goto Y, Yamada O, Igarashi Y (1983) Effect of positive inotropic agents on the relation between oxygen consumption and systolic pressure volume area in canine left ventricle. Circ Res 53:306–318
10. Suga H, Goto Y, Yasumura Y, Nozawa T, Futaki S, Tanaka N, Uenishi M (1988) O$_2$ consumption of dog heart under decreased coronary perfusion and propranolol. Am J Physiol 254:H292–H303
11. Goto Y, Slinker BK, LeWinter MM (1990) Decreased contractile efficiency and increased nonmechanical energy cost in hyperthyroid rabbit heart: relation between O$_2$ consumption and systolic pressure-volume area or force-time integral. Circ Res 66:999–1011
12. Goto, Y, Futaki S, Kawaguchi O, Hata K, Takasago T, Saeki A, Nishioka T, Suga H (1992) Left ventricular contractility and energetic cost in disease models: an approach from the pressure-volume diagram. Jpn Circ J 56:716–721
13. Ohgoshi Y, Goto Y, Futaki S, Yaku H, Kawaguchi O, Suga H (1991) Increased oxygen cost of contractility in stunned myocardium of dog. Circ Res 69:975–988
14. Hata K, Goto Y, Kawaguchi O, Takasago T, Saeki A, Nishioka T, Suga H (1994) Hypercapnic acidosis increases oxygen cost of contractility in the dog left ventricle. Am J Physiol 266:H730–H740

15. Hata K, Takasago T, Saeki A, Nishioka T, Goto Y (1994) Stunned myocardium after rapid correction of acidosis: increased oxygen cost of contractility and the role of the Na^+-H^+ exchange system. Circ Res 74:794–805
16. Tani M, Neely JR (1989) Role of intracellular Na^+ in Ca^{2+} overload and depressed recovery of ventricular function of reperfused ischemic rat hearts: possible involvement of H^+-Na^+ and Na^+-Ca^{2+} exchange. Circ Res 65:1045–1056
17. Murphy E, Perlman M, London RE, Steenbergen C (1991) Amiloride delays the ischemia-induced rise in cytosolic free calcium. Circ Res 68:1250–1258
18. Karmazyn M (1988) Amiloride enhances postischemic ventricular recovery: possible role of Na^+-H^+ exchange. Am J Physiol 255:H608–H615
19. Meng H, Pierce GN (1991) Involvement of sodium in the protective effect of 5-(N,N-dimethyl) amiloride on ischemia-reperfusion injury in isolated rat ventricular wall. J Pharmacol Exp Ther 256:1094–1100
20. Lazdunski M, Frelin C, Vigne P (1985) The sodium/hydrogen exchange system in cardiac cells: its biochemical and pharmacological properties and its role in regulating internal concentrations of sodium and internal pH. J Mol Cell Cardiol 17:1029–1042
21. Kusuoka H, Porterfield JK, Weisman HF, Weisfeldt ML, Marban E (1987) Pathophysiology and pathogenesis of stunned myocardium: depressed Ca^{2+} activation of contraction as a consequence of reperfusion-induced cellular calcium overload in ferret hearts. J Clin Invest 79:950–961
22. Krause SM, Hess ML (1984) Characterization of cardiac sarcoplasmic reticulum dysfunction during short-term, normothermic, global ischemia. Circ Res 55:176–184
23. Goto Y, Slinker BK, LeWinter MM (1988) Similar normalized Emax and O_2 consumption-pressure-volume area relation in rabbit and dog. Am J Physiol 255:H366–H374

Diagnostic Value of the Transient Response of Oxygen Consumption to Exercise in Cardiac Patients: Random Noise Approach

KENJI SUNAGAWA, HIROSHI TAKAKI, and MASARU SUGIMACHI

Abstract. Although peak oxygen uptake (Vo_2) at maximal exercise stress is useful for assessing functional capacity in patients, various factors, including the need to impose strenuous load and the subjectivity of the endpoint, make its utility somewhat limited. To circumvent the limitations we developed a technique where we focused on the transient response of Vo_2 to exercise. In patients with chronic heart failure (NYHA class II–III), we intermittently imposed mild bicycle exercise while measuring breath-by-breath Vo_2 After determining the transfer function from the workload to Vo_2, we computed a Vo_2 response against a hypothetical step exercise. The Vo_2 step response showed an initial immediate increase followed by a slow monotonic rise toward a steady-state level. The amplitude of the response was smaller in patients than in control subjects (182 ± 50 versus 262 ± 58 ml/min at 120 s; $P < 0.001$). The time constant of the slow monotonic rise was longer in patients than in control subjects (48 ± 37 versus 31 ± 8 s; $P < 0.005$). In patients with mitral stenosis the time constant was longer (62 ± 23 s; $P < 0.005$) with a small amplitude (195 ± 76 ml/min; $P < 0.05$). Successful percutaneous transvenous mitral commissurotomy (PTMC) shortened the time constant (40 ± 10 s; $P < 0.05$) without increasing the amplitude. These immediate effects of PTMC were unidentifiable by the peak Vo_2. We conclude that the dynamic Vo_2 response is useful and sensitive for quantitating the functional status of the cardiocirculatory system.

Key words. Exercise testing—Oxygen uptake—Random noise approach—Chronic heart failure—PTMC

Introduction

Peak oxygen uptake (Vo_2) measured at maximal exercise using incremental protocols is useful for assessing the functional status of the cardiocirculatory system [1, 2]. Despite the importance of measuring peak Vo_2, its clinical value has been somewhat limited for various reasons. First, to determine peak Vo_2, we must impose a strenuous workload on patients with heart disease. This condition increases the risk of serious complications [3, 4] and discourages frequent, repetitive serial testings. Second, am-

Department of Cardiovascular Dynamics, National Cardiovascular Center Research Institute, 5-7-1 Fujishiro-dai, Suita, Osaka 565, Japan

biguity associated with defining the endpoint, which depends heavily on one's motivation, makes peak Vo_2 considerably subjective. The variability associated with the subjectivity inevitably makes peak Vo_2 relatively insensitive for identifying a subtle change in cardiocirculatory functional capacity [5–8]. Therefore there is a clear need for a more sensitive, less subjective, less strenuous stress test for assessing the global functional status of the cardiocirculatory system.

Instead of imposing a strenuous load, many investigators have analyzed the Vo_2 response against a submaximum constant workload (i.e., the step response) [1, 9–14]. According to these investigations, Vo_2 rose at the beginning of exercise prior to the widening of the arteriovenous (A-V) oxygen difference [1, 9, 10]. This response was attributed to the increase in pulmonary flow (i.e., the cardiodynamic response). The slow exponential rise following the initial transient response reflected further increases in pulmonary flow and widening the A-V oxygen difference. The time constant of the exponential rise varied with the strength of exercise [1, 11, 12] and the degree of conditioning [11]. Thus the transient response of Vo_2 against exercise appears to characterize functional capacity of the cardiocirculatory system.

The step response of Vo_2 has many limitations as well, the major one being its accuracy. The variability of breath-by-breath Vo_2 is unacceptably large even without exercise. The exercise stress would further increase the variability. Thus to estimate an accurate Vo_2 step response, we must average the response over many trials [1, 13, 14]. If the variability of Vo_2 was consistently coupled with exercise, a simple summation hardly attenuates the variance. Furthermore, even if we could estimate the step response with high precision, the sensitivity of detecting subtle changes in functional status has not been established.

The purpose of this investigation was to develop a submaximum stress test capable of sensitively and objectively analyzing the functional status of the cardiocirculatory system. For this purpose we applied the random noise technique [15] and determined the hypothetical step response. The analysis indicated that the step response of Vo_2 in patients with heart failure was significantly different from that of control subjects. The test was sensitive enough to identify a subtle change associated with acute alterations in hemodynamics [16].

Random Exercise Test

Exercise Protocol

We used an electrically braked ergometer to impose a random workload on the subjects [16]. The subjects bicycled intermittently according to a computer-generated command at a fixed load (50 watts) with a pedaling rate of 50–55 revolutions per minute (rpm). The command signal was a random binary sequence with a minimal interval of 5 s. It was a band-limited white noise with a corner frequency of 6 cycles per minute (cpm). The whiteness is crucial when determining a nonbiased estimate of the step response [15–17]. The average duty ratio was 0.5, which made the average workload 25 watts. The intermittent exercise continued for 20 min while we measured the Vo_2 breath by breath. After applying an antialiasing digital filter, we digitized the command signal and Vo_2 at 4 Hz for subsequent analyses. At the conclusion of each test, we rated the perceived exertion during exercise in terms of the Borg scale (6–20) [18]. As a reference for the random exercise test, we performed a conventional symptom-limited maximal exercise test and determined the peak Vo_2.

Data Analysis

We first estimated the frequency spectra of the time series for the workload (the input) and Vo_2 (the output) (Fig. 1). We divided the time series into multiple segments, each of which consisted of 256 s of the time series. We applied the fast Fourier transform (FFT) for each segment after applying the four-term Blackman-Harris window [19] and obtained power spectra [Sxx(f)]. Second, we obtained crosspower spectra between Vo_2 and the workload [Sxy(f)] by multiplying the spectra of Vo_2 with conjugate of the spectra of workload at corresponding frequencies. We repeated these procedures over the segments and averaged them to minimize variance. Third, we computed the ratio of the crosspower to the power of workload and determined the transfer function from the workload to Vo_2. Fourth, transforming the transfer function to the time domain yielded the impulse response. Finally, we integrated the impulse response with respect to time and obtained the step response. The step response represents the transient Vo_2 response against a hypothetical step increase in workload from rest to 50 watts. Because the Vo_2 step response, after the initial transient, approximated a monoexponential curve, we estimated its time constant.

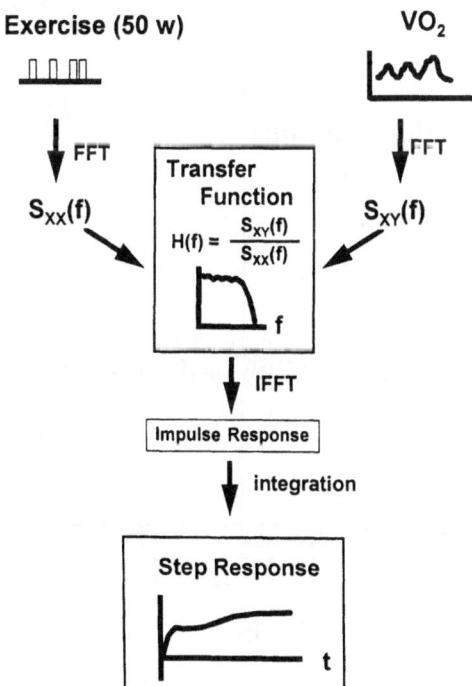

FIG. 1. Estimation of the Vo_2 step response. First, we computed the spectrum of the exercise sequence [$S_x(f)$] and Vo_2 [$S_y(f)$] by the fast Fourier transform (FFT). Taking the ratio of the cross-power spectrum between the exercise and Vo_2 [$S_{xy}(f)$] to the power spectrum of exercise [$S_{xx}(f)$] yields the transfer function [H(f)]. We estimated the Vo_2 impulse response by transforming H(f) to the time domain through the inverse FFT. The time integral of the impulse response gives the Vo_2 step response

Control Subjects Versus Patients with Chronic Heart Failure

We examined 21 patients with chronic heart failure (CHF), of whom 17 were NYHA class II and 4 were class III. For comparison, we examined 23 age-matched control

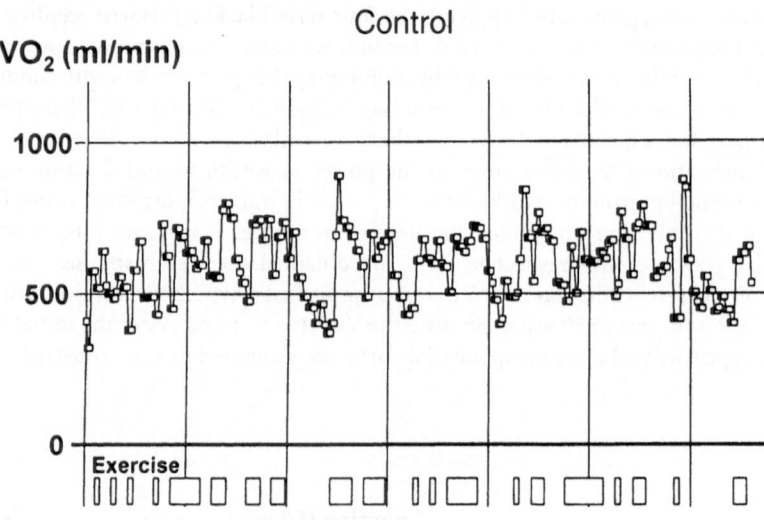

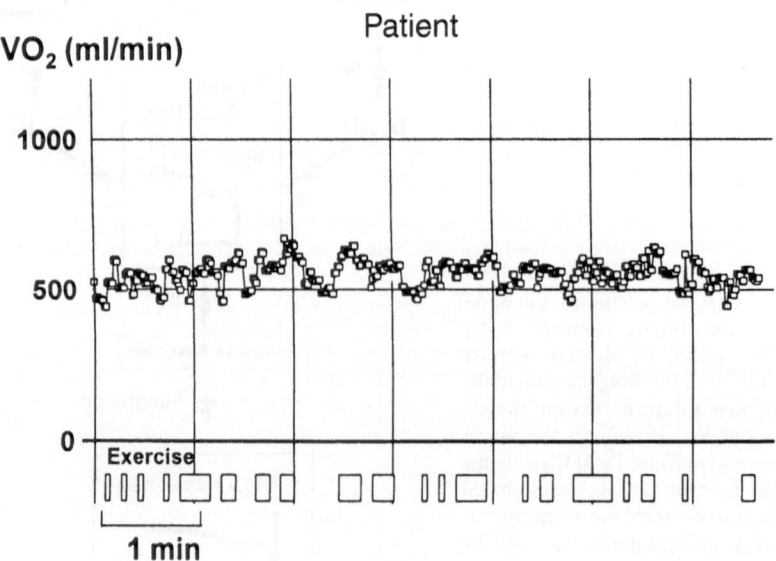

FIG. 2. Time trend of Vo_2 during the random exercise test in a control subject (*top*) and a patient with chronic heart failure (*bottom*). The block bars at the bottom of each panel indicate the exercise command

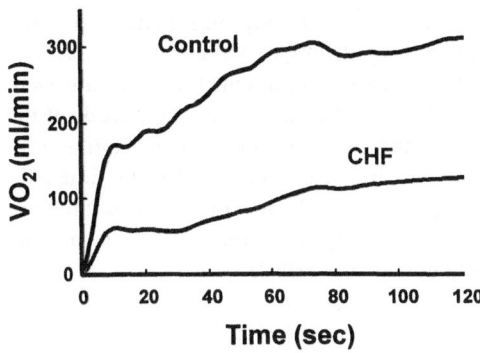

FIG. 3. Step responses of Vo₂ in the same two subjects as in Fig. 2. There are marked differences in the responses between the control subject and the patient with chronic heart failure (*CHF*)

sedentary subjects (16 men, 7 women, age 55 ± 12 years). All subjects completed the random exercise test without significant symptoms. The maximal value of the Borg scale during the test ranged from 11 to 17 (controls 11.0 ± 1.7, patients 12.6 ± 1.9; $P < 0.01$).

Representative examples of the time series of breath-by-breath Vo_2 and workload during the random exercise are illustrated in Fig. 2. The mean value of Vo_2 did not sizably differ between the patient and the control subject. In contrast, changes in Vo_2 associated with workload were significantly larger in the control subject than in the patient.

Illustrated in Fig. 3 are the Vo_2 step responses of the same subjects shown in Figure 2. The Vo_2 step responses increased immediately after the onset of exercise, remained constant until about 30 s, and then slowly increased again toward a steady-state level. The Vo_2 step response was larger in the control subjects than in the patients.

The pooled data indicated that the Vo_2 step response was significantly larger in the control subjects than in the patients between 5 and 120 s ($P < 0.050$–0.001). The amplitude of the step response at 120 s was 262 ± 58 ml/min in the control subjects and 182 ± 50 ml/min in the CHF patients ($P < 0.05$). The average amplitude over 120 s correlated well with the peak Vo_2 ($r = 0.72$, $P < 0.001$). The average time constant of the slow response after the initial transient was longer in the patients than in the control subjects (31 ± 8 s versus 48 ± 37 s; $P < 0.005$).

Effects of PTMC on the Transient Vo₂ Response

We evaluated how the acute hemodynamic improvement affected Vo_2 kinetics in response to exercise. We analyzed the transient Vo_2 response in 11 patients with mitral stenosis before and after successful percutaneous transvenous mitral commissurotomy (PTMC). The mean mitral valve area was 1.1 ± 0.2 cm² before PTMC and 1.8 ± 0.3 cm² after PTMC ($P < 0.001$). The mean left atrial pressure decreased after PTMC (17.8 ± 5.2 versus 13.2 ± 3.4 mm Hg; $P < 0.001$). Before PTMC, eight patients were NYHA class II and three were class III. After PTMC, nine patients became asymptomatic (NYHA class I), with only two remaining symptomatic (class II).

Despite improvements in resting hemodynamics and symptoms, neither the peak Vo_2 (994 ± 303 versus 1069 ± 377 ml/min; not significant, or NS) nor the $\Delta Vo_2/\Delta WR$ (7.6 ± 1.4 versus 7.9 ± 1.1 ml/min/W; NS), where WR represents the work rate, were improved within a few days after successful PTMC. In contrast, the amplitude of the Vo_2 step response significantly increased in the early-to-mid portion (34–65 s; $P <$ 0.02–0.05). The following portion remained unchanged. Consequently, the time constant shortened from 62 ± 23 s to 40 ± 10 s ($P < 0.02$). The maximal value of the Borg scale during the random exercise test decreased by more than one scale in nine patients and was unaltered in the remaining two ($P < 0.002$).

Discussion

Diagnostic Value of the Vo_2 Step Response

We have shown that the Vo_2 response to a hypothetical step exercise using the random exercise protocol was capable of differentiating patients with CHF from control subjects [16]. The step response was lower and slower in patients than in control subjects. The difference manifested most obviously at 20–120 s after the initial transient response. Because the estimation of the Vo_2 step response does not require any judgment about the endpoint, unlike the estimation of peak Vo_2 [6, 7], the interpretation is objective. Furthermore, the mean work rate imposed on the subjects was only 25 watts, which was lower than their peak capacity. The submaximality of the workload makes it possible to serially, repetitively evaluate given patients.

In addition to these unique advantages, what made this method even more useful was its ability to detect subtle changes in the Vo_2 response against exercise. As we demonstrated, conventional peak Vo_2 failed to detect the immediate effect of PTMC despite the fact that the patients' symptoms and hemodynamics were improved. This observation was in line with that previously reported [8, 20]. Marzo et al. demonstrated that PTMC improved the maximal exercise capacity chronically (3 months) but improved it little acutely [20]. In contrast, the Vo_2 step response demonstrated a significant acceleration of the early monotonic rise soon after PTMC. The statistical nature and the lack of subjectivity, both of which are inherent in this method, made the Vo_2 step response a sensitive, objective index of cardiocirculatory function.

Determinants of the Transient Response of Vo_2

We evaluated the transient Vo_2 response to a hypothetical step exercise in patients with impaired pump function. The Vo_2 rose immediately and reached a first plateau. It stayed there for 20 s or so and then increased monotonically with mild oscillation toward a steady state. These general features of the step response resembled those that were directly determined [1, 9–14]. The details were different, however. During the actual step response, the variability associated with the measurement obscured the clear transition from the initial transient to the subsequent slow response. Because of the statistical nature of the random exercise protocol [16], details of the initial transient response were disclosed. Blood flow from the exercising muscle does not return to the lung during the first several seconds after the onset of exercise; therefore the initial rise in Vo_2 cannot be attributed to the increase in muscle Vo_2 [1, 9, 10]. The increase in stroke volume and thus cardiac output immediately after the onset of exercise [9, 21] would be responsible for the initial rise of V_{O_2}.

The major factors that determine the slow rise of V_{O_2} after the initial transient would be the increase in muscle V_{O_2}. Previous investigations using a step exercise of moderate intensity indicated that V_{O_2} increased monoexponentially [9, 11, 13]. This increase was achieved by a further increase in pulmonary flow and widening of the A-V oxygen difference. The time constant of the exponential rise paralleled more the A-V oxygen difference than the cardiac output [9]. Because the time constant has been known to be shorter in well-trained subjects than in poorly trained ones [11], our observations were consistent with those reported elsewhere.

The hypothetical V_{O_2} step response indicated that its response after the initial transient was lower in patients than in control subjects. The difference became smaller during the latter portion of the step response and disappeared after 220s, suggesting that the apparent difference observed during the first 120s was due to premature termination of the estimation of the system step response. In other words, the long time constant of the patients made the apparent response smaller during the first 120 s.

Effects of PTMC

The mechanism responsible for improvement of the V_{O_2} step response immediately after PTMC was not clear. As demonstrated by Doppler technique in another cohort who had undertaken PTMC in our institute [22], a widened mitral valve area might facilitate the rapid increase of cardiac output after the onset of exercise, resulting in the quick rise of V_{O_2} and the diminished oxygen deficit. These changes in hemodynamics may contribute to immediate symptomatic improvement. The remaining peripheral dysfunction that probably resulted from the deconditioning [8] may account for the unaltered amplitude of the latter portion of the step response.

V_{O_2} Response to Step Exercise and Ramp Exercise

Figure 4 shows the relation among the impulse response, step response, and ramp response. The impulse response is the time domain expression of the transfer fuction [15–17, 23]. It represents the transient response of a given system to a hypothetical, large impulse-like input. The time integral of the impulse response is the step response. The time integral of the step response yields the ramp response. As we have shown, the V_{O_2} step response was attenuated and slowed in patients compared to that in the control subjects. This finding implies that the corresponding ramp response of V_{O_2} should be lower in patients than in the control subjects for any given moment (bottom panel of Fig. 4), which was indeed the case. In other words, the oxygen deficit was larger in patients than in control subjects.

As shown in the bottom panel of Fig. 4, the attenuated response of V_{O_2} in the patients resulted in the decreased slope of the ramp response. It has been observed by others [24] and accounts for the decreased $\Delta V_{O_2}/\Delta WR$ in the patients. Thus the decreased $\Delta V_{O_2}/\Delta WR$ in the ramp protocol observed in the patients was a manifestation of their attenuated V_{O_2} response.

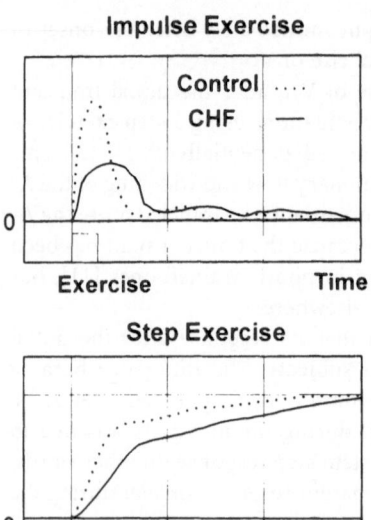

FIG. 4. Relation between the impulse response (*top*) step response (*middle*), and ramp response (*bottom*)

Advantages of Computing the Step Response Using the Random Exercise Protocol

We have shown that the step response of Vo_2 using the random exercise protocol carries useful information for assessing patients. The transient response of Vo_2 can be obtained by imposing an actual step workload. This method is limited by the fact that the amplitude and temporal resolution obtained with a single measurement are unacceptably poor [1, 13, 25]. Although some investigators improved the accuracy by ensembling repeated measurements [1, 13, 14], the requirement for numerous measurements makes this technique impractical for clinical use, accounting for the constant workload test not being widely applied as a clinical tool despite its potential for assessing the functional status of patients [1, 6, 7].

In contrast, because of the statistical nature of the random exercise method [16], we can obtain a precise step response of Vo_2 with a high amplitude and temporal resolution. The average of the spectra and the randomness of the exercise were essential for estimating the unbiased step response.

Despite the many advantages to the random exercise test, it had limitations. In this investigation, we used the frequency domain approach for estimating the step response. Because the exercise input had a limited bandwidth (i.e., up to 6 cpm), the finite bandwidth inevitably enlarged the estimation variance of the step response in the high frequency range. If we could widen the bandwidth of the exercise, the Vo_2 step response would have less variance. Additional investigations are needed to obtain a more precise step response. In this investigation, we focused on the linear response of Vo_2, ignoring a potential nonlinear response. The fact that the averaged Vo_2 (by imposing many step exercises) resembled that obtained by random exercise suggested that the nonlinear response in the tested condition was relatively insignificant. Furthermore, if we truly need to analyze the nonlinear response, the random noise approach is still applicable for nonlinear system analysis [17].

Conclusion

Patients with CHF showed a markedly attenuated, slow increase in the Vo_2 step response to mild exercise. The subtle change in Vo_2 kinetics associated with successful PTMC was identifiable with the step response but unidentifiable by measuring peak Vo_2. Thus the Vo_2 step response using random exercise is useful and sensitive for quantitating functional capacity [16].

References

1. Wasserman K (1988) New concepts in assessing cardiovascular function. Circulation 78:1060–1071
2. Weber KT, Kinasewits GT, Janicki JS, Fishman AP (1982) Oxygen utilization and ventilation during exercise in patients with chronic cardiac failure. Circulation 65:1213–1223
3. Atterhög J-H, Jonsson B, Samuelsson R (1979) Exercise testing: a prospective study of complication rates. Am Heart J 98:572–579
4. Rochmia P, Blackburn H (1971) Exercise tests: a survey of procedures, safety, and litigation experience in approximately 170 000 tests. JAMA 217:1061–1066
5. Maskin CS, Forman R, Sonnenblick EH, Frishman WH, LeJemtel TH (1983) Failure of dobutamine to increase exercise capacity despite hemodynamic improvement in severe chronic heart failure. Am J Cardiol 51:177–182
6. LeJemtel TH, Mancini D, Gumbardo D, Chadwick B (1985) Pitfalls and limitations of "maximal" oxygen uptake as an index of cardiovascular functional capacity in patients with chronic heart failure. Heart Failure 1:112–124
7. Solal AC, Gourgon R (1991) Assessment of exercise tolerance in chronic congestive heart failure. Am J Cardiol 67:36C–40C
8. Tanabe Y, Suzuki M, Takahashi M, Oshima M, Yamazaki Y, Yamaguchi T, Igarashi Y, Tamura Y, Yamazoe M, Shibata A (1993) Acute effect of percutaneous transvenous mitral commissurotomy on ventilatory and hemodynamic responses to exercise: pathophysiological basis for early symptomatic improvement. Circulation 88:1770–1778
9. DeCort SC, Innes JA, Barstow TJ, Guz A (1991) Cardiac output, oxygen consumption and arteriovenous oxygen difference following a sudden rise in exercise level in humans. J Physiol (Lond) 441:501–512
10. Weissman ML, Jones PW, Oren A, Lamarra N, Whipp BJ, Wasserman K (1982) Cardiac output increase and gas exchange at start of exercise. J Appl Physiol 52:236–244
11. Whipp BJ, Wasserman K (1972) Oxygen uptake kinetics for various intensities of constant-load work. J Appl Physiol 33:351–356
12. Hagberg JM, Mullin JP, Nagle FJ (1978) Oxygen consumption during constant-load exercise. J Appl Physiol 45:381–384

13. Whipp BJ, Ward SA, Lamarra N, Davis JA, Wasserman K (1982) Parameters of ventilatory and gas exchange dynamics during exercise. J Appl Physiol 52:1506–1513
14. Sietsema KE, Cooper DM, Perloff JK, Rosove MH, Child JS, Canobbio MM, Whipp BJ, Wasserman K (1986) Dynamics of oxygen uptake during exercise in adults with cyanotic congenital heart disease. Circulation 73:1137–1144
15. Suyama A, Sunagawa K, Hayashida K, Sugimachi M, Todaka K, Nose Y, Nakamura M (1988) Random exercise stress test in diagnosing effort angina. Circulation 78:825–830
16. Takaki H, Sunagawa K (1994) Abnormal transient response of VO_2 to exercise in patients with heart failure: random noise approach [abstract]. Circulation 90:1–16
17. Marmarelis PZ, Marmarelis VZ (1978) Analysis of physiological system. Plenum, New York
18. Borg G (1970) Perceived exertion as an indicator of somatic stress. Scand J Rehabil Med 2–3:92–98
19. Harris FJ (1978) On the use of windows for harmonic analysis with the discrete Fourier transform. Proc IEEE 66:51–83
20. Marzo KP, Herrmann HC, Mancini DM (1993) Effect of balloon mitral valvuloplasty on exercise capacity, ventilation and skeletal muscle oxygenation. J Am Coll Cardiol 21:856–865
21. Loeppky JA, Greene ER, Hoekenga DE, Caprihan A, Luft UC (1981) Beat-by-beat stroke volume assessment by pulsed Doppler in upright and supine exercise. J Appl Physiol 50:1173–1182
22. Tamai J, Nagata S, Akaike M, Ishikura F, Kimura K, Takamiya M, Miyatake K, Nimura Y (1990) Improvement in mitral flow dynamics during exercise after percutaneous transvenous mitral commissurotomy: noninvasive evaluation using continuous wave Doppler technique. Circulation 81:46–51
23. Hughson RL (1990) Exploring cardiorespiratory control mechanisms through gas exchange dynamics. Med Sci Sports Exerc 22:72–79
24. Hansen JE, Sue DY, Oren A, Wasserman K (1987) Relation of oxygen uptake to work rate in normal men and men with circulatory disorders. Am J Cardiol 59:669–674
25. Sietsema KE, Ben-Dov I, Zhang YY, Sullivan C, Wasserman K (1994) Dynamics of oxygen uptake for submaximal exercise and recovery in patients with chronic heart failure. Chest 105:1693–1700

Part 4
Medical Treatment of Heart Failure

Mechanisms of Novel Cardiotonic Agents Developed to Treat the Failing Heart Syndrome

Masao Endoh

Abstract. Several cardiotonic drugs have been developed as potential therapeutic agents for patients with the failing heart syndrome. These agents act through different but relatively limited subcellular signal-transduction pathways. Accumulation of $3',5'$-cyclic adenosine monophosphate (cyclic AMP) plays a main role in mediating the cardiotonic effects of most of these agents. Cyclic AMP promotes mobilization of intracellular Ca^{2+} in association with a decrease in myofibrillar responsiveness to Ca^{2+}, leading to the characteristic positive inotropic and lusitropic effects of these agents. The quantitative relation between the accumulation of cyclic AMP and a positive inotropic effect, however, differs among agents that act on cyclic AMP metabolism via different mechanisms: For a given increase in contractile force, accumulation of cyclic AMP induced by selective cyclic nucleotide phosphodiesterase (PDE) III inhibitors and β_1-adrenoceptor partial agonists is much less than that produced by nonselective β-adrenoceptor agonists or nonselective PDE inhibitors (or both). The relation between the amplitude of Ca^{2+} transients and the positive inotropic effect differs between selective PDE III inhibitors on the one hand and the β_1-adrenoceptor partial agonist denopamine on the other, suggesting intracellular compartmentation of cyclic AMP in myocardial cells. Newly developed Ca^{2+} sensitizers are expected to be therapeutic agents because of their benefits in cardiac energetics and the absence of potential Ca^{2+} overload. It became evident from motility assays, in vitro binding of Ca^{2+} to troponin C, and Ca^{2+}-dependent actomyosin ATPase activity that the processes responsible for the sensitization of myofibrils to Ca^{2+} involve multiple sites: (1) the binding of Ca^{2+} to troponin C; (2) thin filament interaction involving Ca^{2+} regulation sites; and (3) the actin–myosin interface leading to changes in crossbridge cycling in the absence of Ca^{2+}. In addition, (4) the environments where myofibrils are located may play a crucial role. The therapeutic relevance of these Ca^{2+} sensitizers and a novel Ca^{2+} channel promoter awaits the outcome of clinical application of these agents.

Key words. Cardiotonic agents—PDE III inhibitors—β_1-Adrenoceptor partial agonist—Ca^{2+} sensitizers—Ca^{2+} promoters

Department of Pharmacology, Yamagata University School of Medicine, 2-2-2 Iida-nishi, Yamagata 990-23, Japan

187

Introduction

Cardiac glycosides and catecholamines have long been used clinically as cardiotonic agents to treat the hemodynamic syndromes resulting from myocardial failure. Although these agents have been found to be effective in most clinical situations, their drawbacks, including narrow margins of safety and adverse effects such as an arrhythmogenic property, have imposed restrictions in their clinical application. Moreover, certain patients do not respond favorably to these agents. During the late 1970s Farah and co-workers carried out screening tests with a series of compounds having a positive inotropic effect in search of new cardiotonic agents that could replace cardiac glycosides and catecholamines in the treatment of heart failure [1, 2]. During the years since amrinone was first introduced [3], novel cardiotonic agents, structurally and mechanistically different from previous agents, have been developed and have become available for clinical trials on the treatment of heart failure.

Newly developed cardiotonic agents include compounds belonging to several classes with different chemical structures (Table 1). Agents that act through accumulation of $3',5'$-cyclic adenosine monophosphate (cyclic AMP) and the resultant increase in mobilization of cytoplasmic Ca^{2+} comprise an important class. The cyclic AMP is accumulated either by increased generation due to activation of adenylate cyclase or by a decrease in the rate of breakdown induced by inhibition of cyclic nucleotide phosphodiesterase (PDE). New agents such as selective PDE III (an isoenzyme selective for cyclic AMP, with a low Km and inhibited by cyclic GMP) inhibitors and β_1-adrenoceptor partial agonists elicit a positive inotropic effect with cyclic AMP accumulation that is less than that produced by the nonselective β-adrenoceptor agonist isoproterenol or nonselective PDE inhibitors such as 3-isopropyl-1-methylxanthine (IBMX) and theophylline [4–7]. In this respect newly developed agents possess an advantage because an excessive accumulation of cyclic AMP in myocardial cells, which leads to intracellular Ca^{2+} overload, is considered responsible for the generation of arrhythmia and ultimately myocardial cell death.

Short-term administration of new agents successfully ameliorated hemodynamic syndromes associated with heart failure. In addition, however, new orally available cardiotonic agents must provide a mechanism to decrease the morbidity and mortality of patients with congestive heart failure. The newly developed PDE III inhibitors,

---

TABLE 1. Mechanism of action of inotropic agents

Agents that act via a cyclic AMP-dependent mechanism
  Selective PDE III inhibitors
    Pyridinones: amrinone, milrinone, loprinone (E-1020)
    Imidazoles: enoximone (MDL 17,043), piroximone (MDL 19,205)
    Pyridazinones: pimobendan (UD-GG 115 BS), UD-CG 212 Cl, MCI-154, imazodan, indolidan
      (LY 195115), LY 186126
    Quinolinones: vesnarinone (OPC-8212), Y-20487, OPC-18790
  β_1-Adrenoceptor partial agonists: prenalterol, denopamine, xamoterol

Agents that act via a cyclic AMP-independent mechanism
  Ca^{2+} sensitizers: EMD 53998, Org 30029, pimobendan, MCI-154
  Ca^{2+} promoters: Bay k 8644, CGP 28392, YC-170, H 160/51, ($\pm$)202–791, Bay y 5959

---

such as amrinone, milrinone, enoximone, and piroximone, and the β_1-adrenoceptor partial agonist xamoterol failed to prolong the lives of patients with severe heart failure [8-12]. Although the prognosis of the patients with congestive heart failure has been shown to be improved by vasodilators and angiotensin-converting enzyme (ACE) inhibitors, which may act partially by decreasing the energy expenditure of the heart [13-15], congestive heart failure is still a severe disease with a high mortality rate.

It was once believed that long-term administration of cardiotonic agents that achieve their effects by increasing $[Ca^{2+}]_i$ actually worsen the prognosis of the patients with congestive heart failure. However, we must interpret previous clinical findings with caution because it is too early to draw conclusions. There is a need for further accumulation of basic and clinical information. First, in most previous trials digitalis (and ACE inhibitors) were administered beforehand, which may have provided the condition that would readily lead to intracellular Ca^{2+} overload by adding new cardiotonic agents that increase $[Ca^{2+}]_i$. Second, the dose of the new agents was selected based on their acute hemodynamic effects, which might have been overdoses for long-term administration. There is a definite difference in the concentrations of PDE III inhibitors that enhance the positive inotropic effect mediated by β-adrenoceptor stimulation and those that elicit a direct positive inotropic effect, indicating that the respective effects may be exerted via different subcellular mechanisms in respect to cyclic AMP metabolism; the former effect requires lower concentrations of PDE III inhibitors than the latter [16-18].

The rapid, transient increase in $[Ca^{2+}]_i$ that occurs prior to the generation of force plays a central role in excitation-contraction (E-C) coupling in intact cardiac muscle [19]. Termed the Ca^{2+} transient, which occurs subsequent to excitation, it is an essential determinant of the time course of cardiac contraction-relaxation. The amplitude and duration of Ca^{2+} transients are determined by several transmembrane and intracellular events that are pertinent to mobilization and handling of intracellular Ca^{2+}, including the actions of voltage-dependent L-type Ca^{2+} channels, Na^+-Ca^{2+} exchange and the Ca^{2+} pump of the sarcolemma, the Ca^{2+} pump and Ca^{2+}-release channels of the sarcoplasmic reticulum (SR), calcium-binding proteins such as calmodulin and, troponin C, and mitochondria. In particular, the release of Ca^{2+} from the SR makes the largest contribution to the amplitude of Ca^{2+} transients in mammalian cardiac muscle. The uptake of Ca^{2+} by the SR (mediated by the Ca^{2+} pump) and the binding of Ca^{2+} to and their release from troponin C play an important role in determining the shape of Ca^{2+} transients. A number of inotropic drugs and interventions modulate both of these processes, which are termed upstream mechanisms [20]. The overall regulatory mechanism of individual inotropic interventions in intact myocardial cells can be analyzed by simultaneously assessing the strength and time course of single contractions and Ca^{2+} transients [21, 22]. Biochemical and electrophysiological findings, as well as those from experiments with skinned cardiac fibers and the in vitro motility assay, provide a molecular basis for interpretation of the integrated regulation of contractility in intact cardiac muscle.

Cardiotonic agents such as EMD 53998 and Org 30029, which act via a novel mechanism to increase myofibrillar responsiveness to Ca^{2+}, have received attention in terms of their potential usefulness clinically [23, 24]. These agents either increase the affinity of troponin C for Ca^{2+} (central mechanism) or act on the processes subsequent to the binding of Ca^{2+} to troponin C, including thin filament interaction and the cycling rate of crossbridges (downstream mechanisms) (Table 2) [20, 25].

TABLE 2. Steps of cardiac excitation-contraction coupling involved in the mechanisms for altering Ca^{2+} sensitivity

Step	Central mechanism	Downstream mechanism	
	I	II	III
Contractile proteins	Troponin C	Tropomyosin Troponin C Troponin I Troponin T (Tm-Tn complex)	Actin Myosin
Ca^{2+} regulation	+	+	−
Drug	Caffeine	MCI-154	(+)EMD 53886

Tm-Tn, tropomyosin-troponin.

Selective PDE III Inhibitors

Cloning of cDNA indicates that there are at least seven genes encoding the various PDE isozymes (Table 3) [26]. Classical isozyme-nonselective PDE inhibitors such as theophylline and IBMX enhance and mimic the effects of β-adrenoceptor agonists on the electrical characteristics of membranes, Ca^{2+} transients, and contractile force. PDEs may similarly be compartmentalized in myocardial cells because selective inhibition of PDE III bound to the SR, which may lead to localized increases in levels of cyclic AMP and activation of protein kinase A (PKA), has been shown to be relevant to the positive inotropic effect of PDE inhibitors in most mammalian cardiac muscles

TABLE 3. Classification of phosphodiesterase (PDE): substrate specificity, functional relevance, selective inhibitors

PDE isozyme	Substrate specificity and functional relevance	Selective inhibitor
I	Low Km for cAMP and cGMP Ca^{2+}/calmodulin-stimulated	Vinpocetine
II	High Km for cAMP and cGMP Stimulated by cGMP Lowers cAMP via cGMP in frog heart	No
III	Low Km for cAMP Inhibited by cGMP Positive inotropic effect Vasodilatation	Novel cardiotonic agents (amrinone, milrinone)
IV	Relatively low Km for cAMP Plays roles in bronchial asthma, atopic dermatitis, infectious diseases	Ro 20-1724, rolipram
V	Low Km for cGMP Vasodilatation	Zaprinast (M&B 22,948), MY 5445, dipyridamole
VI	Low Km for cGMP (retina) Similar to PDE V	No
VII	Relatively low Km for cAMP Similar to PDE IV, but insensitive to rolipram	No

[22, 27–30]. Newly developed cardiotonic agents, such as amrinone, milrinone, enoximone, piroximone, imazodan, and LY 195115, selectively inhibit the PDE III isozyme, which has a low Km for cyclic AMP and can be inhibited by cyclic guanosine monophosphate (cGMP) [21, 22, 27] bound to the cardiac SR membrane. Selective inhibition of this type of isozyme has been shown to be relevant to the positive inotropic effect and vasodilatation induced by these agents [28–31].

It also appears that localization of PDE III shows a wide range of variation among species of animals [17, 22, 26, 27]. Selective PDE III inhibitors elicit a pronounced positive inotropic effect in the dog, rabbit, monkey, and human; a moderate positive inotropic effect in the guinea pig and hamster; and no positive inotropic effect in the rat. Thus PDE III bound to the SR membrane shows a wide range of species-dependent variation that is considered responsible for species differences in positive inotropic effect. In contrast to other species, in the rat selective inhibitors of PDE IV, such as rolipram and Ro 20-1724, markedly enhance cyclic AMP accumulation induced by isoproterenol [17], an indication that PDE IV plays a crucial role in cyclic AMP metabolism in the rat.

Pyridinones

Amrinone, milrinone, and loprinone belong to the pyridinone family (Fig. 1), and the effects of these agents on the cardiovascular system are similar [32]. They have a selective inhibitory action on PDE III in vitro, and the positive inotropic effect of these agents is associated with cyclic AMP accumulation in cardiac tissue. The maximal inotropic response to these agents is approximately 50%–60% of that of isoproterenol (ISOmax) [16, 32, 33]. The positive inotropic effect of milrinone, amrinone, enoximone, and piroximone was accompanied by increases in the peak Ca^{2+} transient

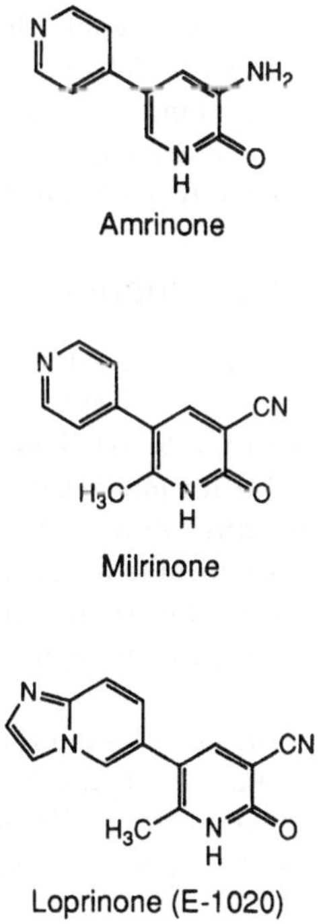

Amrinone

Milrinone

Loprinone (E-1020)

FIG. 1. Chemical structures of pyridinone derivatives

in association with increases in the rate of uptake of Ca^{2+} ions by the SR [33, 34]. Accumulation of cyclic AMP and the increase in peak Ca^{2+} transients and force induced by these agents in dog ventricular muscle can be abolished by carbachol, an indication that their effects are mediated by a cyclic AMP-dependent mechanism [33]. Milrinone at higher concentrations has a direct inhibitory action on PKA [35], which may contribute to the negative inotropic effect observed at high concentrations [36]. It is reported that milrinone exerts an effect on Ca^{2+} handling in myocardial cells [37, 38] but it does not affect Ca^{2+} sensitivity of contractile proteins [39].

The phosphorylation of functional proteins induced by milrinone has been compared with that induced by isoproterenol in intact guinea pig cardiac muscle [40]. For a given increase in cardiac contraction, phospholamban phosphorylation was less with milrinone than with isoproterenol; milrinone and IBMX did not cause significant phosphorylation of either troponin I or C protein, which were phosphorylated by isoproterenol. These findings suggest the presence of a cyclic AMP compartment in intact myocardial cells that leads to differential regulation of SR Ca^{2+} pump activity and Ca^{2+} sensitivity induced by these agents acting at different levels of cyclic AMP metabolism. The following observations further indicate that these differences in phosphorylation of functional proteins may result in differential modulation of the relation between Ca^{2+} transients and contractile force.

The regulation of Ca^{2+} transients and contractility by selective inhibitors of PDE III was examined in a comparison with those induced by isoproterenol in the aequorin-injected ventricular muscle of the dog. The curves representing the relation between peak Ca^{2+} transients and force during induction of the positive inotropic effect by two selective inhibitors of PDE III (i.e., OPC-18790 [41] and Org 7931 [42]) were superimposable on the curve obtained when $[Ca^{2+}]_o$ was elevated, a result that indicates that the inhibitors of PDE III did not cause a decrease in myofibrillar responsiveness to Ca^{2+} ions. The effects of these inhibitors differed from those of denopamine and isoproterenol, which caused a shift of the relation to the direction indicating a decrease in Ca^{2+} sensitivity [43, 44]. These findings support the proposed existence of different intracellular compartments of cyclic AMP, in which the levels of cyclic AMP may be regulated differentially by facilitating the generation of cyclic AMP or by selectively inhibiting its breakdown.

Pyridazinones

Pyridazinones comprise another class of PDE III inhibitors [18]. Pimobendan (UD-CG 115 BS), UD-CG 212 Cl, imazodan (CI-914), MCI-154, indolidan (LY 195115), and LY 186126 belong to this class (Fig. 2). In addition to their inhibitory action on PDE III, some pyridazinones are able to increase the Ca^{2+} sensitivity of contractile proteins. Among the pyridazinones, the extent of contribution of the latter mechanism to the positive inotropic effect is considered to be the greatest with MCI-154. The functional relevance of the Ca^{2+}-sensitizing effect in the cardiotonic action of these agents in animal models of heart failure or the clinical setting remains to be clarified.

The maximal inotropic response to pimobendan was 60% of ISOmax; pimobendan accumulates cyclic AMP during induction of the positive inotropic effect, but the extent of cyclic AMP accumulation for a given increase in contractile force is much less than that induced by isoproterenol [5, 45]. Pimobendan is rapidly demethylated

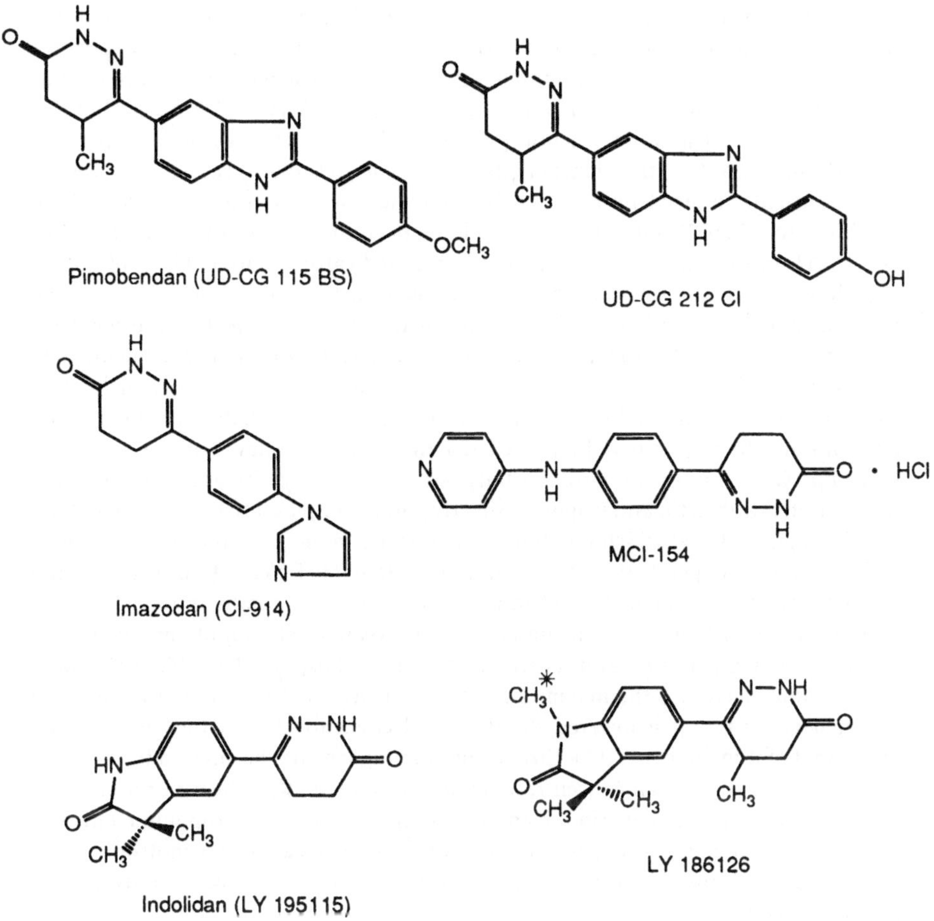

FIG. 2. Chemical structures of pyridazinone derivatives

to UD-CG 212 Cl (Fig. 2) [46, 47]. Because UD-CG 212 Cl elicits a positive inotropic effect at concentrations much lower than pimobendan, the active metabolite UD-CG 212 Cl may contribute to the positive inotropic effect of the parent compound in vivo [5, 48]. Carbachol only partially inhibited the positive inotropic effect of pimobendan, whereas it abolished the positive inotropic effect of UD-CG 212 Cl [5, 49], an indication that the positive inotropic effect of the demethylated metabolite UD-CG 212 Cl is exclusively mediated by cyclic AMP [5]. Pimobendan prolongs the action potential duration [45], and it increases Ca^{2+} sensitivity in skinned cardiac fibers [50–52], both of which may contribute to the high inotropic/chronotropic ratio of the compound compared with other PDE III inhibitors such as milrinone [49, 53]. It is shown that the l-isomer of pimobendan is more active than the d-isomer in producing a Ca^{2+}-sensitizing effect [52]. Whereas PDE III inhibitors failed to induce a positive inotropic effect in human failing heart [54, 55], pimobendan effectively increased the contractile force under such conditions, indicating that the Ca^{2+}-sensitizing effect of pimobendan may have some functional relevance in the failing human heart [55].

Another pyridazinone derivative, MCI-154 (6-[4-(4'-pyridylamino)phenyl]-4,5-dihydro-3(2H)pyridazinone hydrochloride trihydrate) (Fig. 2), elicits a positive inotropic effect and vasodilatation in anesthetized or conscious dogs and in cardiac muscle isolated from various mammalian species [56–59]. MCI-154 is a cardiotonic agent with PDE III inhibitory action [56] and Ca^{2+}-sensitizing action [57]. Because MCI-154 increases Ca^{2+} transients in intact cardiac muscle [60, 61] and the increase in Ca^{2+} transients induced by MCI-154 is attenuated by carbachol [61], cyclic AMP resulting from PDE III inhibition is considered to contribute to its positive inotropic effect [61]. In experiments with chemically skinned cardiac muscle fibers of guinea pigs, however, it was suggested that the increase in Ca^{2+} sensitivity of contractile proteins may significantly contribute to its positive inotropic effect [57]. It has been reported that MCI-154 is 100 times more potent than sulmazole in increasing the Ca^{2+} sensitivity in skinned cardiac muscle fibers from guinea pigs [56]. This original observation has been confirmed by other investigators [58, 59, 62–65]. Because it enhanced Ca^{2+} binding to troponin C [65], MCI-154 may act at the level of E–C coupling involving Ca^{2+}. In the in vitro motility assay using myosin and thin filament reconstituted with actin and tropomyosin–troponin complex, MCI-154 increased the threshold pCa value at which the thin filament starts to move on the myosin layer in a concentration-dependent manner, indicating that MCI-154 acts directly on the reconstituted thin filament to lead to an increase in Ca^{2+} sensitivity [66]. MCI-154 exerted a similar effect even under pathophysiological conditions, including acidosis, low temperature, and increased inorganic phosphate level [62, 63]. These interventions decreased the maximum sliding velocity; MCI-154 did not recover the maximal velocity, but it lowered the threshold concentration of Ca^{2+} to start the movement of thin filaments [66]. Crossbridge cycling may not be affected by MCI-154 because MCI-154 at a high concentration (10^{-4}M) did not affect the maximum velocity of simple actin filaments (in the absence of the tropomyosin–troponin complex). Perreault and co-workers [67] showed that MCI-154 elicits a positive inotropic effect even in cardiac muscle isolated from patients with end-stage heart failure due to cardiomyopathy.

Among agents belonging to pyridazinones, the positive inotropic effect of imazodan [27, 68], LY 195115 [28, 69], and LY 186126 [29, 70] (Fig. 2) is essentially due to cyclic AMP accumulation resulting from selective PDE III inhibition.

Quinolinones

Quinolinones (Fig. 3), such as vesnarinone (OPC-8212) [71, 72], Y-20487 [17], and OPC-18790 [33, 73], selectively inhibit PDE III and thereby elicit a positive inotropic effect in association with cyclic AMP accumulation. In addition, quinolinones exert direct action on membrane K^+ and Na^+ channels via a cyclic AMP-independent mechanism. For example, although the effects of vesnarinone to facilitate L-type Ca^{2+} channels are mediated by cyclic AMP [74], this agent does not increase (or only slightly increases) heart rate because of the inhibitory action on K^+ channels [75]. Furthermore, vesnarinone inhibited the positive chronotropic effect of isoproterenol and histamine [76], and it has been shown to increase the intracellular Na^+ concentration by suppressing Na^+ channel inactivation [77, 78]. The less chronotropic activity of vesnarinone may contribute to its causing beneficial hemodynamic improvement during short-term treatment [79, 80] and therapeutic effectiveness during long-term treatment of chronic heart failure [81, 82]. Modulation of blood levels of cytokines,

FIG. 3. Chemical structures of quinolinone derivatives

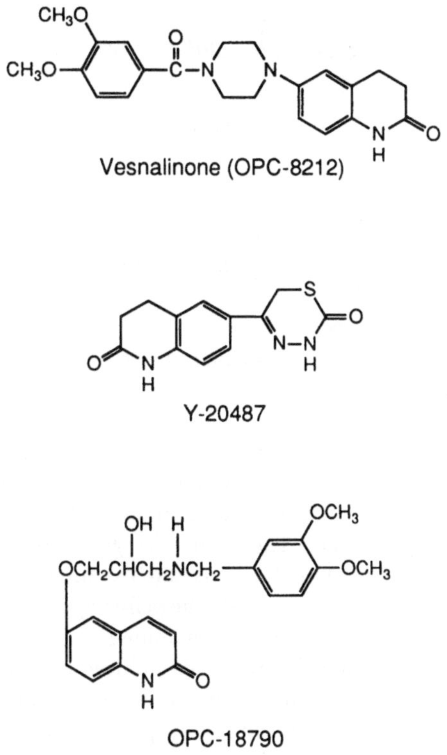

Vesnalinone (OPC-8212)

Y-20487

OPC-18790

such as tumor necrosis factor α (TNF-α), has likewise been proposed to be responsible for the beneficial effect of vesnarinone on the morbidity and mortality of patients with severe heart failure [83].

β₁ Partial Agonists

β_1-Adrenoceptor partial agonists, such as prenalterol [4, 84], xamoterol [6, 85], and denopamine [86] (Fig. 4), are much less effective than isoproterenol with respect to the accumulation of cyclic AMP. However, the inotropic response to these partial agonists is much greater than that expected from the extent of accumulation of cyclic AMP in cardiac tissue. In the perfused guinea pig heart, denopamine ($3\mu M$) and isoproterenol ($0.1\mu M$) exerted an equivalent positive inotropic effect, whereas the increases in heart rate and tissue cyclic AMP levels produced by denopamine were significantly smaller than those produced by isoproterenol [87]. Another β_1-partial agonist (i.e., prenalterol) increased free and bound cyclic AMP levels proportionately, whereas isoproterenol caused a greater increase in free than in bound cyclic AMP levels in the rat perfused heart [4]. At functionally equieffective concentrations, prenalterol and isoproterenol increased bound cyclic AMP levels to the same extent, whereas the increase in free cyclic AMP level was much greater with isoproterenol. These findings support the proposed compartmentation of cyclic AMP in myocardial cells and may indicate that β_1-partial agonists elevate cyclic AMP levels in the functionally relevant compartment(s) more effectively than isoproterenol.

FIG. 4. Chemical structures of β_1-adrenoceptor partial agonists

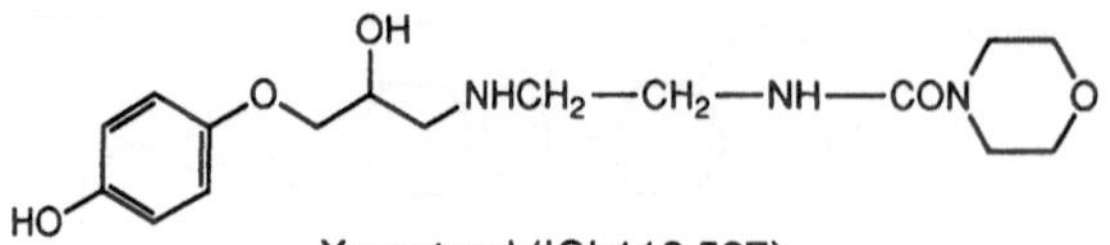

Xamoterol (ICI 118,587)

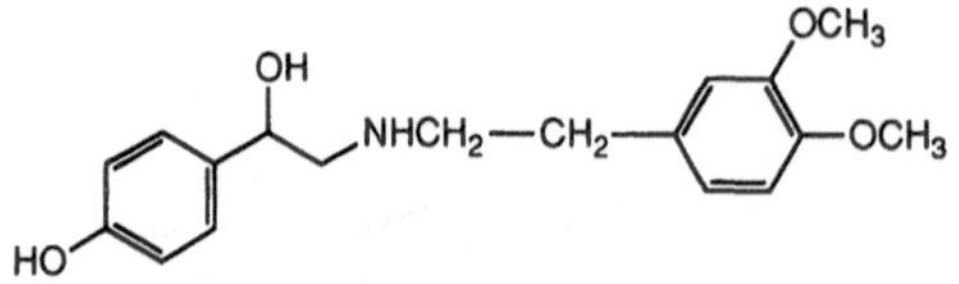

Denopamine (TA-064)

Although β_1-partial agonists caused the accumulation of much less cyclic AMP than isoproterenol for a given increase in force, it was unclear if the nature of the regulation of Ca^{2+} transients and contractility by these agents is different from that exerted by isoproterenol. The partial β_1-agonist denopamine, with an intrinsic activity of 0.9 (versus ISOmax), was used to examine this question in aequorin-injected ventricular muscle of the dog [44]. The bell-shaped concentration–response curve for the positive inotropic effect of denopamine [7] was associated with the bell-shaped curve for an increase in Ca^{2+} transients induced by denopamine [44]. The relation between peak force and the amplitude of Ca^{2+} transients induced by denopamine was no different from that induced by isoproterenol. This equivalence indicates that although denopamine, a partial agonist of β_1-adrenoceptors, causes the accumulation of cyclic AMP to a much lesser extent than the full agonist isoproterenol, the extent of accumulation of cyclic AMP in the functionally relevant compartment(s) may be identical; hence the myofibrillar responsiveness to Ca^{2+} ions is decreased by denopamine in a manner similar to the decrease caused by isoproterenol [44].

These agents are available in oral preparations. They are less arrhythmogenic than isoproterenol because they cause less accumulation of cyclic AMP [6]. Pharmacologically, β_1-partial agonists exert their chronotropic and inotropic effects depending on the extent of intrinsic sympathetic activation in individual patients: When sympathetic activity is high they act as β_1-blocking agents, whereas they act as β_1-adrenoceptor agonists when sympathetic activity is low [85]. After the administration of sufficient doses, inotropy and chronotropy are buffered to the level of intrinsic sympathomimetic activity (ISA) of individual partial agonists, indicating that the desired level of β-adrenoceptor stimulation could be achieved by the development of partial agonists with different ISAs. The ISA of denopamine is 0.9 and those of xamoterol and pindolol are 0.43 and 0.2, respectively [85], indicating that denopamine acts as a full β_1-agonist, whereas pindolol acts as a β-blocker in most clinical situations. It is still controversial whether β_1-partial agonists induce β_1-adrenoceptor down-regulation during long-term administration [88–90].

Clinical development of xamoterol has been abandoned because it increased the incidence of cardiac deaths compared with placebo during the course of treatment of severe congestive heart failure patients [10]. When β-receptor down-regulation occurs in patients with severe congestive heart failure, β-partial agonists act as β-blockers [91], which may have been a reason for the adverse effects reported with acute administration of relatively large doses of xamoterol to severe heart failure patients [10]. It is probable that β_1-partial agonists inhibit the development of β_1-adrenoceptor down-regulation induced with the progression of heart failure [92, 93].

Selective β_2-agonists, such as pirbuterolol [94] and dopexamine [95], which have been shown to be effective for the treatment of congestive heart failure, likewise caused a positive inotropic effect. These agents, however, are considered to be effective largely by reducing the afterload to the heart due to vasodilation via β_2-adrenoceptor activation rather than their positive inotropic effect.

Ca^{2+} Sensitizers

The relation between $[Ca^{2+}]_i$ and developed tension has been studied extensively using skinned cardiac muscle fibers. Some interventions, including hypoxia [96, 97], acidosis [98], accumulation of inorganic phosphate in myocardial cells [99], experimentally lowering temperature [100], and phosphorylation of troponin I induced by cyclic AMP generation due to β-adrenoceptor stimulation [101, 102], alter the relation, which is defined as an "alteration of myofibrillar responsiveness to Ca^{2+}" or "alteration of Ca^{2+} sensitivity of the contractile apparatus" [20]. The development of experimental methods by means of various intracellular Ca^{2+} indicators, such as aequorin, indo-1, and fura-2, made it possible to examine the relation between $[Ca^{2+}]_i$ transient and twitch contraction in intact cardiac preparations. In addition, a novel method that makes it possible to identify directly the mechanism of action involved in the alteration of Ca^{2+} sensitivity has been developed: With this new technique, cardiac actomyosin interaction can be observed with the in vitro motility assay, using reconstituted native thin filament by adding the cardiac tropomyosin-troponin complex to actin filament and myosin filament. The immediate environment around the crossbridges can be controlled, and the effect of various factors including cardiotonic agents on the movement of thin filaments on the myosin layer is observable. By comparing the mechanical response to Ca^{2+} of the reconstituted thin filament (with tropomyosin–troponin complex) and the simple actin filament (without tropomyosin–troponin complex), the site of drug action can be differentiated by investigating if its action requires the presence of the whole regulatory system [23, 66]. The relation between actin-activated myosin ATPase activity and $[Ca^{2+}]$ while changing the condition of the reaction solution provides useful information to explain the modulation of Ca^{2+} sensitivity, although the myosin ATPase activity in vitro is not always a good index of changes in mechanical properties of contractile proteins [103, 104].

It has long been known that caffeine and theophylline, in addition to their non-selective inhibitory action on PDE, possess the ability to increase Ca^{2+} sensitivity of contractile proteins in skinned cardiac fibers. This effect is shown to be due to their ability to increase the affinity of troponin C to Ca^{2+} ions by reduction of the off-rate of Ca^{2+} from troponin C [105]. However, because methylxanthines have multiple actions on different sites of E–C coupling and receptor-mediated regulatory processes, the ultimate response to these agents is complex. In addition to the effect of inhibiting PDE activity nonselectively, they inhibit the amplitude of Ca^{2+} transients by attenuating the uptake and release of Ca^{2+} ions by the SR in intact cardiac muscle [106]. As a whole, the effects of caffeine and theophylline in preparations of intact myocardium are consistent with those in skinned or hyperpermeable cardiac muscle [105, 107]. In addition, theophylline acts simultaneously by inhibiting adenosine A_1 receptors in the cardiovascular system.

Calcium sensitivity of the contractile apparatus has been shown to be modulated by a new class of cardiotonic agents termed Ca^{2+} sensitizers. In the early studies, sulmazole was shown to be more efficient than other newly developed cardiotonic drugs, such as milrinone, amrinone, isomazole, imazodan, or piroximone, when tested in the rabbit papillary muscle [30]. A significant portion of the contractile response to sulmazole is believed to result from an increase in myofibrillar responsiveness to Ca^{2+} ions, as observed in in vitro studies [108, 109]. In dog ventricular muscle, the positive inotropic effect of sulmazole was mediated by both cyclic AMP-dependent and cyclic AMP-independent mechanisms, whereas that of enoximone was exerted exclusively via the former mechanism [110]. In aequorin-injected ventricular trabeculae of the dog, the increase in peak Ca^{2+} transients, the positive inotropic effect, and the accumulation of cyclic AMP produced by enoximone are abolished by carbachol. The effects of sulmazole on the Ca^{2+} transient and its interaction with carbachol are more complicated: At concentrations up to 0.3 mM, sulmazole increases the peak Ca^{2+} transient and contractile force in parallel in a concentration-dependent manner, and these effects are antagonized by carbachol. At concentrations of 1 mM and higher, sulmazole decreases the peak Ca^{2+} transient in association with a slight reduction in the rate of decline of Ca^{2+} transients, but it increases the force still further with prolongation of the time to peak tension [33]. Because the effects of high concentrations of sulmazole are resistant to carbachol, it appears that sulmazole elicits its positive inotropic effect via a cyclic AMP-dependent mechanism at low concentrations and via an increase in the responsiveness of myofilaments to Ca^{2+} ions at high concentrations in dog ventricular muscle. The reduction in peak Ca^{2+} transients elicited by high concentrations of sulmazole may be due in part to inhibition of the uptake of Ca^{2+} ions by the SR, as is also observed with other inhibitors of PDE, such as caffeine and theophylline in cardiac muscles [e.g., 106].

Among Ca^{2+} sensitizers, the effect of a derivative of diazinone designated EMD 53998 (Fig. 5) has been studied most extensively. It has been reported that EMD 53998

EMD 53 998

Org 30029   FIG. 5. Chemical structures of novel Ca^{2+} sensitizers

improves the economy of chemomechanical energy transduction in cardiac muscle [111]. In other studies the positive inotropic effect of EMD 53998 was not associated with a change in Ca^{2+} transients, or with only a small increase or decrease in Ca^{2+} transients [112, 113]. Available preparations of EMD 53998 consist of a racemic mixture with both PDE-inhibitory action and Ca^{2+}-sensitizing action. It has been shown that the (+)isomer has a predominantly Ca^{2+}-sensitizing action, whereas the (−)isomer inhibits PDE [113, 114]. These findings are important and intriguing because a number of classical and new agents, such as caffeine, theophylline, sulmazole, pimobendan, MCI-154, and Org 30029, have both PDE-inhibitory and Ca^{2+}-sensitizing actions. The selective actions of the enantiomers of EMD 53998 suggest that the binding sites or sites of action on PDE and contractile proteins may be structurally closely interrelated. EMD 53998 or MCI-154 have been shown to be able to reverse the contractile depression induced by anoxia [112], acidosis [59, 115], and inorganic phosphate [116], which may have a critical modulatory effect on cardiac contractility under ischemic conditions.

Although the mechanism of the drug-induced myofibrillar sensitization to Ca^{2+} ions has not been unequivocally elucidated, it appears that, in addition to modulating the affinity of troponin C for Ca^{2+} ions, EMD 53998 may exploit the actin–myosin interface as its potential site of action and cause a change in cycling of crossbridges [23]. Solaro and co-workers [23] showed that EMD 53998 activates actomyosin ATPase in the absence of Ca^{2+}-regulatory proteins and increases the rate of movement of actin–myosin in the motility assay in the absence of Ca^{2+} ions. The latter effect does not involve Ca^{2+} ions or is operative at a site beyond Ca^{2+}-signaling events; therefore the term "Ca^{2+} sensitizer" is no longer applicable.

The novel agent Org 30029 (Fig. 5) acts also through PDE inhibition and Ca^{2+} sensitization, but the latter mechanism is much more pronounced than the former. In the aequorin-injected ventricular trabeculae of the dog, even in the presence of carbachol, which selectively inhibits the changes induced via cyclic AMP, Org 30029 increased the isometric contraction to a level even higher than the maximum response to isoproterenol; moreover, the positive inotropic effect of Org 30029 was associated with decreases in Ca^{2+} transients [24].

The relation of $[Ca^{2+}]_i$ and the force developed by cardiac myofilaments has been shown to be modified by pathophysiological conditions such as hypoxia, ischemia, and congestive heart failure. Under these situations, which are commonly encountered in the clinical setting, Ca^{2+} transients are scarcely affected, but the force is suppressed, indicating that Ca^{2+} sensitivity is decreased. For example, Allen and Orchard [97] showed in aequorin-loaded ferret papillary muscle that during the early phase of hypoxia the developed tension decreased quickly whereas $[Ca^{2+}]_i$ remained unchanged.

The change in Ca^{2+} sensitivity during hypoxia or ischemia has been shown to be associated with an accumulation or a decrease in myocardial metabolic products, including increased H^+ [98], decreased phosphocreatine [99], or increased inorganic phosphate [99]. The situation in respect to changes in Ca^{2+} sensitivity is more complicated in the failing heart. Although a decrease in Ca^{2+} sensitivity has been demonstrated in papillary muscle isolated from an experimentally induced heart failure model [117], no change or an increase in Ca^{2+} sensitivity was detected in skinned fibers of ventricular muscle isolated from the human failing heart [118]. It is therefore highly probable that there is a contribution by the environment where the myofibrils are located, which are modulated via a receptor-mediated intracellular messenger system, by cytokines, or by metabolic changes that result from the progression of failing heart symptoms [83, 119].

The Ca^{2+} sensitizers are considered to be attractive as potential therapeutic agents for the treatment of patients with congestive heart failure because (1) the activation energy required for the transport of Ca^{2+} ions may be preserved with this class of agents; (2) Ca^{2+} overload, which may be responsible for the arrhythmogenic actions of cardiac glycosides and catecholamines and the ultimate death of myocardial cells, can be avoided; and (3) these agents provide a potential novel mechanism for reversing the myocardial contractile dysfunction encountered in hypoxia, ischemia and reperfusion, and congestive heart failure.

By applying new techniques, it is now known that the increase in Ca^{2+} sensitivity is due to at least three underlying mechanisms (Table 2): (1) Modulation of the affinity of troponin C to Ca^{2+} has been postulated to be the primary mechanism of some drug actions, such as caffeine (causing an increase) or cyclic AMP (causing a decrease), mostly based on the findings in skinned cardiac muscle fibers. (2) Facilitation of thin filament interaction (troponin, tropomyosin, actin) may result in facilitated interaction with myosin. This mechanism can be differentiated by combining experimental techniques: First, the drug acting through this mechanism requires a complete thin filament system (tropomyosin–troponin complex) in the motility assay; and second, the drug does not facilitate the binding of Ca^{2+} to troponin C in the in vitro experimental system. (3) Modulation of crossbridge cycling by the drug is postulated by the experimental evidence, which can be provided by a motility assay system that includes simply actin and myosin. Because this system lacks a site for Ca^{2+} regulation, the drug that acts via this mechanism cannot be termed a "Ca^{2+} sensitizer" and may be named in a novel category, such as "crossbridge promoter" or "crossbridge enhancer". The (+)isomer of EMD 53996 (EMD 51378) has been shown to act via this mechanism [20]. It has been shown in intact tetanized ferret papillary muscle by means of perturbation analysis [120] that β-stimulation increases the crossbridge cycling rate [121], but the effect of Ca^{2+} sensitizers has not yet been analyzed by this technique. (4) The influence of the environment in which myofibrils are located is also crucial. Under pathophysiological conditions, intracellular metabolites (creatine phosphate, inorganic phosphate) and ions such as H^+ may modulated Ca^{2+} sensitivity in intact cardiac muscle. In addition, receptor-mediated regulation and cytokines due to elevated levels in the blood under pathophysiological conditions may likewise modulate Ca^{2+} sensitivity [18, 119].

The energetic advantage expected to be associated with the drugs acting through different subcellular mechanisms is not experimentally evident when analyzed by sophisticated techniques meticulously provided to detect the cardiac efficacy in canine perfused heart [122]. The reason for this lack is not clear, but at least two reasons may be involved. First, when the relation of cardiac work and heat production, which represents "cardiac economy" (but not "cardiac efficacy") is measured, the Ca^{2+} sensitizers show a definite advantage in that they produce less heat for a comparable increase in cardiac work compared with catecholamines, and therefore cardiac economy may be a more sensitive indicator for revealing the underlying mechanistic difference [123, 124]. Second, energetic advantages may be realized in the failing heart more easily than in the normal heart because cardiotonic agents exert their effects in concert with other hemodynamic improvements encountered only under pathophysiological conditions.

Clinical trials for these Ca^{2+} sensitizers have started, and it must be determined whether these drugs exert beneficial clinical actions with their novel mechanisms.

Ca^{2+} Promoters

Calcium promoters such as Bay k 8644, YC-170, H160/51, ($\pm$)202-791, and CGP 28392 bind directly to the specific binding sites on L-type Ca^{2+} channels and thereby increase cardiac contractile function through facilitation of the open probability of Ca$^+$ channels [125, 126]. It is reported that Bay k 8644 is less oxygen-consuming than other inotropic agents (e.g., isoproterenol, amrinone, pimobendan) in the isolated guinea pig working heart [126]. Ca^{2+} promoters also exert constrictor effects on the peripheral and coronary vasculature, causing increased afterload to the heart and elevated coronary vascular resistance. Therefore it is necessary to increase their cardioselective activity for clinical application. Some Ca^{2+} agonist enantiomers, such as ($\pm$)202-791, act differentially with Ca$^+$ agonistic and antagonistic properties on cardiac muscle and vascular smooth muscle. The development of clinically beneficial agents based on this peculiar characteristic of enantiomers has been proposed [126]. More recently a Ca^{2+} promotor with highly cardioselective characteristics has been developed. Bay y 5959 [(R)-isopropyl 2-amino-5-cyano-6-methyl-1,4-dihydro-4-(3-phenyl-quinoline-5-yl)-pyridine-3-carboxylate] has been shown to be energetically as efficient as ouabain, Bay k 8644, and calcium, which are more efficient than the agents that cause cyclic AMP accumulation, such as catecholamines or PDE III inhibitors (amrinone, milrinone, pimobendan) [127]. Furthermore, Bay y 5959 has accelerated the functional recovery of the myocardium from ischemia more effectively than isoproterenol in the anesthetized dog [128]. It is going to be examined in clinical settings.

Acknowledgments. This work was supported in part by a Grant-in-Aid for Developmental Scientific Research (B) (04557009, 1992–1994; 07557193, 1995) from the Ministry of Education, Science, and Culture, Japan.

References

1. Farah AE, Alousi AA (1978) New cardiotonic agents: a search for digitalis substitute. Life Sci 22:1139–1148
2. Farah AE, Alousi AA, Schwarz RP Jr (1984) Positive inotropic agents. Annu Rev Pharmacol Toxicol 24:275–328
3. Alousi AA, Farah AE, Lesher GY, Opalka CJ Jr (1979) Cardiotonic activity of amrinone— Win 40680 [5-amino 3,4'-bipyridin-6(1H)-one]. Circ Res 45:666–677
4. Aass H, Skomedal T, Osnes JB (1988) Increase of cyclic AMP in subcellular fractions of rat heart muscle after β-adrenergic stimulation: prenalterol and isoprenaline caused different distribution of bound cyclic AMP. J Mol Cell Cardiol 20:847–860
5. Endoh M, Shibasaki T, Satoh H, Norota I, Ishihata A (1991) Different mechanisms involved in the positive inotropic effects of benzimidazole derivative UD-CG 115 BS (pimobendan) and its demethylated metabolite UD-CG 212 Cl in canine ventricular myocardium. J Cardiovasc Pharmacol 17:365–375
6. Main BG (1982) Structure-activity relations of β-adrenergic agents. J Chem Tech Biotechnol 32:617–626
7. Yokoyama H, Yanagisawa T, Taira N (1988) Details of mode and mechanism of action of denopamine, a new orally active cardiotonic agent with affinity for β$_1$-receptors. J Cardiovasc Pharmacol 12:323–331

8. DiBianco R, Shabetai R, Kostuk W, Moran J, Schlant RC, Wright RA (1989) A comparison of oral milrinone, digoxin, and their combination in the treatment of patients with chronic heart failure. N Engl J Med 320:677–683

9. Packer M, Carver JR, Rodeheffer RJ, et al, for PROMIS Study Research Group (1991) Effect of oral milrinone on mortality in severe chronic heart failure. N Engl J Med 325:1468–1475

10. Xamoterol in Severe Heart Failure Study Group (1990) Xamoterol in severe heart failure. Lancet 336:1–6 [Erratum, Lancet (1990) 336:698]

11. Uretskey BF, Jessup M, Konstam MA, Dec W, Leier CV, Benotti J, Murali S, Herrmann HC, Sandberg JA for the Enoximone Multicenter Trial Group (1990) Multicenter trial of oral enoximone in patients with moderate to moderately severe congestive heart failure: lack of benefit compared with placebo. Circulation 82:774–780

12. Massie B, Bourassa M, DiBianco R, Hess M, Kostam M, Likoff M, Packer M (1985) Long-term oral administration of amrinone for congestive heart failure: lack of efficiency in a multicenter controlled trial. Circulation 71:963–971

13. Veterans Administration Study Group (1986) Effect of vasodilator therapy on mortality in chronic congestive heart failure. N Engl J Med 314:1547–1552

14. CONSENSUS Trial Study Group (1987) Effect of enalapril on mortality in severe congestive heart failure. N Engl J Med 316:1429–1435

15. Solved Investigators (1991) Effect of enalapril on survival in patients with reduced left ventricular ejections and congestive heart failure. N Engl J Med 325:293–302

16. Endoh M, Yamashita S, Taira N (1982) Positive inotropic effect of amrinone in relation to cyclic nucleotide metabolism in the canine ventricular muscle. J Pharmacol Exp Ther 221:775–783

17. Katano Y, Endoh M (1992) Effects of a cardiotonic quinolinone derivative Y-20487 on the isoproterenol-induced positive inotropic action and cyclic AMP accumulation in rat ventricular myocardium: comparison with rolipram, Ro 20-1724, milrinone, and isobutylmethylxanthine. J Cardiovasc Pharmacol 20:715–722

18. Endoh M, Hori M (1993) Basic pharmacology and clinical application of new positive inotropic agents. Drugs Today 29:29–56

19. Reiter M (1988) Calcium mobilization and cardiac inotropic mechanisms. Pharmacol Rev 40:189–217

20. Blinks JR, Endoh M (1986) Modification of myofibrillar responsiveness to Ca^{++} as an inotropic mechanism. Circulation 73(suppl III):85–98

21. Harrison SA, Reifsnyder DH, Gallis B, Cadd GG, Beavo JA (1986) Isolation and characterization of bovine cardiac muscle cGMP-inhibited phosphodiesterase: a receptor for new cardiotonic drugs. Mol Pharmacol 29:506–514

22. Weishaar RE, Burrows SD, Kobylarz DC, Quade MM, Evans DB (1986) Multiple molecular forms of cyclic nucleotide phosphodiesterase in cardiac and smooth muscle and in platelets: isolation, characterization, and effects of various reference phosphodiesterase inhibitors and cardiotonic agents. Biochem Pharmacol 35:787–800

23. Solaro RJ, Gambassi G, Warshaw DM, Keller MR, Spurgeon HA, Beier N, Lakatta EG (1993) Stereoselective actions of thiadiazinones on canine cardiac myocytes and myofilaments. Circ Res 73:981–990

24. Kawabata Y, Endoh M (1993) Effects of the positive inotropic agent Org 30029 on developed force and aequorin light transients in intact canine ventricular myocardium. Circ Res 72:597–606

25. Blinks JR (1993) Analysis of the effects of drugs on myofibrillar Ca^{2+} sensitivity in intact cardiac muscle. In: Lee JA, Allen DG (eds) Modulation of cardiac calcium sensitivity: a new approach to increasing the strength of the heart. Oxford University Press, Oxford, pp 242–282

26. Beavo JA, Conti M, Heaslip RJ (1994) Multiple cyclic nucleotide phosphodiesterases. Mol Pharmacol 46:399–405

27. Weishaar RE, Kobylarz-Singer DC, Steffen RP, Kaplan HR (1987) Subclasses of cyclic AMP-specific phospodiesterase in left ventricular muscle and their involvement in regulating myocardial contractility. Circ Res 61:539–547

28. Kauffman RF, Crowe VG, Utterback BG, Robertson DW. (1986) LY195115: a potent, selective inhibitor of cyclic nucleotide phosphodiesterase located in the sarcoplasmic reticulum. Mol Pharmacol 30:609–616

29. Kauffman RF, Utterback BG, Robertson DW (1989) Specific binding of [³H]LY186126, an analogue of indolidan (LY195115), to cardiac membranes enriched in sarcoplasmic reticulum vesicles. Circ Res 64:1037–1040

30. Kithas PA, Artman M, Thompson WJ, Strada SJ (1988) Subcellular distribution of high-affinity type IV cyclic AMP phosphodiesterase activity in rabbit ventricular myocardium: relations to the effects of cardiotonic drugs. Circ Res 62:782–789

31. Silver PJ (1989) Biochemical aspects of inhibition of cardiovascular low (Km) cyclic adenosine monophosphate phosphodiesterase. Am J Cardiol 63:2A–8A

32. Endoh M (1993) Pharmacology of loprinone (E-1020), a new pyridinone inodilator, as a therapeutic agent for acute heart failure. Cardiovasc Drug Rev 11:432–450

33. Endoh M, Yanagisawa T, Taira N, Blinks JR (1986) Effects of new inotropic agents on cyclic nucleotide metabolism and calcium transients in canine ventricular muscle. Circulation 73(suppl III):117–133

34. Gwathmey JK, Morgan JP (1985) The effects of milrinone and piroximone on intracellular calcium handling in working myocardium from the ferret. Br J Pharmacol 85:97–108

35. Earl CQ, Linden J, Weglicki WB (1986) Inhibition of cyclic AMP-dependent protein kinase activity by the cardiotonic drugs amrinone and milrinone. Life Sci 39:1901–1908

36. Rapundalo ST, Grupp I, Grupp G, Matlib MA, Solaro RJ, Schwartz A (1986) Myocardial actions of milrinone: characterization of its mechanism of action. Circulation 73(suppl III):134–144

37. Malecot CO, Bers DM, Katzung BG (1986) Biphasic contractions induced by milrinone at low temperature in ferret ventricular muscle: role of the sarcoplasmic reticulum and transmembrane calcium influx. Circ Res 59:151–162

38. Holmberg SRM, Williams AJ (1991) Phosphodiesterase inhibitors and the cardiac sarcoplasmic reticulum calcium release channel: differential effects of milrinone and enoximone. Cardiovasc Res 25:537–545

39. Alousi AA, Grant AM, Allen PD, Pagani ED (1988) Effects of milrinone on Ca⁺⁺-sensitivity of myofibrillar Mg-adenosine triphosphatase isolated from normal human and canine hearts. J Pharmacol Exp Ther 246:30–37

40. Rapundalo ST, Solaro RJ, Kranias EG (1989) Inotropic responses to isoproterenol and phosphodiesterase inhibitors in intact guinea pig hearts: comparison of cyclic AMP levels and phosphorylation of sarcoplasmic reticulum and myofibrillar proteins. Circ Res 64:104–111

41. Endoh M, Kawabata Y, Katano Y, Norota I (1994) Effects of a novel cardiotonic agent (±)-6-[3-(3,4-dimethoxybenzylamino)-2-hydroxypropoxy] 2(1H)-quinolinone (OPC-18790) on contractile force, cyclic AMP level, and aequorin light transients in dog ventricular myocardium. J Cardiovasc Pharmacol 23:723–730

42. Kawabata Y, Endoh M (1995) Effects of a novel cardiotonic agent, Org 9731, on force and aequorin light transients in intact ventricular myocardium of the dog: involvement of a cyclic AMP-mediated mechanism and myofibrillar responsiveness to Ca²⁺ ions. J Cardiac Failure 1:143–153

43. Endoh M, Blinks JR (1988) Actions of sympathomimetic amines on the Ca²⁺ transients and contractions of rabbit myocardium: reciprocal changes in myofibrillar responsiveness to Ca²⁺ mediated through α- and β-adrenoceptors. Circ Res 62:247–265

44. Kohi M, Norota I, Takanashi M, Endoh M (1993) On the mechanism of action of the beta-1 partial agonist denopamine in regulation of myocardial contractility: effects on myocardial alpha adrenoceptors and intracellular Ca⁺⁺ transients. J Pharmacol Exp Ther 265:1292–1300

45. Honerjäger P, Heiss A, Schäfer-Korting M, Schönsteiner G, Reiter M (1984) UD-CG 115—a cardiotonic pyridinone which elevates cyclic AMP and prolongs the action potential in guinea-pig papillary muscle. Naunyn Schmiedebergs Arch Pharmacol 325:259–269

46. Verdouw PD, Hartog JM, Duncker DJ, Roth W, Saxena PR (1986) Cardiovascular profile of pimobendan, a benzimidazole-pyridazinone derivative with vasodilating and inotropic properties. Eur J Pharmacol 126:21–30

47. Duncker DJ, Hartog JM, Levinsky L, Verdouw PD (1987) Systemic haemodynamic actions of pimobendan (UD-CG 115 BS) and its O-demethylmetabolite UD-CG 212 Cl in the conscious pig. Br J Pharmacol 91:609–615

48. Westfall MV, Wahler GM, Fujino K, Solaro RJ (1992) Electrophysiological actions of the pimobendan metabolite, UD-CG 212 Cl, in guinea pig myocardium. J Pharmacol Exp Ther 260:58–63
49. Berger C, Meyer W, Scholz H, Starbatty J (1985) Effects of the benzimidazole derivatives pimobendan and 2-(4-hydroxy-phenyl)-5-(5-methyl-3-oxo-4,5-dihydro-2H-6-pyridazinyl) benzimidazole HCl on phosphodiesterase activity and force of contraction in guinea-pig hearts. Arzneimittelforschung 35(II):1668–1673
50. Rüegg JC, Pfitzer G, Eubler D, Zeugner C (1984) Effect on contractility of skinned fibers from mammalian heart and smooth muscle by a new benzimidazole derivative, 4,5-dihydro-6-[2-(4-methoxyphenyl)-1H-benzimidazol-5-yl]-5-methyl-3(2H)-pyridazinone. Arzneimittelforschung 34(II):1736–1738
51. Fujino K, Sperelakis N, Solaro RJ (1988) Sensitization of dog and guinea pig heart myofilaments to Ca^{2+} activation and the inotropic effect of pimobendan: comparison with milrinone. Circ Res 63:911–922
52. Fujino K, Sperelakis N, Solaro RJ (1988) Differential effects of d- and l-pimobendan on cardiac myofilament calcium sensitivity. J Pharmacol Exp Ther 247:519–523
53. Brunkhorst D, Von der Leyen H, Meyer W, Nigbur R, Schmidt-Schumacher C, Scholz H (1989) Relation of positive inotropic and chronotropic effects of pimobendan, UD-CG 212 Cl, milrinone and other phosphodiesterase inhibitors to phosphodiesterase III inhibition in guinea-pig heart. Naunyn Schmiedebergs Arch Pharmacol 339:575–583
54. Von der Leyen H, Mende U, Meyer W, et al (1991) Mechanism underlying the reduced positive inotropic effects of the phosphodiesterase III inhibitors pimobendan, adibendan and saterinone in failing as compared to nonfailing human cardiac muscle preparations. Naunyn Schmiedebergs Arch Pharmacol 334:90–100
55. Böhm M, Morano I, Pieske B, Rüegg JC, Wankerl M, Zimmermann R, Erdmann E (1991) Contribution of cAMP-phosphodiesterase inhibition and sensitization of the contractile proteins for calcium to the inotropic effect of pimobendan in the failing human myocardium. Circ Res 68:689–701
56. Kitada Y, Narimatsu A, Suzuki R, Endoh M, Taira N (1987) Does the positive inotropic action of a novel cardiotonic agent, MCI-154, involve mechanisms other than cyclic AMP? J Pharmacol Exp Ther 243:639–645
57. Kitada Y, Narimatsu A, Matsumura N, Endo M (1987) Increase in Ca^{++} sensitivity of the contractile system by MCI-154, a novel cardiotonic agent, in chemically skinned fibers from the guinea pig papillary muscles. J Pharmacol Exp Ther 243:633–638
58. Hosono M, Taira N (1987) Cardiac and coronary vasodilator effects of the novel cardiotonic agent, MCI-154, assessed in isolated, blood-perfused dog heart preparations. J Cardiovasc Pharmacol 10:692–698
59. Allert JA, Adams HR (1990) Inotropic and chronotropic profile of MCI-154: comparison with isoproterenol and imazodan in guinea pig cardiac preparations. J Cardiovasc Pharmacol 16:59–67
60. Warren SE, Kihara Y, Pesaturo J, Gwathmey JK, Phillips P, Morgan JP (1989) Inotropic and lusitropic effects of MCI-154 (6-[4-(4-pyridyl)aminophenyl]-4,5-dihydro-3(2H)-pyridazinone) on human myocardium. J Mol Cell Cardiol 21:1037–1045
61. Endoh M (1990) Characteristics of regulation of intracellular calcium mobilization and sensitivity by beta-adrenoceptor and muscarinic agonists, and a novel inotropic agent, MCI-154 in canine ventricular myocardium. In: Yamada K, Shibata S (eds) Recent advances in calcium channels and calcium-antagonists. Pergamon, New York, pp 51–59
62. Kitada Y, Abe Y, Narimatsu A, Tobe A (1991) MCI-154, a novel cardiotonic agent, reverses the acidic pH-induced decrease in responses of cardiac myofilaments to Ca^{++}: comparison with sulmazole and pimobendan. J Pharmacol Exp Ther 257:812–819
63. Abe Y, Kitada Y, Narimatsu A (1992) Beneficial effect of MCI-154, a cardiotonic agent, on ischemic contractile failure and myocardial acidosis of dog hearts: comparison with dobutamine, milrinone and pimobendan. J Pharmacol Exp Ther 261:1087–1095
64. Narimatsu A, Kitada Y, Satoh N, Suzuki R, Okushima H (1987) Cardiovascular pharmacology of 6-[4-(4'-pyridyl)aminophenyl]-4,5-dihydro-3(2H)-pyridazinone hydrochloride, a

novel and potent cardiotonic agent with vasodilator properties. Arzneimittelforschung 37:398–406

65. Kitada Y, Kobayashi M, Narimatsu A, Ohizumi Y (1989) Potent stimulation of myofilament force and adenosine triphosphatase activity of canine cardiac muscle through a direct enhancement of troponin C Ca^{++} binding by MCI-154, a novel cardiotonic agent. J Pharmacol Exp Ther 250:272–277

66. Sata M, Sugiura S, Yamashita H, Fujita H, Momomura S, Serizawa T (1995) MCI-154 increases Ca^{2+} sensitivity of the reconstituted thin filament: a study using a novel in vitro motility assay technique. Circ Res 76:626–633

67. Perreault C, Brozovich FV, Ransil Bj, Morgan JP (1989) Effects of MCI-154 on Ca^{2+} activation of skinned human myocardium. Eur J Pharmacol 165:305–308

68. Steffen RP, Eldon CM, Evans DB (1986) The effect of the cardiotonic imazodan (CI-914) on myocardial and peripheral hemodynamics in the anesthetized dog. J Cardiovasc Pharmacol 8:520–526

69. Hayes JS, Pollock GD, Wilson H, Bowling N, Robertson DW (1987) Pharmacology of LY195115, a potent, orally active cardiotonic with a long duration of action. J Cardiovasc Pharmacol 9:425–434

70. Kauffman RF, Utterback BG, Robertson DW (1989) Characterization and pharmacological relevance of high affinity binding sites for [^{3}H]LY186126, a cardiotonic phosphodiesterase inhibitor, in canine cardiac membranes. Circ Res 65:154–163

71. Taira N, Endoh M, Iijima T, Satoh K, Yanagisawa T, Yamashita S, Maruyama M, Kawada M, Morita T, Wada Y (1984) Mode and mechanism of action of 3, 4-dihydro-6-[4-(3,4-dimethoxybenzoyl)-1-piperazinyl]-2(1H)-quinolinone (OPC-8212), a novel positive inotropic drug, on the dog heart. Arzneimittelforschung 34(I):347–355

72. Yanagisawa T, Endoh M, Taira N (1984) Involvement of cyclic AMP in the positive inotropic effect of OPC-8212, a new cardiotonic agent, on canine ventricular muscle. Jpn J Pharmacol 36:379–388

73. Hosokawa T, Mori T, Fujiki H, et al (1992) Cardiovascular actions of OPC-18790: a novel positive inotropic agent with little chronotropic action. Heart Vessels 7:66–75

74. Yatani A, Imoto Y, Schwartz A, Brown AM (1989) New positive inotropic agent OPC-8212 modulates single Ca^{2+} channels in ventricular myocytes of guinea pig. J Cardiovasc Pharmacol 13:812–819

75. Iijima T, Taira N (1987) Membrane current changes responsible for the positive inotropic effect of OPC-8212, a new positive inotropic agent, in single ventricular cells of the guinea pig heart. J Pharmacol Exp Ther 240:657–662

76. Yanagisawa T, Ishii K, Taira N (1987) Antitachycardiac effect of OPC-8212, a novel cardiotonic agent, on tachycardiac response of guinea pig isolated right atria to isoproterenol and histamine. J Cardiovasc Pharmacol 10:47–54

77. Lathrop DA, Schwartz A (1985) Evidence for possible increase of sodium channel open time and involvement of Na/Ca exchange by a new positive inotropic drug: OPC-8212. Eur J Pharmacol 117:391–392

78. Rapundalo ST, Lathrop DA, Harrison SA, Beavo JA, Schwartz A (1988) Cyclic AMP-dependent and cyclic AMP-independent actions of a novel cardiotonic agent, OPC-8212. Naunyn Schmiedebergs Arch Pharmacol 338:692–698

79. Asanoi H, Sasayama S, Iuchi K, Kameyama T (1987) Acute hemodynamic effects of a new inotropic agent (OPC-8212) in patients with congestive heart failure. J Am Coll Cardiol 9:865–871

80. Inoue M, Hori M, Yasuda H, Takishima T, Sugimoto T, Sasayama S, Sakurai T, Nonogi H, Kodama K, Kusukawa R, Nakamura M, Kawai C (1987) A multicenter study of a new inotropic agent, piperanometozine (OPC-8212) in congestive heart failure: clinical improvement during short-term treatment. Cardiovasc Drugs Ther 1:169–175

81. OPC-8212 Multicenter Research Group (1990) A placebo-controlled, randomized, double-blind study of OPC-8212 in patients with mild chronic heart failure. Cardiovasc Drugs Ther 4:419–426

82. Feldman AM, Bristow MR, Parmley WW, et al (1993) Effects of vesnarinone on morbidity and mortality in patients with heart failure. N Engl J Med 328:149–155

83. Shioi T, Matsumori A, Matsui S, Sasayama S (1994) Inhibition of cytokine production by a new inotropic agent, vesnarinone, in human lymphocytes, T cell line, and monocytic cell line. Life Sci 54:11–16

84. Hedberg A, Carlsson E, Fellenius E, Lundgren B (1982) Cardiostimulatory effects of prenalterol, a beta-1 adrenoceptor partial agonist, in vivo and in vitro: correlation between physiological effects and adenylate cyclase activity. Naunyn Schmiedebergs Arch Pharmacol 318:185–191

85. Nuttall A, Snow HM (1982) The cardiovascular effects of ICI 118,587: a β_1-adrenoceptor partial agonist. Br J Pharmacol 77:381–388

86. Inamasu M, Totsuka T, Ikeo T, Nagao T, Takayama S (1987) Beta$_1$-adrenergic selectivity of the new cardiotonic agent denopamine in its stimulating effects on adenylate cyclase. Biochem Pharmacol 36:1947–1954

87. Sasaki Y, Yabana H, Nagao T, Takayama S (1988) Effect of denopamine on the phosphorylation of cardiac muscle proteins in the perfused guinea-pig heart. Biochem Pharmacol 37:679–686

88. Reithmann C, Wieland F, Jakobs KH, Werdan K (1989) Intrinsic sympathomimetic activity of beta-adrenoceptor antagonists: down-regulation of cardiac beta$_1$- and beta$_2$-adrenoceptors. Eur J Pharmacol 170:243–255

89. Yabana H, Naito K, Nagao T (1986) Effect of chronic administration of denopamine (TA-064), a new positive inotropic agent, on cardiac response of rats to denopamine. Jpn J Pharmacol 42:87–97

90. Barnett DB, Lu X (1991) Cardiac beta-adrenoceptor regulation and the effects of partial agonism. Am J Cardiol 67:18C–19C

91. Kenakin TP, Ferris RM (1983) Effects of in vivo beta-adrenoceptor down-regulation on cardiac responses to prenalterol and pirbuterol. J Cardiovasc Pharmacol 5:90–97

92. Bristow MR, Ginsburg R, Umans V, et al (1986) Beta$_1$- and beta$_2$-adrenergic-receptor subpopulations in nonfailing and failing human ventricular myocardium: coupling of both receptor subtypes to muscle contraction and selective beta$_1$-receptor down-regulation in heart failure. Circ Res 59:297–309

93. Brodde OE (1991) Beta$_1$- and beta$_2$-adrenoceptors in the human heart: properties, function, and alterations in chronic heart failure. Pharmacol Rev 43:203–242

94. Moore PF, Constantine JW, Barth WE (1978) Pirbuterol, a selective beta$_2$-adrenergic bronchodilator. J Pharmacol Exp Ther 207:410–418

95. Brown RA, Dixon J, Farmer JB, et al (1985) Dopexamine: a novel agonist at peripheral dopamine receptors and beta$_2$-adrenoceptors. Br J Pharmacol 85:599–608

96. Kusuoka H, Weisfeld ML, Zweier JL, Jacobus WE, Marban E (1986) Mechanism of early contractile failure during hypoxia in intact ferret heart: evidence for modulation of maximal Ca^{2+}-activated force by inorganic phosphate. Circ Res 59:270–282

97. Allen DG, Orchard CH (1987) Myocardial contractile function during ischaemia and hypoxia. Circ Res 60:153–168

98. Allen DG, Orchard CH (1983) The effect of changes in pH on intracellular calcium transients in mammalian cardiac muscle. J Physiol (Lond) 335:555–567

99. Kentish JC (1986) The effect of inorganic phosphate and creatine phosphate on force production in skinned muscles from rat ventricle. J Physiol (Lond) 370:585–604

100. Harrison SM, Bers DM (1990) Temperature-dependence of myofilament Ca sensitivity of rat, guinea pig and frog ventricular muscle. Am J Physiol 258:C274–C281

101. Endoh M, Blinks JR (1988) Actions of sympathomimetic amines on the Ca^{2+} transients and contractions of rabbit myocardium: reciprocal changes in myofibrillar responsiveness to Ca^{2+} mediated through α- and β-adrenoceptors. Circ Res 62:247–265

102. Okazaki O, Suda N, Hongo K, Konishi M, Kurihara S (1990) Modulation of ca^{2+} transients and contractile properties by β-adrenoceptor stimulation in ferret ventricular muscles. J Physiol (Lond) 423:221–240

103. Sata M, Sugiura S, Yamashita H, Momomura S, Serizawa T (1993) Dynamic interaction between cardiac myosin isoforms modifies velocity of actomyosin sliding in vitro. Circ Res 73:696–704

104. Honda H, Asakura S (1989) Calcium-triggered movement of regulated actin in vitro: a fluorescence microscopy study. J Mol Biol 205:677–683
105. Wendt IR, Stephenson DG (1983) Effects of caffeine on Ca-activated force production in skinned cardiac and skeletal muscle fibers of the rat. Pflugers Arch 398:210–216
106. Endoh M (1994) The effects of theophylline on aequorin light transients and force in the isolated dog right ventricular myocardium. J Mol Cell Cardiol 26:87–98
107. Fabiato A, Fabiato F (1976) Techniques of skinned cardiac cells and of isolated cardiac fibers with disrupted sarcolemmas with reference to the effects of catecholamines and of caffeine. In: Roy PE, Dhalla NS (eds) Recent advances in studies on cardiac structure and metabolism. Vol 9: The sarcolemma. University Park Press, Baltimore, pp 71–94
108. Herzig JW, Feile K, Rüegg JC (1981) Activating effects of AR-L 115 BS on the Ca^{2+} sensitive force, stiffness and unloaded shortening velocity (V_{max}) in isolated contractile structures from mammalian heart muscle. Arzneimittelforschung 31(I): 188–191
109. Solaro RJ, Rüegg JC (1982) Stimulation of Ca^{++} binding and ATPase activity of dog cardiac myofibrils by AR-L 115 BS, a novel cardiotonic agent. Circ Res 51:290–294
110. Endoh M, Yanagisawa T, Morita T, Taira N (1985) Differential effects of sulmazole (AR-L 115 BS) on contractile force and cyclic AMP levels in canine ventricular muscle: comparison with MDL 17,043. J Pharmacol Exp Ther 234:267–273
111. Gross T, Lues I, Daut J (1993) A new cardiotonic drug reduces the energy cost of active tension in cardiac muscle. J Mol Cell Cardiol 25:239–244
112. Lee JA, Allen DG (1991) EMD 53998 sensitizes the contractile proteins to calcium in intact ferret ventricular muscle. Circ Res 69:927–936
113. Gambassi G, Capogrossi MC, Klockow M, Lakatta EG (1993) Enantiomeric dissection of the effects of the inotropic agent, EMD 53998, in single cardiac myocytes. Am J Physiol 264: H728–H738
114. White J, Lee JA, Shah N, Orchard CH (1993) Differential effects of the optical isomers of EMD 53998 on contraction and cytoplasmic Ca^{2+} in isolated ferret cardiac muscle. Circ Res 73:61–70
115. Lee JA, Shah N, White J, Orchard CH (1993) A novel thiadiazinone derivative fully reverses acidosis-induced depression of force in cardiac muscle by a calcium-sensitizing effect. Clin Sci 84:141–144
116. Strauss JD, Zeugmer C, Rüegg JC (1992) The positive inotropic calcium sensitizer EMD 53998 antagonizes phosphate action on cross-bridges in cardiac skinned fibers. Eur J Pharmacol 227:437–441
117. Wang JX, Flemal K, Qiu Z, Ablin L, Grossman W, Morgan JP (1994) Ca^{2+} handling and myofibrillar Ca^{2+} sensitivity in ferret cardiac myocytes with pressure-overload hypertrophy. Am J Physiol 267: H918–H924
118. Schwinger RHG, Böhm M, Koch A, Schmidt U, Morano I, Eissner HJ, Uberfuhr P, Reichart B, Erdmann E (1994) The failing human heart is unable to use the Frank-Starling mechanism. Circ Res 74:959–969
119. Matsumori A, Shioi T, Yamada T, Matsui S, Sasayama S (1994) Vesnarinone, a new inotropic agent, inhibits cytokine production by stimulated human blood from patients with heart failure. Circulation 89:955–958
120. Saeki Y, Sagawa K, Suga H (1978) Dynamic stiffness of cat heart muscle in Ba^{2+} contracture. Circ Res 42:324–333
121. Hongo K, Tanaka E, Kurihara S (1993) Alterations in contractile properties and Ca^{2+} transients by β- and muscarinic receptor stimulation in ferret myocardium. J Physiol (Lond) 461:167–184
122. Suga H (1990) Ventricular energetics. Physiol Rev 70:247–277
123. Holubarsch C, Hasenfuss G, Just H, Blanchard EM, Mulieri LA, Alpert NR (1990) Modulation of myothermal economy of isometric force generation by positive inotropic interventions in the guinea pig myocardium. Cardioscience 1:33–41
124. Holubarsch C, Hasenfuss G, Just H, Alpert NR (1994) Positive inotropism and myocardial energetics: influence of β receptor agonist stimulation, phosphodiesterase inhibition, and ouabain. Cardiovasc Res 28:994–1002

125. Schramm M, Thomas G, Towart R, Franckowiak G (1983) Novel dihydropyridines with positive inotropic action through activation of Ca^{2+} channels. Nature 303:535–537
126. Bechem M, Hebisch S, Schramm M (1988) Ca^{2+} agonists: new sensitive probes for Ca^{2+} channels. Trends Pharmacol Sci 9:257–261
127. Dembowsky K, Bechem M, Goldmann S, Gross R, Hebisch S, Hütter J, Rounding P, Schramm M, Stoltefuss J, Straub A (1994) The calcium promotor BAY y 5959 increases cardiac contractility without an oxygen wasting effect in vitro as well as in vivo. Circulation 90:I-483
128. Rounding P, Bechem M, Goldmann S, Gross R, Hebisch S, Hütter J, Schramm M, Stoltefuss J, Straub A (1994) BAY y 5959 prevents myocardial stunning in the anesthetized dog. Circulation 90:I-645

Positive Inotropic Therapy for Chronic Heart Failure: New Perspective on Therapeutic Strategies

HIDETSUGU ASANOI, SHINJI ISHIZAKA, TOMOKI KAMEYAMA[1],
and SHIGETAKE SASAYAMA[2]

Abstract. Despite enthusiasm for the clinical benefits of converting enzyme inhibitors, many patients fail to respond to this therapy. Although positive inotropic therapy can lead to symptomatic relief, a pressing therapeutic goal at the late stage of congestive heart failure, numerous attempts to utilize cyclic AMP-enhancing positive inotropic agents to increase life expectancy have been disappointing. Recently, however, promising results were introduced with digitalis glycoside and agents with mixed mechanisms of inotropic actions. These experiences have led to the concept that to be clinically beneficial and well tolerated, positive inotropic agents should enhance myocardial contractility to only a modest degree without activating the sympathetic and renin-angiotensin systems. In terms of the prognostic benefit from positive inotropic therapy, a little hemodynamic improvement seems to go a long way. Therefore consideration of the mechanism of inotropic action, selection of the proper drug dose, and the influence on autonomic balance may ultimately make critical contributions to the long-term clinical effects of positive inotropic agents.

Key words. Neurohumoral concept—Mechanical efficiency—Left ventricular relaxation—Ca^{2+} sensitizer—Optimal dosage

Introduction

Despite the dramatic benefits of angiotensin-converting enzyme inhibitors for chronic heart failure, many patients fail to respond favorably to these drugs [1, 2]. It is expected that this therapeutic void could be filled by the new inotropic agents. Augmentation of cardiac pumping ability with new inotropic agents contributes to the alleviation of symptoms and improvement in the prognosis of patients with acute heart failure. However, introduction of this hemodynamic concept into chronic heart failure has revealed that the concept is no longer enough for the long-term treatment of most patients. Activation of pressure-elevating mechanisms, such as the sympathetic nervous system and the renin–angiotensin system, serves to maintain arterial

---

[1] Second Department of Internal Medicine, Toyama Medical and Pharmaceutical University, 2630 Sugitani, Toyama 930-01, Japan
[2] Third Division, Department of Internal Medicine, Kyoto University School of Medicine, 54 Shogoin Kawahara-cho, Sakyo-ku, Kyoto, 606 Japan

209

pressure within the normal range, but it imposes a burden on the failing heart and comes to have deleterious long-term effects. Therapeutic strategies for chronic heart failure must take into account this neurohumoral concept. Although the new inotropic agents could be expected to negate the influence of the sympathetic nervous system by increasing cardiac performance, an increase in intracellular cyclic adenosine monophosphate (AMP) directly damages the myocardium and stiumlates the pressure-elevating mechanisms. Thus from the viewpoint of hemodynamic and neurohumoral concepts, most of the inotropic agents are a double-edged sword that might be crucially relevant to long-term outcome in the treatment of chronic heart failure. Some drugs with new or mixed mechanisms of inotropic action have been introduced, with the result of a growing body of evidence of long-term usefulness of inotropic agents [3–5].

Theoretical and Practical Considerations for Inotropic Therapy

Adverse reactions to inotropic therapy might not be related to changes in contractility per se; they include tachycardia, arrhythmogenesis, increased energy expenditure, impaired relaxation, excessive peripheral dilatation, and sympathetic activation (Fig. 1). In many cases these adverse effects have a common subcellular pathway with positive inotropic effects. Therefore some believe that inotropic stimulation is inherently deleterious for the failing heart [6]. Yet others believe that positive inotropic agents failed not because of how they acted but how they were used [7]. Therefore it is a fundamental issue that a positive inotropic agent could improve cardiac pump function without causing these adverse effects.

Importance of the Neurohumoral Concept

Although vasodilators and positive inotropic agents exert favorable hemodynamic effects during acute heart failure, the long-term effects of these drugs on chronic heart failure differ [1, 2, 8–12]. What are the mechanisms for this controversy? The adverse clinical reactions to vasodilators (direct arterial dilators and calcium channel blockers) during chronic heart failure may be related to the activation of endogenous neurohumoral systems (sympathetic nervous system and renin–angiotensin system) that occurs in response to the hypotensive effects of these drugs [13]. Among the therapeutic agents available for the management of chronic heart failure, digitalis and angiotensin-converting enzyme exert beneficial influences on both hemodynamics and neurohumoral pathways at a variety of levels. Angiotensin-converting enzyme unloads the failing heart while centrally and peripherally suppressing sympathetic nervous activity and increasing parasympatheic tone. The CONSENSUS study [14] documented that neurohumoral activation was inhibited by enalapril, suggesting that the effect of enalapril on mortality is related partly to the suppression of the sympathetic and renin–angiotensin systems. The SOLVD study [15] also demonstrated that the positive effects of long-term converting enzyme inhibition on survival were observed in subjects with the highest norepinephrine concentrations. Although short-term treatment with digitalis has beneficial hemodynamic and autonomic effects in patients with chronic hear failure [16], whether these short-term autonomic changes are characteristic of long-term digoxin administration requires further investigation. One clinical trial, the Prospective Randomized Flosequinan Longevity Evaluation (PROFILE), was terminated early due to excess mortality in patients treated with

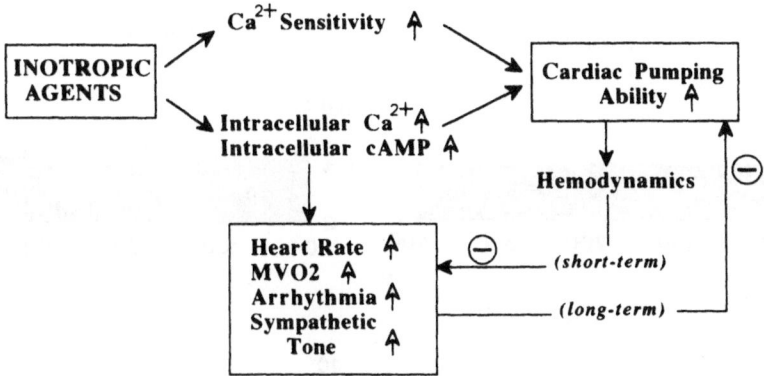

FIG. 1. Positive inotropic agents as a double-edged sword. Positive inotropic agents enhance cardiac pumping ability and improve peripheral organ function largely through increases in intracellular calcium, cyclic adenosine monophosphate (AMP), or both or by augmentation of calcium affinity to contractile protein. At the same time, these inotropic actions have the potential to cause serious adverse effects, which could result in a terminal ventricular event over time. Overall clinical effects appear to depend on the relative magnitude of the counteracting actions of these agents

flosequinan versus placebo. The treatment with flosequinan was associated with reduced atrial natriuretic peptide (improved hemodynamics) but increased norepinephrine (sympathoexcitation), which could override the hemodynamic effect, with a potentially unfavorable impact on survival [17]. These findings suggest that neurohumoral modulation plays a crucial role in the prognosis of patients with chronic heart failure. From the viewpoint of the neurohumoral concept, the drug that improves cardiac function but shifts the autonomic balance toward sympathetic tone appears to have an unfavorable outcome during long-term treatment.

Improvement of the pump function with inotropic agents could, in turn, result in amelioration of the secondary consequences of pump failure, such as neurohumoral activation (Fig. 1). However, most clinical trials with the β-adrenergic agonists and the phosphodiesterase inhibitors have demonstrated that prolonged inotropic stimulation of the failing heart would increase the risk of death in severely ill patients [11, 12, 18]. An increase in intracellular cyclic AMP and a resultant increase in endogenous neurohumoral activity could undermine the beneficial effects of enhanced contractility over time and provoke life-threatening arrhythmias. These adverse experiences are not seen with all inotropic agents, particularly those with mechanisms in addition to or independent of intracellular cyclic AMP. Inotropic agents with unique mixed mechanisms of action have been developed and tested clinically. For example, vesnarinone affects ion channels and the phosphodiesterase enzyme and improves cardiac function during acute and chronic heart failure [19, 20]. This agent has been shown to improve the quality of life and decrease morbidity and mortality among patients with heart failure [3]. Pimobendan, which sensitizes the contractile proteins to intracellular calcium and inhibits phosphodiesterase, also appears to be beneficial for long-term treatment [4, 5]. Clinical trials of both vesnarinone and pimobendan suggest that with the use of appropriate doses these drugs might decrease morbidity and mortality in patients with heart failure, minimizing the adverse effects of increased cyclic AMP concentration and endogenous neurohumoral activation [4]. Indeed, we have examined the acute effects of the Ca^{2+} sensitizer pimobendan on the

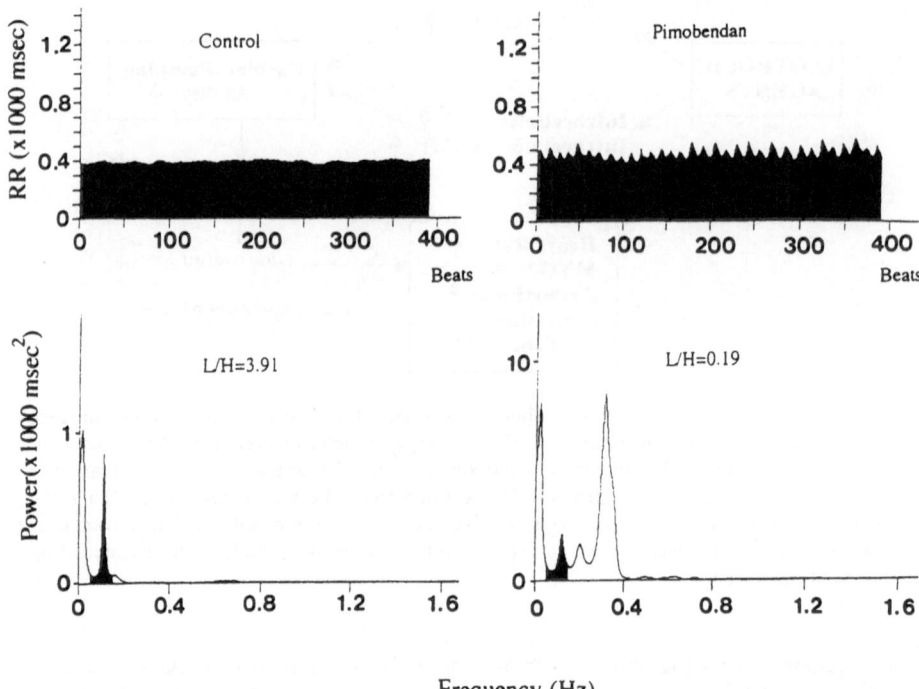

FIG. 2. Power spectral analysis of the heart rate variability of conscious dogs with tachycardia-induced heart failure. The most distinct profile of heart rate variability with heart failure is a substantial reduction in the parasympathetically mediated high-frequency component (>0.15 Hz) and a relative increase in the low-frequency component. This situation is the condition for dominant sympathetic tone (*left*). After administration of pimobendan, the high-frequency fluctuation increased substantially, suggesting a shift of autonomic balance toward parasympathetic tone (*right*)

autonomic balance assessed by the power spectral analysis of heart rate variability; we found that an appropriate dose of this agent shifted the autonomic balance toward parasympathetic tone (Fig. 2). To date, there have been no studies that systematically evaluated hemodynamic and neurohumoral effects of the new inotropic agents for long-term treatment of chronic heart failure.

Energy Expenditure and Mechanical Efficiency of the Failing Heart

The mechanism underlying chronic heart failure is considered to be partly related to the lack of chemical energy needed to sustain the high levels of mechanical work. Most of the known positive inotropic agents require energy expenditure to increase contractility; and they might accelerate progressive myocardial cell death insofar as the failing heart is energy-starved [21]. It is of note that administration of an inotropic agent to the failing heart may not increase energy expenditure (i.e., myocardial oxygen consumption at the organ level) because the metabolic cost of increasing contractility is offset by a concomitant fall in left ventricular (LV) wall stress [22, 23]. Thus an effective transfer from chemical energy to mechanical work might critically affect the long-term prognosis when inotropic agents are applied to chronic heart failure. We have examined the relation of baseline inotropic conditions and the optimal mechanical efficiency of the failing heart and found the cardiovascular system is normally regulated to maximize mechanical efficiency [24, 25]. In the failing heart, however, the working point of the left ventricle deviated from optimal mechanical efficiency. In patients with less compromised ventricular function (the slope of the end-systolic pressure–volume relation; Ees $\geq$ 3.0 mm Hg/ml), the operating end-systolic pressure was close to the optimal pressure (109 mm Hg), achieving nearly maximal mechanical efficiency (82% of maximal). As the heart deteriorated (Ees < 3.0 mm Hg/ml), however, the optimal end-systolic pressure became significantly lower (39 mm Hg) than normal, whereas the actual end-systolic pressure remained within the normal range. This discrepancy between optimal and operating pressures in the failing heart may be responsible for deviation of the mechanical efficiency from the maximal level (68% of maximal). These findings suggest two strategies for optimizing the mechanical efficiency of the failing left ventricle. One is to reduce the operating arterial pressure toward the optimal pressure without changing contractility by the use of vasodilators. Under circumstances where pressure-elevating mechanisms are strongly activated, drugs that directly interfere with these systems—angiotensin-converting enzyme (ACE) inhibitors or β-blockers—seem to be more reasonable for decreasing arterial pressure toward the maximal mechanical efficiency. Another strategy to optimize the mechanical efficiency of the failing heart is to increase the optimal arterial pressure toward normal with inotropic agents. Augmentation of contractility could optimize mechanical efficiency of the failing heart while maintaining normal arterial pressure and potentially attenuate endogenous neurohumoral activity (Fig. 1) [26]. We have demonstrated in an open-chest canine model that augmentation of contractility with dobutamine can restore the afterload-induced deterioration of mechanical efficiency toward the maximal level [27]. Among drugs currently available for the treatment of heart failure, digitalis has ideal properties in terms of optimizing the mechanical efficiency of the failing heart, as this agent attenuates pressure-elevating mechanisms by restoring the sympathetic–parasympathetic autonomic balance and reducing renin secretion; it also increases the optimal end-systolic pressure toward normal by enhancing LV contractility.

Effects on Left Ventricular Relaxation

Several experimental studies have shown that the effects of phosphodiesterase inhibitors are markedly attenuated because of the diminished basal production of cyclic AMP in failing hearts [28, 29]. Failing myocardium also has a diminished capacity to take up cytosolic calcium into sarcoplasmic reticulum and a decreased affinity of troponin C for calcium, which could potentially depress cardiac contractility. Under these circumstances the calcium-sensitizing effect of pimobendan might further compromise the relaxation and filling of a failing heart while augmenting contractility. Accordingly, to determine if pimobendan deteriorates LV diastolic properties in the failing heart we examined the effect of this drug before and after the development of tachycardia-induced heart failure in conscious dogs [30].

Pimobendan dose-dependently increased the Ees in both normal and failing hearts, although its magnitude was markedly attenuated in failing hearts. Heart rate was increased by pimobendan in normal hearts but did not change in failing hearts. LV

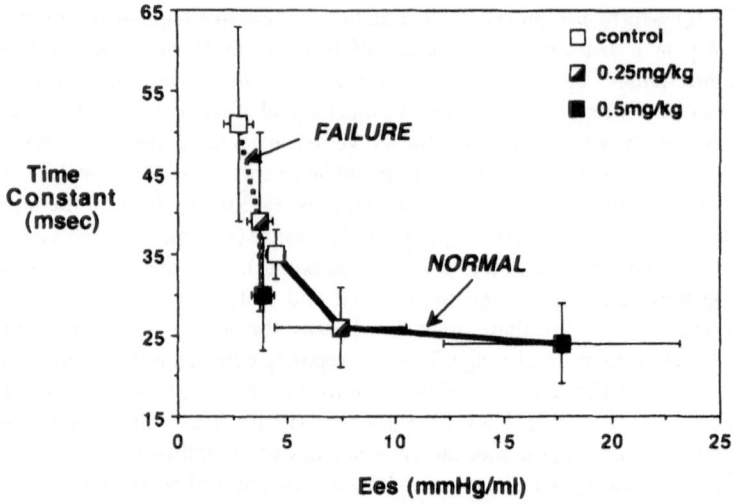

Fig. 3. Changes in the time constant of isovolumic relaxation as a function of ventricular elastance (*Ees*) with intravenous injection of pimobendan. A hyperbolic relation is maintained, suggesting that the failing heart undergoes large changes in relaxation with small changes in contractility compared with normal hearts. (From [30], with permission)

relaxation, assessed by peak $-dP/dt$ and the time constant of isovolumic pressure decay, was substantially improved to the same extent in failing and normal hearts. Consequently, Ees and the time constant exhibited a hyperbolic relation over a wide range of contractility states (Fig. 3). In normal hearts pimobendan caused a leftward shift of the diastolic pressure–volume relation while maintaining a similar curve. In failing hearts this relation shifted directly downward with a concomitant increase in end-diastolic volume, indicating a reduction in the constraints on LV distension and a resultant increase in preload reserve. Thus pimobendan accelerated LV isovolumic relaxation and improved distensibility in conscious dogs with tachycardia-induced heart failure despite the marked attenuation of inotropic responses.

Long-Term Effects of Pimobendan on Chronic Heart Failure

Multicenter trials have demonstrated that pimobendan is beneficial as adjunctive therapy with digitalis, diuretics, and a vasodilator in patients who have had heart failure for at least 12 weeks. We designed a double-blind placebo-controlled trial to assess the long-term efficacy of pimobendan [5]. Twenty-one patients with chronic heart failure [New York Heart Association (NYHA) class IIm–III] were recruited for the study. After the baseline assessment, patients were randomly assigned to treatment with pimobendan or a matching placebo in a double-blind fashion. Pimobendan was available in low-dose capsules (1.25 mg; $n = 7$) and high-dose capsules (2.5 mg; $n = 3$), and the initial dosage was taken twice daily. Both doses were effective, but an imbalance in the number of patients who received the two doses precluded analysis of dose-related effects. Clinical evaluation, including a quality-of-life assessment, was repeated every 4 weeks throughout the study period. Of the placebo-treated patients, five were withdrawn from the study because of deterioration of their heart failure, whereas none of the treated group was withdrawn owing to increased symptoms. Quality of life, assessed by the specific activity scale derived

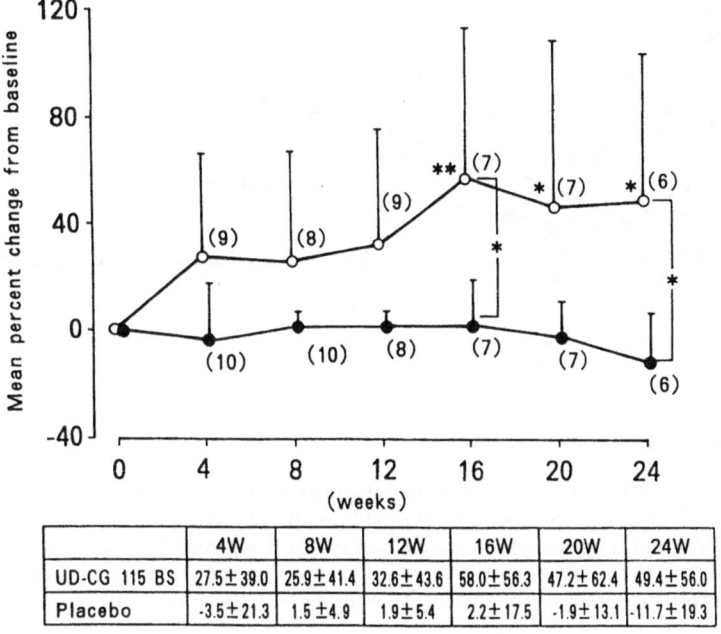

FIG. 4. Specific activity scale derived from the energy cost of physical activities. Percentage changes in comparison to baseline values are plotted for the placebo (*solid circles*) and pimobendan (*open circles*) group. Values are expressed as the mean ± SD; numbers in parentheses indicate numbers of patients. *$P < 0.05$; **$P < 0.01$

	4W	8W	12W	16W	20W	24W
UD-CG 115 BS	27.5±39.0	25.9±41.4	32.6±43.6	58.0±56.3	47.2±62.4	49.4±56.0
Placebo	-3.5±21.3	1.5 ±4.9	1.9±5.4	2.2±17.5	-1.9±13.1	-11.7±19.3

from metabolic costs of individual physical activity, was 3.5 ± 0.9 mets in the baseline state and increased significantly at week 16, averaging 5.1 ± 1.4 and 4.7 ± 1.5 mets at weeks 16 and 24, respectively (Fig. 4). In the placebo-treated group, however, the specific activity scale was 3.3 ± 1.2 mets at baseline and remained unchanged throughout the study period. Patients treated with pimobendan were able to increase their exercise duration significantly. Thus in contrast to the pessimistic view of the long-term efficacy of cardiotonic drugs, pimobendan and vesnarinone seem beneficial for long-term treatment of patients with congestive heart failure and may favorably modify their prognosis.

Optimal Dosage, Therapeutic Duration, Clinical Effects

The results of vesnarinone and pimobendan therapy provided important clinical information regarding the risks and benefits of inotropic agents for long-term use [3–5]. These two drugs exerted different inotropic actions but produced a similar clinical outcome in terms of dose-related effects. In the vesnarinone trial [3], at a dose of 60 mg/day vesnarinone caused a 50% reduction in the combined endpoints of worsening heart failure and death, 62% reduction in deaths, and significant improvement in the quality of life. In striking contrast, the high dose of vesnarinone (120 mg/day) caused a more than two-fold increase in deaths. Kubo et al. [4] reported dose-related effects of pimobendan in 198 patients randomized to placebo or to 2.5, 5.0, or 10.0 mg of pimobendan for 12 weeks. The greatest improvements in quality-of-life scores and exercise tolerance were found for the 5 mg/day dose and, to a lesser extent, the 10.0 mg/

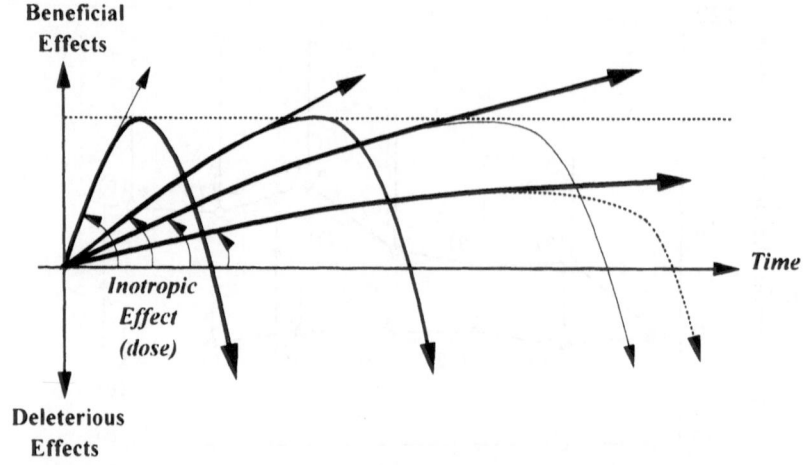

FIG. 5. Relation between clinical effects and the therapeutic doses and duration of inotropic therapy. High-dose inotropic agents exert great hemodynamic changes (large angle) and rapid symptomatic improvements (distance from baseline), accompanied by a high risk of overdose and death. Low doses, which only little or mildly affect hemodynamics (small angle), would potentially produce gradual clinical benefits over time with few adverse effects

day dose. There were no significant improvements in quality of life for the 2.5 mg/day dose within 12 weeks. In our study, however, most of the patients who received pimobendan of 2.5 mg/day improved significantly after 16 weeks of treatment [5]. The clinical improvements with these drugs were not associated with an apparent increase in LV ejection fraction. Therefore some clinicians have proposed that these agents do not elicit positive inotropic properties. However, more contractility-specific indices, such as the slope of the end-systolic pressure–volume relation clearly demonstrated that vesnarinone at 60 mg/day could clearly augment LV contractility [20, 31]. This finding is in contrast to the results of the PROMISE study [11] and the enoximone trial [12], where high doses of phosphodiesterase inhibitors were selected to maximally enhance systolic function of the left ventricle on the basis of the hemodynamic concept. Despite immediate and marked hemodynamic improvements, these agents increased the mortality of patients with chronic heart failure. These studies suggest a narrow toxic/therapeutic ratio, with the dose relations for clinical effects exhibiting a J-shaped curve with decreasing prognostic benefit at higher doses of inotropic agents. Figure 5 shows the relation between clinical effects and therapeutic doses and duration. Higher doses of inotropic agents exert greater hemodynamic changes and more rapid symptomatic improvements but are accompanied by a high risk of overdose and death. Lower doses, which only mildly affect hemodynamics, potentially produce gradual clinical benefits over time with few adverse effects.

Conclusions

Positive inotropic therapy can lead to symptomatic improvement, which is likely to result from greater cardiac output and the consequent improvement in organ function. Whether such symptomatic improvement is associated with increased life expectancy is unclear at present. However, symptomatic relief at the late stage of congestive heart failure is a pressing therapeutic goal. Clinical trials of new inotropic agents demonstrated that selection of the proper drug dose and the influence on autonomic balance seem critical to the long-term clinical effects. Excessive administration of a positive inotropic agent most often results in a terminal ventricular event in contrast to the major adverse effects of vasodilators, which include symptomatic hypotension and worsening renal function, which are easily detectable. Additional investigations are warranted to define the rationale to select safe, effective therapeutic doses for individual patients with chronic heart failure.

References

1. CONSENSUS trial study group (1987) Effects of enalapril on mortality in severe congestive heart failure: results of the Cooperative North Scandinavian Enalapril Survival Study (CONSENSUS). N Engl J Med 316:1429–1435
2. SOLVD investigators (1991) Effect of enalapril on survival in patients with reduced left ventricular ejection fractions and congestive heart failure. N Engl J Med 325: 293–302
3. Feldman AM, Bristow MR, Parmly WW, Carson PE, Pepin CJ, Gilbert EM, Strobeck JE, Hendrix GH, Powers ER, Bain RP, White BG, for the vesnarinone study group (1993) Effects of vesnarinone on morbidity and mortality in patients with heart failure. N Engl J Med 329:149–155
4. Kubo SH, Gollub S, Bourge R, Rahko P, Cobb F, Jessup M, Brozena S, Brodsky M, Kirlin P, Shanes J, Konstam M, Gradman A, Morledge J, Cinquegrani M, Singh S, LeJemtel T, Nicklas J, Troha J, Cohn J, for the pimobendan multicenter research group (1992) Beneficial effects of pimobendan on exercise tolerance and quality of life in patients with heart failure, results of a multicenter trial. Circulation 85:942–949
5. Sasayama S, Asanoi H, Kihara Y, Yokawa S, Terada Y, Yoshida S, Ejiri M, Horikoshi I (1992) Clinical effects of long-term administration of pimobendan in patients with moderate congestive heart failure. Heart Vessels 9:113–120
6. Katz AM (1986) Potential deleterious effects of inotropic agents in the therapy of chronic heart failure. Circulation 73(suppl III):184–188
7. Colucci WS (1993) What is the role of orally-active, non-glycoside positive inotropic agents in the treatment of congestive heart failure. Heart Failure 9:126–135
8. Cohn JN, Archbald DG, Ziesche S, Franciosa JA, Harston WE, Tristani FE, Dunkman WB, Jacobs W, Francis GS, Flohr KH, Goldman S, Cobb FR, Shah PM, Saunders R, Fletcher RD, Loeb FR, Hughes VC, Baker B (1986) Effect of vasodilator therapy on motality in chronic congestive heart failure; results of a Veterans Administration cooperative study. N Engl J Med 314:1547–1552
9. Franciosa JA, Jordan RA, Wilen MM, Ledy CL (1984) Minoxidil in patients with chronic heart failure: contrasting hemodynamic and clinical effects in a controlled trial. Circulation 70:63–68
10. Elkayam U, Amin J, Mehra A, Vesquez J, Weber L, Rahimtoola SH (1990) A prospective, randomized, double-blind, crossover study to compare the efficacy and safety of chronic nifedipine therapy with that of isosorbide dinitrate and their combination in the treatment of chronic congestive heart failure. Circulation 82:1954–1961
11. Packer M, Carver JR, Rodeheffer RJ, Ivanhoe RJ, DiBianco R, Zeldis SM, Hendrix GH, Bommer WJ, Elkayam U, Kukin ML, Mallis GI, Sollano JA, Shannon J, Tandon PK, DeMets DL, for the PROMISE study research group (1991) Effect of oral milrinone on mortality in severe chronic heart failure. N Engl J Med 325:1468–1475
12. Uretsky BF, Jessup M, Konstam MA, Dee GW, Leier CV, Bemotti J, Murali S, Herrmann HC, Sandberg JA, for the enoximone multicenter trial group (1990) Multicenter trial of oral enoximone in patients with moderate to moderately severe congestive heart failure: lack of benefit compared with placebo. Circulation 82:774–780

13. Packer M (1990) Calcium channel blockers in chronic heart falure: the risks of "physiologically rational" therapy. Circulation 82:2254-2247

14. Swedberg K, Eneroth P, Kjekshus J, Wilhelmsen L, for the CONSENSUS trial study group (1990) Hormones regulating cardiovascular function in patients with severe congestive heart failure and their relation to mortality. Circulation 82:1730-1736

15. Benedict CR, Weiner DH, Johnston DE, Bourassa MG, Ghali JK, Nicklas J, Kirlin P, Greenberg B, Quinones MA, Yusuf A, for the SOLVD investigators (1993) Comparative neurohormonal responses in patients with preserved and impaired left ventricular ejection fraction: results of the studies of left ventricular dysfunction (SOLVD) registry. J Am Coll Cardiol 22(suppl A):146A-153A

16. Packer M, Gheoghiade M, Young JB, Constantini PJ, Adams KF, Cody RJ, Smith LK, Voorhees LV, Gourly LA, Jolly MK, for the RADIANCE study (1993) Withdrawal of digoxin from patients with chronic heart failure treated with angiotensin-converting enzyme inhibitors. N Engl J Med 329:1-7

17. Moe GW, Rouleau JL, Proulx G, Arnold M, Sestier F, on behalf of the Canadian PROFILE investigators (1994) Increased mortality of flosequinan in patients with failure is accompanied by increased plasma norepinephrine. Circulation 90(suppl I):380

18. Dies F, Lilly E, Whitlow P, et al (1986) Intermittent dobutamine in ambulatory out-patients with chronic heart failure [abstract]. Circulation 74(suppl II):38

19. Asanoi H, Sasayama S, Iuchi K, Kameyama T (1987) Acute hemodynamic effects of a new inotropic agent (OPC-8212) in patients with congestive heart failure. J Am Coll Cardiol 9:865-871

20. Asanoi H, Sasayama S, Kameyama T, Ishizaka S, Iuchi K (1989) Sustained inotropic effects of a new cardiotonic agent: OPC-8212 in patients with chronic heart failure. Clin Cardiol 12:133-138

21. Katz AM (1990) Cardiomyopathy of overload: a major determinant of prognosis in congestive heart failure. N Engl J Med 322:100-110

22. Kameyama T, Asanoi H, Ishizaka S, Yamanishi K, Fujita M, Sasayama S (1992) Energy conversion efficiency in human left ventricle. Circulation 85:988-996

23. Sakai O, Fujita M, Sasayama S, Asanoi H, Nakajima H, Yokawa S (1988) Effect of xamoterol on myocardial energetics in man. Jpn Circ J 52:149-154

24. Asanoi H, Sasayama S, Kameyama T (1989) Ventriculoarterial coupling in normal and failing heart in humans. Circ Res 65:483-493

25. Asanoi H, Kameyama T, Ishizaka S, Nozawa T, Inoue H (1995) Energetically optimal left ventricular pressure for the failing human heart. Circulation (in press)

26. Colucci WS, Denniss AR, Leatherman GF, Quigg RJ, Ludmer PL, Marsh JD, Gauthier DE (1988) Intracoronary infusion of dobutamine to patients with and without severe congestive heart failure: dose-response relationships, correlation with circulating catecholamine, and effect of phosphodiesterase inhibition. J Clin Invest 81:1103-1110

27. Nozawa T, Wada O, Ishizaka S, Asanoi H, Fujita M, Sasayama S (1992) Dobutamine improves afterload-induced deterioration of mechanical efficiency toward maximal. Am J Physiol 263:H1201-H1207

28. Feldman MD, Copelas L, Gwathmey JK, Phillips P, Warren SE, Schoen FJ, Grossman W, Morgan JP (1987) Deficient production of cyclic AMP: pharmacologic evidence of an important cause of contractile dysfunction in patients with end-stage heart failure. Circulation 75:331-339

29. Perreault CL, Shannon RP, Komamura K, Vatner SF, Morgan JP (1992) Abnormalities in intracellular calcium regulation and contraction function in myocardium from dogs with pacing-induced heart failure. J Clin Invest 89:932-938

30. Asanoi H, Ishizaka S, Kameyama T, Ishise H, Sasayama S (1994) Disparate inotropic and lusitropic responses to pimobendan in conscious dogs with tachycardia-induced heart failure. J Cardiovasc Pharmacol 23:268-274

31. Kass DA, Anden EV, Pownall KK, Carnivale K, White WG, Feldman AM (1994) Positive inotropic activity of vesnarinone in patients with dilated cardiomyopathy. Circulation 90(suppl I):111

Cytokines and Heart Failure: Immunomodulating Agents for the Management of Heart Failure

Akira Matsumori, Takehiko Yamada, Shigeo Matsui, Tetsuo Shioi, and Shigetake Sasayama

Abstract. To elucidate the potential role of cytokines in the pathogenesis of heart failure, we measured circulating cytokines in patients with myocarditis and cardiomyopathies. Plasma concentrations of interleukin 1α (IL-1α), interleukin 1β (IL-1β), and tumor necrosis factor α (TNF-α) were increased in patients with acute myocarditis. TNF-α was also increased in those with dilated cardiomyopathy and hypertrophic cardiomyopathy. These results suggest that cytokines play an important role in the pathogenesis of myocardial injury in patients with cardiomyopathy and myocarditis. Vesnarinone, a quinolinone derivative, has been confirmed to improve the prognosis of patients with chronic heart failure, although the precise mechanism of this beneficial effect is not yet clear. In our murine model of acute viral myocarditis resulting from encephalomyocarditis virus infection, survival and myocardial damage were markedly improved by treatment with vesnarinone. Vesnarinone inhibited the increase in natural killer cell activity and production of TNF-α in this animal model. We also studied the effects of vesnarinone on cytokine production by lipopolysaccharide-stimulated whole blood from patients with heart failure and healthy volunteers. Vesnarinone inhibited the production of IL 1α and IL-1β, TNF-α, and interleukin γ (IL-γ). These findings provide evidence that vesnarinone plays an important role in the regulation of cytokines and suggest that the reduction of cytokine release may contribute to the beneficial effects of the drug for the treatment of heart failure.

Key words. Cytokines—Heart failure—Myocarditis—Vesnarinone—Virus

Introduction

Cytokines are being increasingly recognized as essential mediators of normal and pathological immune responses. It is widely accepted that cytokines are involved in the cascade of events that lead to the wide range of biological responses to exogenous and endogenous pathogens. An elevated concentration of tumor necrosis factor α (TNF-α) has been reported in some patients with acute myocardial infarction [1]. Patients with chronic heart failure were also found to have high concentrations of

---

Third Division, Department of Internal Medicine, Kyoto University School of Medicine, 54 Shogoin Kawahara-cho, Sakyo-ku, Kyoto, 606 Japan

TNF-α, but some cachectic patients did not [2, 3]. TNF-α is reported to depress myocardial contractility, alter muscle membrane potential, lower blood pressure, and precipitate pulmonary edema [4–6]. In this review, we discuss the potential role of cytokines in the pathophysiology of heart failure and the immunomodulating effects of a new inotropic agent, vesnarinone, which has been shown to improve the prognosis of patients with heart failure.

Increased Circulating Cytokines in Patients with Heart Failure

We studied 13 patients with acute myocarditis, 23 with dilated cardiomyopathy and 51 with hypertrophic cardiomyopathy who were admitted to our hospital. We also studied 18 patients with angina pectoris, 9 with acute myocardial infarction, 12 with essential hypertension, and 17 healthy volunteers [7].

Interleukin 1α (IL-1α), interleukin 1β (IL-1β), interleukin 2 (IL-2), interleukin 6 (IL-6), TNF-α, TNF-β, granulocyte/macrophage colony-stimulating factor (GM-CSF), granulocyte colony-stimulating factor (G-CSF), interferon α (IFN-α), and IFN-γ were measured by enzyme-linked immunosorbent assay (ELISA). Macrophage colony-stimulating factor (M-CSF) was measured by radiommunoassay. Cytokines were measured with commercial kits originally developed by Otsuka Pharmaceutical Company (Tokushima, Japan), according to the manufacturer's protocols. The sensitivity of the kits for each cytokine was 10 pg/ml for IL-1α, 20 pg/ml for IL-1β, 78 pg/ml for IL-2, 32 pg/ml for IL-6, 20 pg/ml for TNF-α, 1 U/ml for TNF-β, 20 pg/ml for GM-CSF, 10 pg/ml for G-CSF, 0.2 ng/ml for M-CSF, 100 pg/ml for IFN-α, and 10 pg/ml for IFN-γ.

Interleukins

In the controls, IL-1α, IL-1β, IL-2, IL-6, TNF-α, TNF-β, G-CSF, IFN-α, and IFN-γ were below the threshold of detection of our method; M-CSF was 1.9 ± 0.4 ng/ml in normal controls. IL-1α was detected in plasma from 3 of 13 (23.1%, detected value 25 ± 11 pg/ml, mean ± SD) patients with acute myocarditis, in 1 of 23 (4.3%, 14 pg/ml) with dilated cardiomyopathy, and in 4 of 51 (7.8%, 38 ± 15 pg/ml) with hypertrophic cardiomyopathy (Table 1). IL-1β was detected in 30.8% (56 ± 34 pg/ml) of patients with acute myocarditis. Detectable concentrations of IL-1α and IL-1β were more common in patients with acute myocarditis than in controls. IL-2 was detected in 13.7% (2318 ± 4738 pg/ml) of patients with hypertrophic cardiomyopathy and was more commonly found there than in patients with acute myocarditis or dilated cardiomyopathy (the difference was not statistically significant). IL-6 was not often detected in patients with acute myocarditis or cardiomyopathy.

Tumor Necrosis Factor α

Tumor necrosis factor α was detected in 6 of 13 (46.1%, 61 ± 31 pg/ml) patients with acute myocarditis, in 7 of 23 (30.4%, 402 ± 555 pg/ml) with dilated cardiomyopathy, in 10 of 51 (19.6%, 992 ± 1517 pg/ml) with hypertrophic cardiomyopathy, in 1 of 9 (11.1%, 113 pg/ml) with acute myocardial infarction, and in 3 of 18 (16.7%, 146 ± 159 pg/ml) with angina pectoris. It was not detected in plasma from any of the patients

TABLE 1. Frequency of detectable plasma cytokines in cardiac patients

Cytokine	Frequency (%)							Detectable levels, mean ± SD (pg/ml)
	Acute myocarditis	Dilated cardiomyopathy	Hypertrophic cardiomyopathy	Acute myocardial infartion	Angina pectoris	Essential hypertension	Normal volunteers	
	($n = 13$)	($n = 23$)	($n = 51$)	($n = 9$)	($n = 18$)	($n = 12$)	($n = 17$)	
Interleukin 1α	23.1*	4.3	7.8	0	11.1	0	0	>10
Interleukin 1β	30.8***	0	9.8	0	0	0	0	>20
Interleukin 2	7.7	4.3	13.7	0	0	0	0	>78
Interleukin 6	7.7	4.3	3.9	0	0	0	0	>32
Tumor necrosis factor α	46.1****	30.4*	19.6*	11.1	16.7	0	0	>20
Tumor necrosis factor β	7.7	4.3	3.9	0	0	0	0	>1 U/ml
Granulocyte macrophage colony-stimulating factor	7.7	4.3	9.8	11.1	5.5	8.3	0	>20
Granulocyte colony-stimulating factor	46.1*	65.2*	58.8*	22.2*	44.4*	8.3	5.9	>10
Macrophage colony-stimulating factor (ng/ml)	2.5 ± 1.8**	1.5 ± 0.4	1.9 ± 0.4	3.3 ± 1.1*****	2.4 ± 0.9	14.0 ± 0.4	1.9 ± 0.4	>0.2 ng/ml
Interferon α	7.7	0	3.9	0	0	0	0	>100
Interferon γ	7.7	4.3	3.9	0	5.5	0	0	>10

Modified from [7], with permission.

*$P < 0.05$ vs normal volunteers.

**$P < 0.05$ vs dilated cardiomyopathy.

***$P < 0.05$ vs hypertrophic cardiomyopathy.

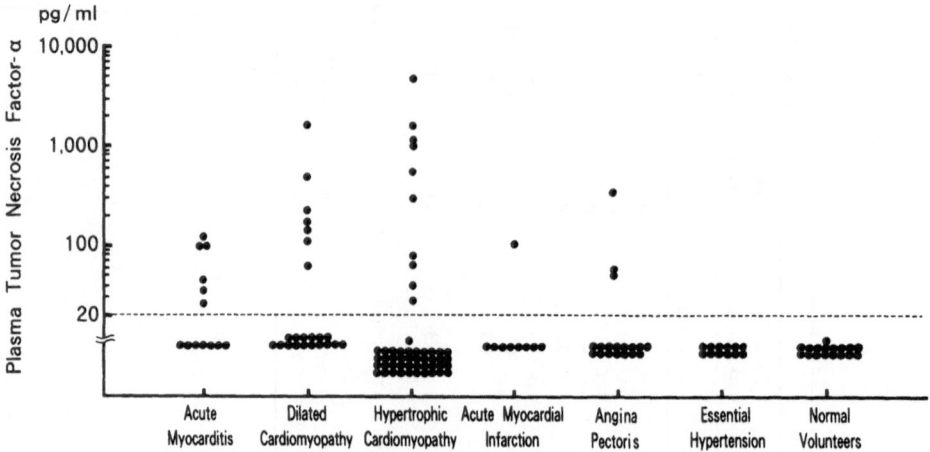

Fig. 1. Plasma tumor necrosis factor α (TNF-α) in patients with acute myocarditis, dilated cardiomyopathy, hypertrophic cardiomyopathy, and other cardiac diseases. Elevated tumor necrosis factor-α (TNF-α) was most commonly seen in patients with acute myocarditis, but the values were higher in those with dilated cardiomyopathy or hypertrophic cardiomyopathy. (From [7], with permission)

with essential hypertension or from normal volunteers. An increased concentration of TNF-α was most commonly seen in patients with acute myocarditis. High values were also seen in those with dilated or hypertrophic cardiomyopathy (Fig. 1). An extremely high concentration of TNF-α ($>1000\,pg/ml$) was seen in a patient with dilated cardiomyopathy who had poor systolic function and congestive heart failure. The severity of the congestive heart failure, however, was not always correlated with the plasma concentrations of TNFα in these subgroups. The concentration of TNF-α was high ($>1000\,pg/ml$) in four patients with hypertrophic cardiomyopathy, although it was not increased in five other such patients in whom a dilated ventricle and poor systolic function developed.

Colony-Stimulating Factors

Tumor necrosis factor β or GM-CSF was detected in only a few of the patients. G-CSF was commonly increased in patients with myocarditis and cardiomyopathies, but no significant differences in frequency were found among the various groups. Elevated concentrations of G-CSF were not correlated with the number of leukocytes.

Macrophage colony-stimulating factor in normal volunteers was $1.9 \pm 0.4\,ng/ml$. Plasma concentrations of M-CSF were $2.5 \pm 1.8\,ng/ml$ in patients with acute myocarditis, $1.5 \pm 0.4\,ng/ml$ in those with dilated cardiomyopathy, $1.9 \pm 0.8\,ng/ml$ in those with hypertrophic cardiomyopathy, $3.3 \pm 1.1\,ng/ml$ in those with acute myocardial infarction, $2.4 \pm 0.9\,ng/ml$ in patients with angina pectoris, and $1.4 \pm 0.4\,ng$ in patients with essential hypertension. The concentration of M-CSF was significantly higher in patients with acute myocarditis and acute myocardial infarction than in those with dilated cardiomyopathy, and the increase was most prominent in those with acute myocardial infarction. GM-CSF, IFN-α, and IFN-γ were uncommonly detected.

Thus concentrations of inflammatory cytokines, such as IL-1α, IL-1β, and TNF-α, were increased in patients with acute myocarditis. In addition, TNF-α was increased in patients with dilated cardiomyopathy and hypertrophic cardiomyopathy.

Treatment of Heart Faiture in the Mouse with the Inotropic Agent Vesnarinone

Vesnarinone, a quinolinone derivative, is a synthesized positive inotropic agent shown to have positive inotropic effects on congestive heart failure [8, 9]. In contrast to the pessimistic views about inotropic agents for treatment of congestive heart failure [10, 11], in one study administration of this agent for 6 months improved the survival of patients with congestive heart failure [12]. Although it has been suggested that the mechanisms of action of vesnarinone are related to slight inhibition of phosphodiesterase III, increased inward calcium current, and reduced potassium current [13, 14], the true mechanism by which the agent reduces mortality has not been determined. We investigated the effects of vesnarinone in an animal model of congestive heart failure due to acute viral myocarditis induced by encephalomyocarditis (EMC) virus [15, 16] and focused on its novel immunomodulating effects [17].

Figure 2 shows that the infected control mice that received no treatment began to die on day 5 after EMC virus inoculation, and that most of the deaths occurred from day 5 to day 8. Mice treated with vesnarinone at 10 mg/kg also started to die on day 5, but the mortality rate was substantially reduced compared with that of the controls. On the other hand, all animals treated with a high dose of vesnarinone survived the first 6 days. The mortality rate was relatively low after the first 7 days in all groups. The cumulative survival rate was significantly increased in a dose-related manner, being 20%, 40%, and 60%, respectively, for the no-treatment group and those treated with vesnarinone at 10 and 50 mg/kg (Fig. 2A) [17]. Treatment with equivalent molar doses of amrinone did not improve the survival rate (Fig. 2B). Thus vesnarinone is considered to exert its beneficial effects at an early stage after viral infection.

Histopathology

The heart weight/body weight ratio correlates closely with the severity of the congestive heart failure, but there were no significant differences between the infected control group and the vesnarinone-treated group. The virus titers in the hearts of mice treated with vesnarinone were similar to those of the infected control mice. Nevertheless, myocardial necrosis of the mice treated with vesnarinone 50 mg/kg was significantly reduced compared with that in the infected control group.

Natural Killer Cell Activity

The natural killer (NK) cell activity of spleen cells obtained from infected mice, expressed as the rate of specific cytotoxicity (the rate of ^{51}Cr release), began to increase from the second day after EMC virus infection. Treatment with vesnarinone at 50 mg/kg inhibited increases in specific cytotoxicity caused by viral infection, but treatment with amrinone 25 mg/kg (a molar dose equal to the dose of vesnarinone) did not inhibit the increase in specific cytotoxicity on day 3 (Fig. 3). At an effector/target (E/T) ratio of 50:1, the rate of specific cytotoxicity obtained for infected control

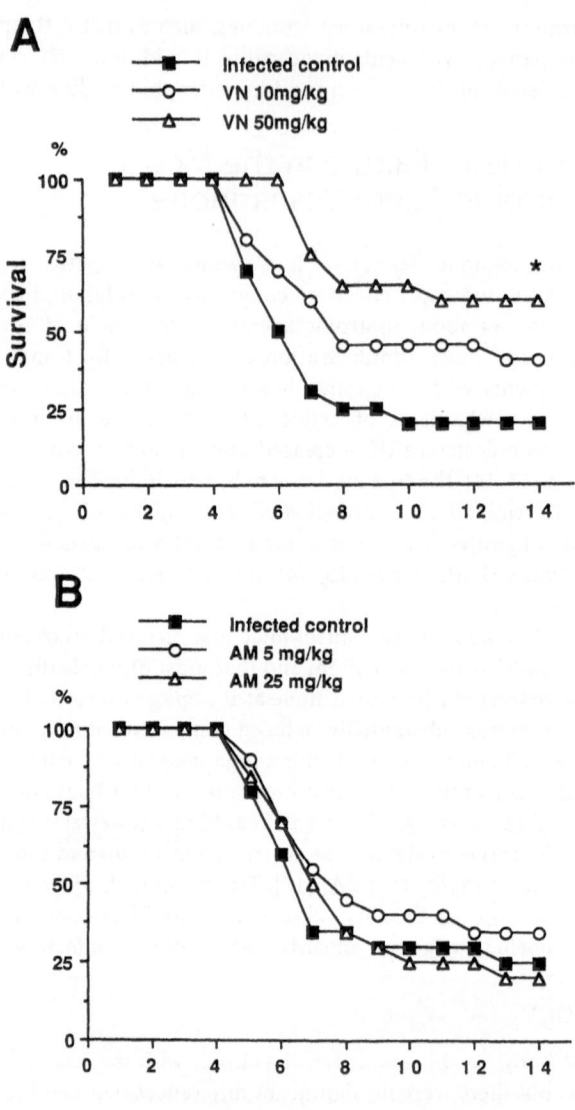

Days after EMCV inoculation

FIG. 2A,B. Effect of vesnarinone and amrinone on survival after encephalomyocarditis virus (EMCV) inoculation. Four-week-old DBA/2 mice were inoculated intraperitoneally with 10 pfu of EMC virus. **A** Two groups were treated with vesnarinone (*VN*) at doses of 10 and 50 mg/kg po daily. Survival of the group treated with vesnarinone at 10 mg/kg was relatively improved compared with the control group, but there was no significant difference. Treatment with vesnarinone 50 mg/kg significantly reduced mortality at an early stage (*$P < 0.01$ versus the control). **B** Mice were also treated with amrinone (*AM*) at doses of 5 and 25 mg/kg po daily. Survival was not improved compared with the control. The vehicle alone was administered to the infected control mice. Each group started with 20 mice. (From [17] with permission)

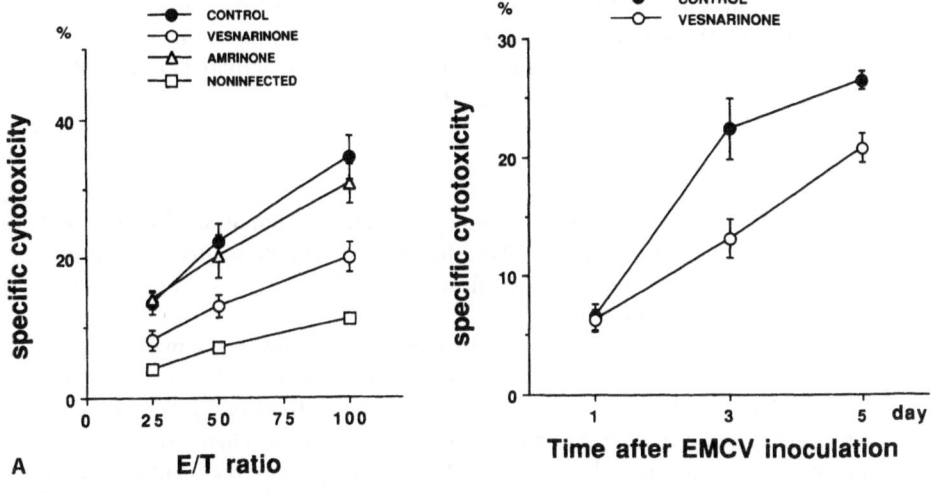

FIG. 3A,B. Effect of vesnarinone and amrinone on natural killer (NK) cell activity after EMC virus infection. Mice were treated as described in Fig. 1 and then sacrificed on days 1, 3, and 5 after EMCV infection. **A** Percent of specific cytotoxicity on day 3 at various E/T ratios. **B** Time course of percent specific cytotoxicity at a fixed effector/target (E/T) ratio of 50:1. (From [17], with permission)

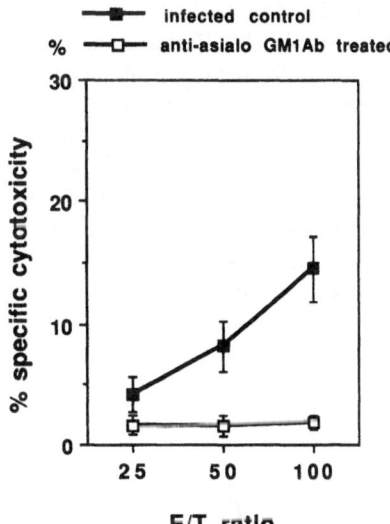

FIG. 4. Effect of anti-asialo GM₁ antibody (*Ab*) on NK cell activity after EMCV infection. Spleen cells obtained from mice treated with rabbit anti-asialo GM₁ antibody by intraperitoneal injection 1 and 3 days before EMCV infection showed no cytotoxicity on the target cells (YAC-1). (From [17], with permission)

mice was $6.5 \pm 1.1\%$ on day 1, $22.4 \pm 2.6\%$ on day 3, and $26.6 \pm 0.7\%$ on day 5; the corresponding values for mice treated with vesnarinone were $6.2 \pm 0.9\%$, $13.1 \pm 1.7\%$, and $20.8 \pm 1.3\%$. The value for mice treated with amrinone was $20.3 \pm 3.0\%$ on day 3, and that for non-infected control mice was $6.6 \pm 2.3\%$ (mean $\pm$ SEM). Lytic units were calculated, and the values for the infected control group were 48 on day 3 and 53 on day 5, those for the vesnarinone-treated group were 21 on day 3 and 42 on day 5, and for the amrinone-treated group the value was 41 on day 3. Vesnarinone significantly reduced this value on days 3 and 5 ($P < 0.05$ versus infected controls), but the effect of amrinone was not significant. Spleen cells obtained from mice pretreated with anti-asialo GM1 antibody showed no response after viral infection (Fig. 4). The increase in specific cytotoxicity was due to the increase in the activity of asialo GM1-bearing NK cells, and vesnarinone inhibited this activity.

Tumor Necrosis Factor α Production

The time course of TNF-α production from spleen cells by lipopolysaccharide (LPS) stimulation showed that the TNF-α level reached almost maximum after 9 h of culture (Fig. 5). Vesnarinone and amrinone significantly suppressed TNF-α production in a dose-dependent manner (Fig. 6).

According to the current concept of heart failure management, the primary goals are to improve the quality of life and prolong life. Newly developed inotropic agents that increase intracellular cyclic AMP by either stimulating β-adrenergic receptors or inhibiting phosphodiesterase have produced dramatic short-term hemodynamic benefits in patients with advanced heart failure. However, long-term treatment with these agents results in an unfavorable outcome, with acceleration of the disease process and an adverse effect on survival [10, 11].

In contrast to these agents, vesnarinone has been shown to improve both the quality of life and the prognosis of the patient with heart failure [8-20]. Particularly, Feldman et al. [12] demonstrated in 238 patients assigned to treatment with vesnarinone (60 mg/day) that the endpoint of death or worsening heart failure was reduced by 50% during the 6-month study period compared with that for 239 patients receiving placebo. Vesnarinone also increases intracellular cyclic AMP by inhibiting a specific isoform of phosphodiesterase. Unlike other phosphodiesterase inhibitors, however, vesnarinone prolongs the action potential duration and slows the heart rate by exerting an effect on ion channels.

A decrease in contractility could be exacerbated by inotropic agents that potentially increase the heart rate of the failing heart, in which case the force-frequency response is attenuated or even reversed [11]. In this regard, in addition to its antiarrhythmic properties, the lack of an increase in heart rate is considered the most likely cause of the beneficial effect of vesnarinone during long-term treatment.

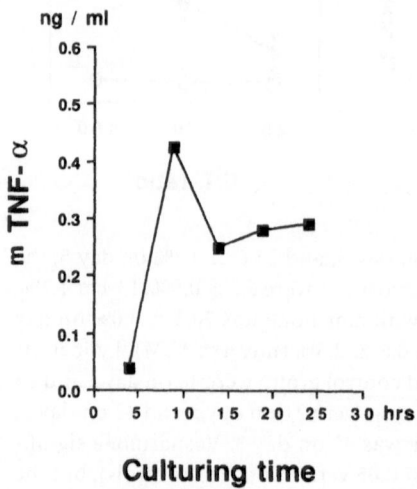

FIG. 5. Time course of TNF-α production after lipopolysacchairde (LPS) stimulation. Spleen cells (1×10^5 cells/well) were stimulated with LPS 1 µg/ml. After serial time incubation, the TNF-α concentration in the supernatant was assayed by enzyme-linked immunosorbent assay (ELISA). Values represent the means of two to four samples. (From [17] with permission)

In the present study we used an animal model of viral myocarditis to investigate the effects of vesnarinone from an immunological point of view. Vesnarinone reduced mortality for the acute stage of viral myocarditis. In this model, myocardial necrosis and cellular infiltration appeared 4–5 days after the viral infection, and some mice began to die on day 5, with others developing severe congestive heart failure after day 7 [15]. Vesnarinone exerted its effect at the stage when most of the deaths were caused by myocardial damage, before congestive heart failure developed. Histopathological examination during the acute stage showed that vesnarinone reduced myocardial damage without having a significant effect on viral replication in the heart. Vesnarinone did not reduce viral replication in cultured myocytes or protect the myocytes from direct virus-mediated cell lysis. Therefore the effect of vesnarinone could be due to altered host immune responses.

We have already reported that circulating TNF-α was increased after EMC virus infection, and pretreatment with anti-TNF-α antibody reduced myocardial damage during the acute stage in this model [21].

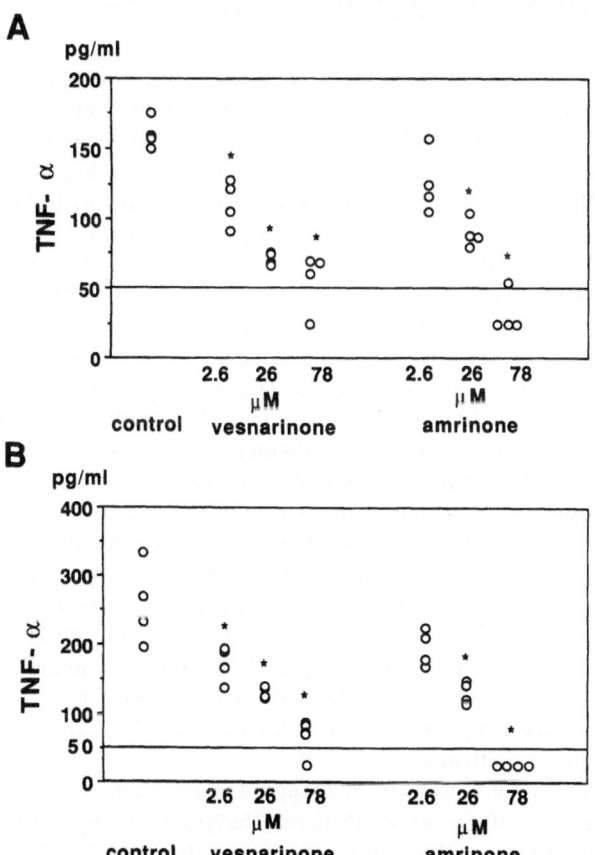

FIG. 6. Suppression of TNF-α production from spleen cells. Spleen cells (1×10^5 cells/well) were stimulated with LPS at doses of 100 ng/ml (A) and 1000 ng/ml (B). Vesnarinone and amrinone were added to the wells at doses of 2.6, 26.0, and 78.0 μM. The control was the vesnarinone vehicle. After 9 h of incubation the TNF-α concentration in the supernatant was assayed by ELISA. The sensitivity was 50 pg/ml. *$P < 0.05$ versus control. (From [17], with permission)

Vesnarinone and amrinone inhibited TNF-α production in cultured spleen cells stimulated by LPS, so the effect on cytokine production might be mediated through phosphodiesterase III inhibition, resulting in an increase in intracellular cyclic AMP [22, 23]. However, the suppression of TNF-α production by vesnarinone and amrinone could not explain the mechanism of increased survival by vesnarinone, as amrinone failed to produce such an improvement. In the acute viral myocarditis model, vesnarinone reduced mortality and myocardial damage by immuno-modulation, without affecting virus replication. In contrast to the inhibitory effect of vesnarinone on NK cell activity, amrinone did not significantly affect the activity. The mechanism of this difference might be produced by differences in the pharmacologi-cal properties of these agents. This additional action might be a major cause for the specific inhibition in NK cell activity, which was related to the improvement of patients with viral myocarditis.

Inhibition of Cytokine Production by Vesnarinone in Blood from Patients with Heart Failure

We studied the effects of vesnarinone on cytokine production by LPS-stimulated human whole blood from seven patients with heart failure and from five normal volunteers [24]. Heparinized blood was diluted in RPMI medium and stimulated with LPS. Vesnarinone (1–30 μg/ml) was added, the blood was incubated for 24 h, and IL-1α, IL-1β, IL-6, TNF-α, TFN-γ, and G-CSF were measured by ELISA.

Figure 7 demonstrates that the markedly suppressed median levels of IL-1α, IL-1β, TNF-α, and IFN-γ release observed at vesnarinone concentrations of 1 to 30 μg/ml were significantly different from the control levels (70 pg/ml for IL-1α, 593 pg/ml for IL-1β, 234 pg/ml for TNF-α, 348 pg/ml for IFN-γ; $P < 0.05$) in healthy volunteers. Vesnarinone caused a dose-dependent reduction in TNF-α release. Reduction of IFN-γ release was prominent and vesnarinone 1 μg/ml suppressed IFN-γ to below the detectable level of 20 pg/ml. Levels of IL-6 (33 pg/ml) and G-CSF (21 pg/ml) were elevated by LPS stimulation in three individuals, and vesnarinone (1 μg/ml) sup-pressed IL-6 and G-CSF to below detectable levels (20 pg/ml).

Because a profound reduction in the release of various cytokines was evident in specimens from normal volunteers containing vesnarinone (10 μg/ml), specimens from patients with heart failure were studied using this vesnarinone dose. Median values for LPS-stimulated cytokines in patients with heart failure were 99 pg/ml for IL-1α, 667 pg/ml for IL-1β, 523 pg/ml for TNF-α, and 64 pg/ml for TFN-γ (Fig. 8). A significant reduction in TNF-α and IFN-γ levels was observed upon incubation with vesnarinone in patients with heart failure ($P < 0.05$). LPS induced an increase of G-CSF in three patients (114 pg/ml), and vesnarinone reduced G-CSF to below detectable levels in two of these patients.

Marked inhibition of G-CSF (from 205 pg/ml to less than 20 pg/ml), IL-1α (from 84 pg/ml to less than 10 pg/ml), IL-1β (from 1589 pg/ml to 58 pg/ml), TNF-α (from 593 pg/ml to 20 pg/ml), and IFN-γ (from 291 pg/ml to less than 20 pg/ml) was observed in one patient with valvular heart disease who had developed neutropenia during vesnarinone therapy and had recovered after treatment with recombinant G-CSF (Fig. 8, *white dots*).

In this study, we demonstrated that vesnarinone inhibited the production of TNF-α and IFN-γ in LPS-stimulated human whole blood from patients with heart failure

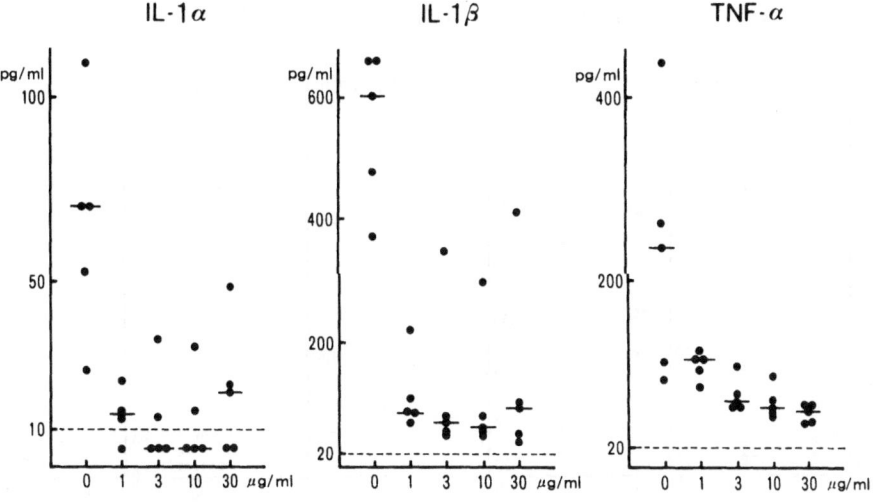

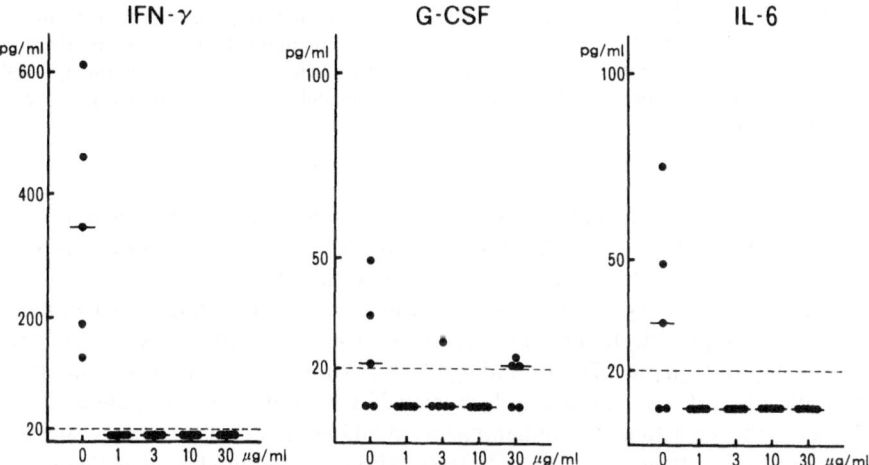

FIG. 7. Effects of vesnarinone on the production of cytokines in LPS-stimulated human whole blood from normal volunteers. Production of interleukin 1 α (IL-1α), IL-1β, TNF-α, and interferon γ (IFN-γ) was significantly suppressed compared with control levels ($P < 0.05$). Induction of IL-6 and granulocyte colony-stimulating factor (G-CSF) in three individuals was reduced to below detectable levels by vesnarinone 1 μg/ml. *Horizontal line* indicates median value. (From [24], with permission)

and from normal volunteers. Although IL-1α and IL-1β were also suppressed in the normal volunteers, significant reduction was not found in patients with heart failure. LPS stimulation induced a more prominent increase in TNF-α in patients with heart failure.

The peak plasma concentration of vesnarinone observed after a single oral dose of 60 mg, which was used in the clinical trial was 3.8 μg/ml (with the 15 mg dose it was 0.9 μg/ml). As 1 μg of vesnarinone per milliliter inhibited this cytokine production, the inhibitory concentration is obtained using a therapeutic dose.

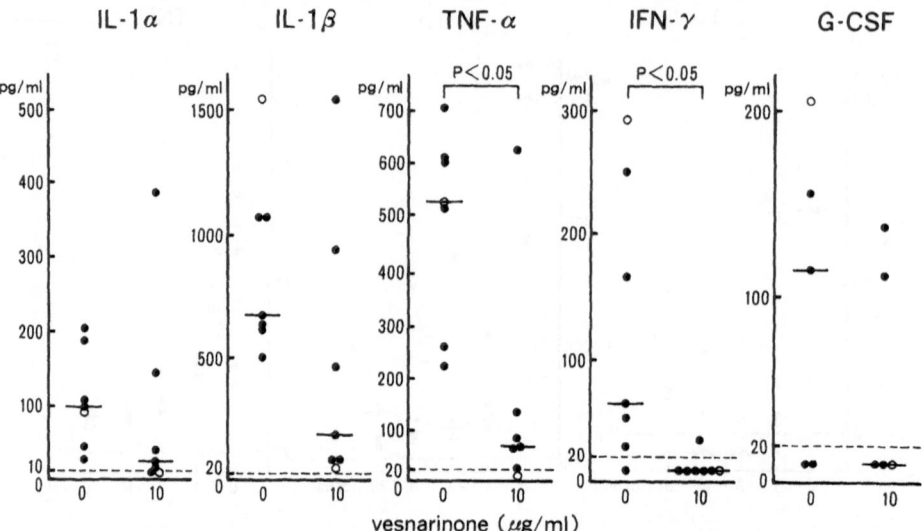

FIG. 8. Effects of vesnarinone on the production of cytokines in LPS-stimulated blood from patients with heart failure. A significant reduction in TNF-α and IFN-γ was seen after treatment with vesnarinone 10 μg/ml. *Open circles* indicate a patient with markedly suppressed production of G-CSF and other cytokines who had developed neutropenia after vesnarinone therapy and had recovered after treatment with G-CSF. *Horizontal line* indicates median value. (From [24], with permission)

The direct effects of proinflammatory cytokines on the contractility of mammalian heart have been studied [25]. TNF-α, IL-6, and IL-2 inhibited the contractility of isolated hamster papillary muscles in a concentration-dependent, reversible manner. The nitric oxide synthase inhibitor NG-monomethyl-L-arginine blocked these negative inotropic effects, and L-Arginine reversed the inhibitory effect of NG-monomethyl-L-arginine. These findings demonstrate that the direct negative inotropic effect of cytokines is largely mediated by myocardial nitric oxide synthase [26]. Thus the regulation of proinflammatory cytokines may provide new therapeutic strategies for treatment of cardiac diseases. Although the number of patients was small and the results preliminary, these findings provide evidence that vesnarinone plays an important role in the regulation of cytokines and suggest that the reduction of cytokine release contributes to the beneficial effects of the drug in the treatment of heart failure.

The marked inhibition of G-CSF observed in one patient with heart failure who had developed neutropenia during vesnarinone therapy suggests that vesnarinone caused neutropenia by suppressing G-CSF. This result suggests that the measurement of cytokines may be useful for predicting the occurrence of neutropenia in patients with heart failure who are treated with vesnarinone.

Acknowledgments. This work was supported in part by a Research Grant from the Ministry of Health and Welfare; a Grant-in-Aid for Developmental Research and for General Scientific Research from the Ministry of Education, Science, and Culture; and by the Kanazawa Research Fund, Japan. We thank Mr. H. Toriyama and Mr. Y. Ohmoto for assistance with the cytokine assays.

References

1. Maury CP, Teppo A-M (1989) Circulating tumor necrosis factor-α (cachectin) in myocardial infarction. J Int Med 225:333–336
2. Levine B, Kalman J, Mayer L, Fillit HM, Packer M (1990) Elevated circulating levels of tumor necrosis factor in severe chronic heart failure. N Engl J Med 323:236–241
3. McMurray J, Abdullah I, Dargie HJ, et al (1991) Increased concentrations of tumor necrosis factor in "cachectic" patients with severe chronic heart failure. Br Heart J 66:356–358
4. Hocking DC, Phillips PG, Ferro TJ, et al (1990) Mechanisms of pulmonary edema induced by tumor necrosis factor-α. Circ Res 67:68–77
5. Tracey KJ, Lowry SF, Beutler B, et al (1986) Cachectin/tumor necrosis factor mediates changes of skeletal muscle plasma membrane potential. J Exp Med 164:1368–1373
6. Cunnion RE, Parillo JE (1989) Myocardial dysfunction in sepsis. Chest 95:941–945
7. Matsumori A, Yamada T, Suzuki H, et al (1994) Increased circulating cytokines in patients with myocarditis and cardiomyopathy. Br Heart J 72:561–566
8. Asanoi H, Sasayama S, Kiuchi K, et al (1987) Acute hemodynamic effects of a new inotropic agent (OPC-8212) in patients with congestive heart failure. J Am Coll Cardiol 9:865–871
9. Sasayama S, Inoue M, Asanoi H, et al (1986) Acute hemodynamic effects of a new inotropic agent, OPC-8212, on severe congestive heart failure. Heart Vessels 2:23–28
10. Packer M (1992) Treatment of chronic heart failure. Lancet 340:92–95
11. Sasayama S (1992) What do the newer inotropic drugs have to offer? Cardiovas Drugs Ther 6:15–18
12. Feldman AM, Bristow MR, Parmley WW, et al (1993) Effects of vesnarinone on morbidity and mortality in patients with heart failure. N Engl J Med 329:149–155
13. Iijima T, Taira N (1987) Membrane current changes responsible for the positive inotropic effect of OPC-8212, a new positive inotropic agent, in single ventricular cells of the guinea pig heart. J Pharmacol Exp Ther 240:657–662
14. Endoh M, Yanagisawa T, Taira N, et al (1986) Effects of new inotropic agents on cyclic nucleotide metabolism and calcium transients in canine ventricular muscle. Circulation 73(suppl III):117–133
15. Matsumori A, Kawai C (1982) An experimental model for congestive heart failure after encephalomyocarditis virus myocarditis in mice. Circulation 65:1230–1235
16. Matsumori A, Kawai C (1982) An animal model of congestive (dilated) cardiomyopathy: dilatation and hypertrophy of the heart in the chronic stage in DBA/2 mice with myocarditis caused by encephalomyocarditis virus. Circulation 66:355–360
17. Matsui S, Matsumori A, Matoba Y, et al (1994) Treatment of virus-induced myocarditis injury with a novel immunomodulating agent, vesnarinone. J Clin Invest 94:1212–1217
18. Feldman AM, Becker LC, Llewellyn MP, et al (1988) Evaluation of a new inotropic agent, OPC-8212, in patients with mild chronic heart failure. Am Heart J 116:771–777
19. OPC-8212 Multicenter Research Group (1990) A placebo-controlled, randomized, double-blind study of OPC-8212 in patients with mild chronic heart failure. Cardiovasc Drugs Ther 4:19–25
20. Feldman AM, Baughman KL, Lee WK, et al (1991) Usefulness of OPC-8212, a quinolinone derivative, for chronic congestive heart failure in patients with ischemic heart disease or idiopathic dilated cardiomyopathy. Am J Cardiol 68:1203–1210
21. Yamada T, Matsumori A, Sasayama S (1994) Therapeutic effect of anti-tumor necrosis factor-α antibody on the murine model of viral myocarditis induced by encephalo-myocarditis virus. Circulation 89:846–851
22. Severn A, Rapson NT, Hunter CA, et al (1992) Regulation of tumor necrosis factor production by adrenaline and β-adrenergic agonists. J Immunol 148:3441–3445
23. Renz H, Gong JH, Schmidt A, et al (1988) Release of tumor necrosis factor-α from macrophages: enhancement and suppression are dose-dependently regulated by prostaglandin E_2 and cyclic nucleotides. J Immunol 141:2388–2393

24. Matsumori A, Shioi T, Yamada T, et al (1994) Vesnarinone, a new inotropic agent, inhibits cytokine production by stimulated human blood from patients with heart failure. Circulation 89:955–958
25. Finkel MS, Oddis CV, Jacob TD, et al (1992) Negative inotropic effects of cytokines on the heart mediated by nitric oxide. Science 257:387–389
26. Balligand J-L, Kelly RA, Marsden PA, et al (1993) Control of cardiac muscle cell function by an endogenous nitric oxide signalling system. Proc Natl Acad Sci USA 90:347–351

Index